Advance Praise

"There is only one person alive who deeply understands the linkages between modern neuroscience, the unconscious mind, and clinical psychology with the academic and practical depth required to effectively teach them to the world. That person is Dr. Allan Schore. *The Right Brain and the Origin of Human Nature* brings forward that understanding so we can all think, feel, and act with more clarity and compassion about who we are and how we can evolve—as individuals, in relationships, and as a species."
—**Andrew D. Huberman, PhD,** Stanford University School of Medicine

"*The Right Brain and the Origin of Human Nature* is the culmination of Allan Schore's pioneering three-decade exploration of the unconscious mind and brain asymmetry. Blending neuroscience, attachment theory, and psychotherapy, Schore invites both clinicians and curious readers into a compelling inquiry of how the right brain shapes our emotional lives, relationships, and sense of self. His integrative approach highlights the vital interplay of cortical and subcortical systems, conscious and unconscious processes, and left–right brain dynamics that underlie our human experience."
—**Stephen W. Porges, PhD,** creator of Polyvagal Theory

"Allan Schore deserves to be congratulated for his important work over many decades on the crucial role played by the right hemisphere in affect regulation. This 'capstone' volume reviews, expands, and consolidates the evidence for the central place of right hemisphere to right hemisphere communication in the development of healthy human beings and a healthy society, and why it is of critical importance to each of us in the world we live in now."
—**Iain McGilchrist, BM, MA, FRCPsych,** author of *The Master and his Emissary* and *The Matter with Things*

"In this latest triumphant tour de force, Allan Schore once again ventures into uncharted territory—a realm in which the enduring wisdom of what it means to be human intersects with the empirical rigor of affective neuroscience and the energetic resonance of the relational fabric that binds us all. A world-renowned, universally revered neuroscientist–clinician–scholar,

Schore's ongoing evidence-based and holistic exploration of the convergence of right brain implicit processes, attachment theory, trauma research, the collective unconscious, and spiritual interconnectedness is gradually unveiling the origin of our shared humanity, firmly establishing him as the undisputed father of affective, relational, and spiritual neuroscience."

—**Martha Stark, MD,** clinical faculty, Harvard Medical
School, and award-winning author of *Relentless Hope: The
Refusal to Grieve* and *Modes of Therapeutic Action*

"Allan Schore offers a compelling foundation for understanding the processes that shape intersubjectivity, affect regulation, and human development. Grounded in decades of clinical and neuroscientific research, this stimulating account resonates with contemporary work about the neurobiological basis of interpersonal dynamics, bridging brain science, mental health, and human relationships."

—**Guillaume Dumas, PhD,** associate professor of
computational psychiatry, Université de Montréal

"Allan Schore has done it again! In yet another masterpiece, he's brought his love of the right brain and impeccable scholarship into what is inarguably his most comprehensive volume to date. *The Right Brain and the Origin of Human Nature* uses the totality of Schore's research to present the highs and lows of being human within mind–body–brain development, relationships, psychotherapy, and culture at large. This book is destined to be a classic."

—**Terry Marks-Tarlow, PhD,** author of *Clinical Intuition in
Psychotherapy, Awakening Clinical Intuition, Mythic Imagination
Today,* and *A Fractal Epistemology for a Scientific Psychology*

THE RIGHT BRAIN AND THE ORIGIN OF HUMAN NATURE

The Norton Series on Interpersonal Neurobiology
Louis Cozolino, PhD, Series Editor
Allan N. Schore, PhD, Series Editor (2007–2014)
Daniel J. Siegel, MD, Founding Editor

The field of mental health is in a tremendously exciting period of growth and conceptual reorganization. Independent findings from a variety of scientific endeavors are converging in an interdisciplinary view of the mind and mental well-being. An interpersonal neurobiology of human development enables us to understand that the structure and function of the mind and brain are shaped by experiences, especially those involving emotional relationships, as well as the relational mechanisms by which interacting and communicating brains synchronize with and align their activities with other individuals.

The Norton Series on Interpersonal Neurobiology provides cutting-edge, multidisciplinary views that further our understanding of the complex neurobiology of the human mind. By drawing on a wide range of traditionally independent fields of research—such as neuroscience, attachment, the unconscious mind, genetics, memory, complex systems, anthropology, and evolutionary science—these texts offer mental health professionals a review and synthesis of scientific findings often inaccessible to clinicians. The books advance our understanding of human experience, identity, and relational connections by finding the unity of knowledge, or consilience, that emerges with the translation of findings from numerous domains of study into a common language and conceptual framework. The series integrates the best of modern science with the healing art of psychotherapy.

THE **RIGHT BRAIN**

AND **THE ORIGIN** OF

HUMAN NATURE

ALLAN SCHORE

Norton Professional Books

An Imprint of W. W. Norton & Company
Independent Publishers Since 1923

Note to Readers: This book is intended as a general information resource for professionals practicing in the field of psychotherapy and mental health. It is not a substitute for appropriate training or clinical supervision. Standards of clinical practice and protocol vary in different practice settings and change over time. No technique or recommendation is guaranteed to be safe or effective in all circumstances, and neither the publisher nor the author(s) can guarantee the complete accuracy, efficacy, or appropriateness of any particular recommendation in every respect or in all settings or circumstances.

Any URLs displayed in this book link or refer to websites that existed as of press time. The publisher is not responsible for, and should not be deemed to endorse or recommend, any website other than its own or any content that it did not create. The author, also, is not responsible for any third-party material.

For information about permission to reproduce selections from this book, write to Permissions, W. W. Norton & Company, Inc., 500 Fifth Avenue, New York, NY 10110

For information about special discounts for bulk purchases, please contact W. W. Norton Special Sales at specialsales@wwnorton.com or 800-233-4830

Manufacturing by Lakeside Book Company
Production manager: Gwen Cullen

ISBN: 978-1-324-08295-8

W. W. Norton & Company, Inc., 500 Fifth Avenue, New York, NY 10110
www.wwnorton.com

W. W. Norton & Company Ltd., 15 Carlisle Street, London W1D 3BS

10 9 8 7 6 5 4 3 2 1

To Judy, over a shared lifetime, wing-to-wing, oar-to-oar.

And to Beth, David, and Amanda, and the future world they'll live in.

Contents

Acknowledgments

In 1994, I overviewed 20th-century developmental neuroscience to offer my first book, *Affect Regulation and the Origin of the Self: The Neurobiology of Emotional Development*. In the opening sentence of that volume, published as a classic edition in 2016, I boldly asserted: "The understanding of early development is one of the fundamental objectives of science. The beginnings of living systems set the stage for every aspect of an organism's internal and external functioning throughout the life span." In that inaugural volume of regulation theory as well as those that followed, I articulated and elaborated the interpersonal neurobiological thesis that runs throughout my work: that events occurring during human infancy, especially transactions with the social environment, are indelibly imprinted into the structures that are maturing in the first years of life. This book further expands the theory, and continues to delve, deeply and widely, into a number of essential brain/mind/body functions that are central to the human condition, and indeed to human nature.

Since my last two volumes in 2019, *Right Brain Psychotherapy* and *The Development of the Unconscious Mind*, I continue to write, research, lecture, and share my work with audiences around the world. I am grateful to a large group of national and international conference organizers for their invitations to present many hundreds of lectures in 22 countries across North and South America, Europe, Asia, and Australia over the last three decades. I'd also like to express my deep appreciation to Wendy

Cherry's video skills and the other members of my Los Angeles Study Group here in my home for our biweekly discussions of the many scientific and clinical literatures that ultimately appear in my writings. I'm indebted to Dr. Robert Bilder for his decades of support of my membership as a UCLA faculty member. This is the ninth volume I've published and I'd like to thank the translators who have made possible editions of my books in many languages including French, Italian, Spanish, German, Romanian, Turkish, Japanese, and Russian, for a total of 28 volumes and counting. For their direct involvement in this book I'd like to thank the Norton staff, especially McKenna Tanner, Jamie Vincent, Mariah Eppes, and Olivia Guarnieri. Most notably, I express deep appreciation to my publisher and valued colleague Deborah Malmud for not only three decades of a productive and gratifying business and personal relationship, but also for her continual advocacy of my work in the Norton Series of Interpersonal Neurobiology.

Once again, I offer love and gratitude to my family: to my son David, for his professional computer skills; and to my daughter Beth, for her truly remarkable creative talents in graphics and the design for the cover and numerous illustrations within this book; and to Judy, for providing so many forms of essential support for my life's work. The words I wrote to her in my first book over thirty years ago still ring true: "Through her intellectual keenness and emotional honesty, she continues to reflect and reveal to me those essential reciprocal emotional processes that are, willingly and unwillingly, most clearly expressed in an intimate loving human relationship."

Introduction

On a daily basis we are continuously exposed to if not bombarded by television, print, and social media with images of the world we're living in going through stressful, accelerated, unpredictable, and seemingly uncontrollable changes. As individuals and as a culture we are now experiencing rapid, dramatic alterations in the physical environment, climate change, extreme weather, and widespread extinction of various species of animals and plants in the natural world, physiological and psychobiological residues of the enduring social isolation of the recent COVID-19 pandemic, and stressful alterations in not just the external social environment but the private psychological internal world. The instability in both the physical and psychological realms of our private and communal lives is inducing increased anxiety at the individual and cultural levels. To attempt to reduce our anxiety and more effectively cope with and make meaning out of these changes, we turn to science to deepen our understanding of these all-too-common stressful events in our everyday lives that impact both our brains and bodies.

Of special interest is neuroscience, with its long history of studies on the brain's reactions to stress, in particular emotional stress from the social environment. As I will show, over the past 30 years a massive body of brain laterality research has documented the critical role of the right brain in the human stress response and its survival strategies that operate across the lifespan, beneath conscious awareness. Neuroscience is now generating a very large body of research on how attachment experiences shape early brain development, and thereby personality variations in stress reactivity and individual differences in coping abilities. These matters bear upon some fundamental questions of science: Exactly how does our first human connection enhance our ability to emotionally and cognitively grow at later stages of life? How does prolonged psychobiological stress in early development induce pain and suffering in human beings? Why do some of us suffer more than others, and how can we enhance our coping abilities, reduce this suffering, and increase the joy of living in more members of our communities?

As for the sources of these individual differences in vulnerability in regulating stress and resilience, current investigations of the structural and functional differences between the two cerebral hemispheres are converging on the essential role of the right brain in early human development. This system is dominant for attachment processes and memories that produce differences in the ability to experience, share, and implicitly regulate our negative and positive emotions, and thereby indelibly shape a variety of basic personality patterns that operate rapidly, and thereby unconsciously, beneath awareness of conscious thought and behavior. The *Oxford English Dictionary* (OED) defines "unconscious" as

> Not conscious or knowing within oneself; unaware. *Psychol.* Designating mental processes of which a person is not aware but which have a powerful effect on his or her attitudes and behavior; *spec.* in Freudian theory, designating processes activated by desires, fears, or memories which are unavailable to the conscious mind and so repressed. Also, designating that part of the mind or psyche in which such processes operate. *Psychol.* The unconscious mind. ("unconscious," n.d.)

In essence, this book, the capstone of three decades of my work, is about the human unconscious mind, an area of great interest to both scientists and clinicians. Recent discoveries of the right-lateralized "emotional brain," the "social brain" are given in every upcoming chapter. The book is also about my own past and ongoing contributions to what has been called "the emotional revolution" in psychology, in which I have been honored to play a significant role, especially my pioneering work on affect regulation and the interpersonal neurobiology of emotion. Neuroscience has been absolutely essential to generating new scientific explorations of emotion, as its methodologies alone allow for direct access into the millisecond-time domain of emotional processes. The perception and complex processing of the smallest change within an emotionally expressive human face occurs within 100 milliseconds, and therefore beneath conscious awareness.

In the upcoming chapters, I show how my work in developmental, affective, and social neuroscience has increased our understanding of how a secure attachment is expressed in a resilience to later life stress, as opposed to an insecure attachment and a vulnerability to stress dysregulation found in various personality and psychiatric disorders. With respect to the latter, a large body of research documents the enduring negative impact of early yet chronic attachment stress on right brain development and how this relational attachment trauma negatively impacts the individual's future stress-regulating capacities over the lifespan. Furthermore, there is now intense clinical interest in the interpersonal neurobiological mechanisms that mediate the intergenerational transmission of both secure and insecure attachments, and thereby more effective models of child-rearing and psychotherapeutic treatment.

Current interdisciplinary studies on the right brain strongly confirm that its early maturation is shaped by maternal-infant attachment experiences, as first described by the child psychiatrist John Bowlby, the creator of attachment theory. But Bowlby was also a psychoanalyst and asserted that internal working models of attachment coping strategies operated outside of awareness, in an unconscious first described by Sigmund Freud. A continuous stream of large bodies of new research has dramatically expanded our knowledge of unconscious processes, underscoring the central role of the right brain in the beginnings of the human experience, and thereby giving us a deeper understanding of the early foundations of a human personality. As I show in the following chapters, attachment imprinting of the right brain and its long-lasting impact over the lifespan is generating heuristic and evidence-based clinical models of normal adaptive human emotional and relational functions.

This interpersonal neurobiological data also offers important new information about the early etiology of deficits of right brain functions in a spectrum of psychopathologies and personality disorders, as well as the symptomatology these individuals bring into psychotherapy. On that matter, as in all my works, I continue to discuss in some detail how the early attachment dynamic plays out in the psychotherapy relationship, beneath conscious awareness of both the patient and psychotherapist. Brain laterality studies now confirm the principle that "the left side is involved with conscious response and the right with the unconscious mind" (Mlot, 1998). These investigations of the early developing right brain can illuminate our understanding of the origin of the subjective core self, and thereby shine a light on the depths of human nature. Authors are now asserting that when processing information about the self, "conscious thought stays firmly under the searchlight, [whereas] unconscious thought ventures out to the dark and dusty nooks and crannies of the mind" (Dijksterhuis & Meurs, 2006, p. 138).

In a 2011 edition of *Scientific American Mind*, the psychoanalytic scholar Jonathan Shedler suggested, "Freud's legacy is not a specific theory but rather a sensibility: an appreciation of the depth and complexity of mental life and a recognition that we do not fully know ourselves. It is also an acknowledgement that what we do not know is nonetheless manifested in our relationships and can cause suffering—or, in a therapy relationship, can be examined and potentially reworked" (p. 54). A few years earlier the Nobel Prize–winning neuroscientist Eric Kandel (1999) asserted, "Psychoanalysis still represents the most coherent and intellectually satisfying view of the mind."

It is important to point out that Freud's psychoanalysis and its central construct of the unconscious has continued to evolve over the last 120 years into its latest iterations, "relational psychoanalysis," which has adopted a two-person face-to-face methodology, and "neuropsychoanalysis," which has incorporated a neurobiological perspective of the unconscious. Both of these clinical and theoretical transformations have been influenced by my work. Although for much of the last century psychoanalysis was criticized for a lack of empirical data, or of not being heuristic, my studies have directly contributed to the foundation of the scientific study of neuropsychoanalysis, the neuroscience of the unconscious mind. As I will show, these clinical investigations and research data continue to be a major contributor to our understanding of the unconscious, the central area of interest to the genius of Freud's mind. It is often forgotten that Freud was trained in and practiced neurology in his early professional career before he created psychoanalysis, the psychology of the unconscious mind. In fact, Freud later suggested that the conscious ego was located in the left hemisphere.

The two greatest early discoveries in the emergent field of neurology in the mid-nineteenth century were the lateralization of language functions in Broca's area in the anterior portion of the left hemisphere and Wernicke's area in the posterior area of the left hemisphere. Soon after, the great English neurologist John Hughlings Jackson identified emotion in the right hemisphere. Over the last three centuries a large volume of brain laterality research has explored the brain's dual cerebral hemispheres. In 1981 the psychologist and maverick brain scientist Roger Sperry won the Nobel Prize in Physiology and Medicine for his studies on the different functions of the left and right hemispheres (Trevarthen, 1994; Berlucchi & Marzi, 2024). Yet even today the majority of images of neuroscience represent the brain as a single image, usually a lateral view of one hemisphere, most commonly the left hemisphere. On the other hand, a top-down (or bottom-up) image of the brain shows a right brain and a left, connected by the corpus callosum. The human brain is thus fundamentally a dual system with unique structures and functions.

Indeed, the large amount of new laterality research generated by recent neuroscience has fueled exponential growth across an array of scientific and clinical disciplines. With the onset of "the Decade of the Brain" and the appearance of neuroimaging technologies in the mid-1990s, research significantly increased, especially brain lateralization studies of the specializations of the right and left hemispheres, which develop at different rates and ages. These studies of hemispheric brain asymmetry have generated valuable insights into the structural and functional specializations of the human early-developing right and later-developing left hemispheres. For example, these findings indicate that while the left hemisphere is associated with the conscious self-concept, the early-maturing right hemisphere generates an enduring unconscious self-image that the person may not want to possess but unconsciously maintains. With respect to new data about the psychodynamics of the human unconscious mind, what is essential is a theoretical model that can not only interpret the research data but also decipher the meaning of the findings and pragmatically apply them to the fundamental problems of the human condition.

Toward that end, over three decades I have elaborated the central role of the right brain's implicit functions in regulation theory, a theory of the development, psychopathogenesis, and treatment of the subjective self. My focus has been on early-evolving right brain implicit, unconscious nonverbal emotion regulation (Schore, 1994/2016), rather than later-maturing explicit left brain conscious verbal emotion regulation and the cognitive control of emotion (e.g., Ochsner & Gross, 2007). It is often overlooked that Gross and Thompson (2007) later added that emotion regulation may be "automatic or controlled, conscious or unconscious" (p. 8). Such separate processes of implicit involuntary and explicit voluntary self-regulation have frequently been conflated by both researchers and clinicians, resulting in impreciseness and confusion, both theoretically and especially clinically. These regulatory functions are lateralized in different hemispheres and operate via distinctive emotional and cognitive neuropsychologies.

Recent authors are now describing a right hemispheric dominance in nonconscious processing, concluding, "The right hemisphere has an advantage in shaping behavior with implicit attention whereas the left hemisphere plays a greater role in expressing explicit knowledge" (Chen & Hsiao, 2014). As I will show in the upcoming chapters, a large body of laterality studies indicates that the implicit, unconscious subjective processing of self-related material and self-awareness, including the recognition of one's own face, voice, and body, are mediated by the nonverbal right hemisphere. That said, brain lateralization remains a blind spot for many researchers and clinicians. There still exists a bias in the mental health field and the psychological sciences for conceptualizing the unconscious human mind and subjective self as solely a silent version of the conscious, objective left brain that can be directly assessed by observations of overt voluntary behavior, verbal measures of self-reports, and self-questionnaires. And yet it is now well established that while explicit measures of self-esteem assess introspectively accessible conscious self-evaluations associated with deliberative responses, measures of implicit self-esteem assess unconscious, introspectively inaccessible aspects of the self associated with automatic responses (Spalding & Hardin, 1999).

McGilchrist (2009, 2021a, 2021b) asserts the left hemisphere is analytic, utilizing focused attention, looking at detail, taking things apart and examining components, and therefore its measures are used to generate and describe rational verbal models of the conscious self. Left brain measures are prominent in what I have termed "classical attachment theory" that focuses on explicit conscious aspects of behavior and affect regulation and completely overlooks Bowlby's foundations in Freud's psychoanalysis. Indeed, it has just about banished the unconscious from developmental psychology. The focus of classical attachment theory is on measures of the child's explicit behavior after a reunion of a dysregulating behavioral separation and the maternal regulation of negative emotion. That said, positive emotion is and continues to be undervalued and underresearched. Frequently, observations of brain activity are not offered, and when they are the emphasis is solely on the higher cortical areas of the left hemisphere. This bias de-emphasizes the importance of right-lateralized subcortical bodily-based processes in both early-evolving positive and negative attachment dynamics, and thereby the foundational origins of human nature. With respect to the central theme of this book, Bowlby (1988) concluded, "The propensity to make strong emotional bonds to a particular individual is a basic component of human nature."

According to classical attachment theory, the original central tenet of Bowlby's theory is that the mother is the cornerstone of her infant's survival, acting as a secure base, encouraging the child to reach out when distressed (note the bias toward negative emotion). As in the maternal attachment context, the therapist acts as a secure base from which the patient explores these early social-emotional experiences, especially distressing ones, and helps the patient understand his or her attachment behavior and create a verbal narrative. The creation of this narrative has been presented as a key element of the patient's therapeutic changes. Note this is a cognitive and not an emotional perspective that doesn't take into account a two-person relational view, in which the nonverbal patient-therapist relationship is the major source of changes in the treatment.

Indeed, a "gold-standard" behavioral measure of attachment used since 1978 is Ainsworth's Strange Situation Procedure, while verbal measures are central in the Adult Attachment Interview (George, Kaplan, et al., 1996) and in self-report questionnaires (Hazan & Shaver, 1987). These explicit behavioral and verbal measures are inappropriately and incorrectly assumed to directly reflect the organizing principles of the early psychobiological preverbal period of attachment. Within the attachment literature, authors have pointed out that these research methodologies have not tapped the less explicit, less conscious implicit aspects of affect regulation, motivation, and mental representations of self and other (Berant et al., 2005), and conclude that self-report measures are unlikely to relate to Bowlby's psychoanalytic processes.

George and Aikins (2023) state these measures are "subject to positive self-report bias where reported attachment dimensions, which for many clients, are sabotaged by unconscious defensive processes." They conclude, "extensive empirical scrutiny of self-report measures shows that the assessment findings are poorly related to childhood experience." On the other hand authors working directly with implicit measures assert, "Because individuals typically have limited conscious control to their motives . . . implicitly measured motives are more powerful than self-report motive measures in predicting spontaneous behavior as compared to planned and consciously controlled behavior" (Quirin, Dusing, et al., 2013).

In fact, decades of studies have emphasized the many insurmountable difficulties associated with self-report research, which is "influenced by cognitive biases and response styles that can render pure self report studies problematic" (Jauk & Kanske, 2021). Self-report measures are commonly used in correlational research methodologies, which are well known to be limited in that they cannot establish or predict causation between variables (Asamoah, 2014). Note also that the verbal measures of left hemispheric self-questionnaires are processed by the linear conscious left mind, and the exclusion of the early-developing preverbal bodily-based emotional nonlinear unconscious right mind. This leads to confounds between verbal explicit and nonverbal implicit functions, and an overemphasis on left hemisphere attachment models in both correlational research and psychotherapy.

Only 10 years ago clinical scientists citing my work were concluding, "The great majority of psychotherapy research studies have stopped short of examining nonverbal dimensions of the therapeutic process. This limitation has arguably precluded a fuller understanding of the therapeutic action of psychotherapy" (Håvås et al., 2015). I would further add that most research studies on emotion use mild to moderate intensities of the left hemisphere, and not the strong emotions of the right that are typical in clinical and real-life contexts. I return to these matters in later chapters.

In contrast to this perspective of "classical attachment theory" that describes the late-developing conscious verbal, behavioral/cognitive functions of the explicit left brain in the third year, what my wife Judith and I have termed "modern attachment theory" (Schore & Schore, 2008) offers models of an early-developing unconscious implicit right brain nonverbal emotional attachment model, that begins in prenatal stages and matures over the course of the first and second years of life. With its emphasis on the beginnings of human development, our neurobiologically informed theory of the evolutionary mechanism of attachment utilizes a biopsychosocial perspective.

This theoretical orientation encompasses not only the infant's inherited genome and its individual biological and bodily-based emotional experiences, but also its relational dynamics and social interactions with the primary caregiver that are embedded in the culture, another central theme of this book. Individual development arises out of the relationship between the brain/mind/body of both infant and caregiver held within a culture and a social environment that supports, inhibits, or even threatens it. These relational experiences are forged in nonverbal attachment experiences in the first two years, "the human brain growth spurt," a critical period of rapid, exponential growth of the right brain. In this manner, they indelibly shape the origin of human nature and the individual's way of being in the world.

Modern attachment theory continues to incorporate new data from neuroscience research. It reveals how these ongoing discoveries of right brain cortical-subcortical attachment processes can give us a more complex knowledge of the essential biological, psychological, and neurochemical processes that fundamentally define human nature, shared by all members of the species, and thereby a common denominator of human beings inclusive of the diversities of culture, gender, and ethnicity/race. Only attending to the mysteries of the early-developing right lateralized unconscious mind and not the later-developing conscious left mind can lead to a more profound understanding of the deeper strata of human nature, the unconscious core of each of us.

The most fundamental question about the human experience is not how does the conscious mind work, but how does the unconscious mind operate? This scientific challenge can only be solved by hemispheric asymmetry methodologies. Citing my work on the right brain (Schore, 2005), current researchers studying the role of attachment and nonverbal communication in the first three years of life now assert, "In comparison to other species, humans process the most asymmetric as well as the most complex brains with a concomitant complexity of behavior" (Leisman et al., 2023, p. 67). A central theme of these chapters is that the depths of human nature are the products of the unique evolution of right brain development.

There is now a consensus that conscious and nonconscious processes operate by different principles and require very different research methodologies. And yet the majority of research on emotion and attachment measures left brain conscious cognitive control of emotional behavior, while it is the right brain that regulates and communicates bodily-based emotion, including strong intense emotion, at unconscious levels. That said, as I will show, it is the early-evolving right brain that generates the human emotional capacity for both love and hate, ecstasy and agony, good and evil, forgiveness and revenge, creativity and destructiveness, the deeper aspects of the human experience, at levels beneath conscious awareness.

In the upcoming chapters, I'll look back over the last 30 years of my work on the fundamental role of the right brain in human development, psychopathology, and psychotherapy, as well as look forward. It began at the end of the last century, with the publication in 1991 of an article on shame in early development, and then in 1994 of my pioneering, ground-breaking book *Affect Regulation and the Origin of the Self: The Neurobiology of Emotional Development* (Schore, 1994/2016; for more on this see the last chapter of *Right Brain Psychotherapy*, Schore, 2019b). Up until its appearance, theories of human development solely focused on cognitive development. It may seem hard to believe, but at that time the problem of emotion was still not being addressed by science. In the book my focus was on emotion, and on the essential constructs that are shared within the overlapping boundaries between psychology and biology, as well as the commonalities that lie beneath what appear on the surface to be unrelated phenomena. A central theme of these chapters was on the adaptive role of the right brain in the subjective experience, communication, and regulation of emotion. At the book's release, I remember thinking that parts of the book would be 20 years ahead of its time.

Grounded in regulation theory, my intention was also to describe the emotional neurobiology of attachment in early development and in adult, adolescent, child, and infant psychotherapy. Toward that end, I elaborated a model of treatment in which the intuitive clinician, like the secure mother, implicitly tracks changes in the patient's emotional state, rather than just linguistically, explicitly attending to the patient's words and conscious thoughts. The book presents the origins of an emotionally focused right brain psychotherapy, an alternative and complement to Freud's insight-oriented "talking cure." The primary focus of the treatment was on emotional changes in the patient-therapist relationship, and the cardinal clinical principle was to "follow the affect, wherever it may lead."

This first volume, published in 1994 and subsequently as a Classic Edition in 2016, acts as a keystone and foundation for my subsequent writings. In 1994 it was essential to the formulation of interpersonal neurobiology, which studies how the brain is shaped by early experiences, especially social and emotional experiences, as well as the relational mechanisms by which interacting, communicating brains intersubjectively synchronize, couple with, and align their activities with other brains. In this cocreated synchronization two psyches "agree" to exchange information (Rabeyron, 2022). All of this is occurring at an implicit level beneath conscious awareness, and thus "people are commonly unaware of their becoming synchronized" (Tschacher et al., 2023).

Here, as in all my work of the last 30 years, I continue to use the term *regulation theory* to explicitly denote what I am offering as a theory, a systematic exposition of the general principles of a science, specifically, a longitudinal formulation of the underlying processes of human development, which I have asserted is one of the fundamental objectives of science. The observations, internal consistency, coherence, scope, pragmatic usefulness, and power of the theory are expressed in its ability to formulate heuristic research hypotheses, as well as to generate evidence-based clinical interventions. In a letter to Werner Heisenberg in 1926 Albert Einstein observed, "On principle, it is quite wrong to try founding a theory on observable magnitudes alone. In reality the very opposite happens. It is the theory which decides what we can observe." The observations of regulation theory focus on the rapid unconscious processes of emotion in human relationships. The hypotheses generated by regulation theory also serve as a source of frequent thought experiments by my scientific imagination, created by my synthetic mind. These thought experiments, fueled by spontaneous brief flashes of insight and body-based emotion are mostly rapid sensory visual, auditory, kinesthetic, and imagistic, as well as nonverbal and visceral and thereby intuitive.

Recent knowledge has greatly amplified our understanding of not only the subjective experience and regulation of emotion within the self but also the nonverbal intersubjective communication of emotion between the self and another self. Toward that end, I continue to describe and elaborate the role of unconscious face-to-face right-brain-to-right-brain attachment emotional communications and regulation in both the mother–infant and therapist–patient relationships, and how these reparative mechanisms can be accessed in all forms of psychotherapy, both short-term symptom-reducing and long-term growth-promoting deep psychotherapy. These ultrarapid right brain processes operate at levels beneath conscious awareness, not only in the therapeutic relationship but fundamentally in everyday life, especially in close human relationships. With respect to my ongoing studies in neuropsychoanalysis, I continue to offer recent brain laterality data supporting the idea that the right hemisphere represents the biological substrate of Freud's human dynamic unconscious. For over a century, the unconscious has been a central focus of classical psychoanalysis, but now it is used as a core theoretical construct in all schools of psychotherapy.

Over the course of my work I have suggested that the integration of psychology and biology has changed the nature of psychotherapy itself, which is now emphasizing the importance of implicit bodily-based emotional and relational subjective processes as much or even more than explicit verbal cognition and overt behavior. Freud's intrapsychic unconscious has returned but transformed into an interpersonal dynamic, a relational unconscious, a "two-person unconscious." This has transformed the lived experience and goal of psychotherapy from an intrapsychic intellectual understanding of the patient's symptomatology and cognitive insight within the patient to the interpersonal experiencing and sharing of emotions, including unconscious emotions, between the patient and therapist. Yet Freud's insight model dominates in the media and cinema and the impressions most people have about psychotherapy.

That said, the ongoing shift from left brain thoughts to right brain emotions has altered our ideas about the therapeutic skills that underlie the science and the art of psychotherapy. As the upcoming chapters show, the focus is no longer just on the verbal narratives over the session, what the patient and therapist say to each other, but on the rapid nonverbal emotional moments of a session that are subjectively experienced and shared by the patient and the empathic therapist and regulated by their dynamic coconstructed relationship. In the following pages, I cite a large number of past and recent studies that support this model.

Throughout this volume, I present my ongoing clinical studies and research on the human unconscious mind, as well as current discoveries of the emotional, relational right brain. My intention is to show the relevance of these discoveries in science to various aspects of the human condition. This exploration of the deeper strata of the human mind, brain, and body includes a focus on rapid unconscious right-brain-to-right-brain nonverbal communications that are invisible but ubiquitous in psychotherapy and in everyday life. Due to the fact that my work bridges many diverse fields of scientific and clinical disciplines, I cite a large number of references over a wide bibliographic spectrum of both the scientific and psychotherapy literatures. The references also serve as a resource to the reader interested in more specific details of a particular citation or field of study.

In my writings I continue to use the device of frequently citing verbatim the current and past voices of master clinicians studying the mind and neuroscientists studying the brain in order to generate a common language that addresses the subjective emotional and social realms of the human experience. These voices are describing the phenomenology of right brain functions, and thereby the psychobiological operations of the unconscious mind. Their evocative direct quotations also serve another very important purpose. They represent an alternative to the usual detached impersonal objective language used in much scientific literature that cannot capture the intensely personal subjective and emotional experience of what Ornstein (1997) calls the human "right mind."

In light of the fact that regulation theory specifically generates both testable research hypotheses and updated clinical interventions grounded in neuroscience, my work has brought me a significant number of both scientific and clinical awards, which I describe at the end of this book. I have received two Lifetime Achievement Awards and induction into Sigma Xi, the Scientific Research Honor Society (https://www.sigmaxi .org/about). It is indeed a great honor to be accepted into this international organization that recognizes eminent scientific researchers, in my case the acknowledgment of my ongoing interdisciplinary work over the last 30 years on the right brain in attachment, early human brain development, trauma, psychotherapy, and psychoanalysis. As the world's largest honor society for scientists and engineers, Sigma Xi recognizes researchers for values held in high esteem: excellence, integrity, leadership, diversity, cooperation, and scholarship. The fact that the body of my work has at this time achieved over 36,000 Google Scholar citations across a broad range of scientific and clinical disciplines tells me, on a daily level, where and how my work penetrates different areas of the sciences, the mental health field, and beyond. In terms of the enduring impact of the first volume, the largest number of citations are from the 1994 book, which continues on a daily basis.

With this introduction in mind, in the upcoming chapters I discuss further clinical, theoretical, and research progressions of regulation theory. To give a brief glimpse of what's to come, in Chapter 1 I offer an overview of the origins and basic constructs of my work on modern attachment theory. I then present highlights of three decades of neurobiological research that validate my studies of the development of the right brain and the interpersonal neurobiology of attachment in the mother–infant relationship. I follow this in Chapter 2 where I discuss basic constructs of my work in neuropsychoanalysis and the early relational origins of Freud's unconscious mind, as well as an interpersonal neurobiological model of the patient-therapist relationship. This right brain system functions as not only a one-person intrapsychic unconscious but a two-person relational conscious that expresses adaptive functions at both the deeper and higher levels of the right brain.

In the middle chapters, I offer newer contributions of regulation theory to what I have termed *relational trauma* and the generation of insecure disorganized attachment, as well as the right brain metabolic defense of dissociation. In Chapter 3 I focus on the role of attachment trauma, dissociation, and the reduced energy dynamics during critical periods of right brain synaptogenesis. In fact, energy is a central theme of this book, and I argue that the biological construct of energy needs to return to psychological theories. I also present clinical applications of this work, including the characterological use of the energy-reducing defense of pathological dissociation in patients with a history of early developmental relational trauma, including borderline personality disorders.

In Chapter 4 I expand my models of the neuropsychoanalysis and hemispheric asymmetry of the repression defense, a left hemispheric blocking of right brain painful affect from reaching explicit conscious awareness. I discuss current advances in the science and the art of psychotherapy, including new interpersonal neurobiological models for working more effectively with "difficult" patients, specifically avoidant dismissive attachments that continually defensively block emotion and intimacy. In Chapter 5 I offer neuropsychoanalytic models of two types of narcissistic personality disorders, grandiose and vulnerable, both of which are now increasing in U.S. culture in men and women. I suggest that the latter disorders reflect an imbalanced left-over-right asymmetry between the hemispheres. I also present a clinical model of right brain psychotherapy for working with repressed affects, and unconscious shame dynamics.

In Chapter 6 I describe in some detail the central role of clinical regressions that allow both the patient and therapist direct access to the right hemispheric depths of human nature, in both short- and long-term treatment, and how these synchronized mutual regressions can lead to a rebalancing of the hemispheres. Offering very recent findings in neuroscience, laterality research, and current neurobiologically informed models of psychotherapeutic change, I show how right brain psychotherapy uncovers and directly impacts the more primitive emotional strata of the human unconscious mind, the origin of human nature.

Following that, in Chapter 7 I present my recent work on the origins of intersubjectivity between the mother and infant, the rapid and unconscious nonverbal right-brain-to-right-brain emotional communication between their minds and bodies, where they synchronize and share emotional states. I then describe how this interpersonal neurobiological mechanism of interbrain synchrony is also involved in the clinical context, in which the empathic therapist and patient (like the psychobiologically attuned mother and infant) can nonverbally communicate and intersubjectively share an emotional state, which then can be interactively regulated. In both social contexts, two interacting right brains couple together and align their activities with other brains. I then discuss the early development of the right brain and its essential role in intersubjectivity, play, and mutual love. Expanding these ideas, I present an interpersonal neurobiological conception of love as a basic human motivational system.

In Chapter 8 I expand my model of right-brain-to-right-brain nonverbal emotional communications in light of recent developmental and clinical advances. I focus on intersubjective emotional communications and interpersonal synchrony in early human development, offering a number of recent international laterality studies on the early structural and functional maturation of the right brain. I then present further clinical applications of the right-brain-to-right-brain model to both short-term symptom-reducing and long-term growth-promoting emotion-focused psychodynamically oriented psychotherapy, directly addressing a number of essential clinical problems and questions:

• How do we work directly with the patient's and our own emotions, and how do we access "primitive" unconscious nonverbal emotional communications within the psychotherapy session?

- How does the clinician shift out of the explicit left hemisphere into the right, the psychobiological substrate of the unconscious mind, in order to have direct access to the patient's and his or her own emotional right brain?
- How can the empathic therapist consciously, explicitly attend to the patient's verbalizations in order to objectively diagnose and rationalize his or her dysregulating symptomatology, while also implicitly listening and interacting at another level, an experience near subjective level, "beneath the words"?
- How can we get inside the patient's subjective experience and then let her know that we have arrived there, without using words?
- How can implicit right brain unconscious communications enable the therapist to know the patient "from the inside out"?
- How does the therapist "follow the affect" and on a moment-to-moment basis track changes in the patient's physiological arousal in order to listen and interact with the preverbal physiological expressions of the earliest unconscious levels of the patient's personality?
- How do we use our own bodily-based subjective self in order to treat the patient's dysregulated self-pathology?
- How does the clinician's interbrain synchrony allow him or her to implicitly psychobiologically attune with, emotionally recognize, intersubjectively share, and interactively regulate the patient, which in turn enables the patient's right brain subjective self to emotionally experience feeling felt by the therapist?
- How does the empathic therapist cocreate a therapeutic alliance of right-brain-to-right-brain nonverbal communications with different types of secure and insecure attachments, and synchronize with an array of different personalities, including various personality and psychiatric disorders?
- How can we use interpersonal neurobiology to describe the right brain change mechanisms of successful psychotherapy?

I end the chapter elaborating upon the preeminent role of rapid, implicit right-brain-to-right-brain communications in the therapeutic alliance, citing a body of current clinical research that demonstrates that the psychotherapy relationship makes substantial and consistent contributions to outcome independent of the treatment, and that the patient-therapist relationship consistently predicts treatment outcome.

In Chapter 9 I describe recent paradigm-shifting hyperscanning research, the simultaneous imaging of two individuals during live interactions. This technological advance allows for the study of two synchronized brains in real-time emotional interactions with each other. We now have a relational technology that measures changes in the patient's and therapist's brains as they are communicating and interacting in a psychotherapy session. These pioneering neuroimaging studies of the patient-therapist relationship show a right-lateralized interbrain synchrony between their right minds, a coupling of their emotional, social right brains, beneath the words. This research directly validates the unconscious right-brain-to-right-brain model that I created in 1994 and have been elaborating for three decades. Indeed, both neuroscience and clinical data in every chapter of this volume support my model of an emotionally focused right brain psychotherapy that engages unconscious processes in both members of the therapeutic relationship in order to promote clinical changes in the patient.

At the end of this book, in Chapter 10, I offer thoughts about the application of my neurobiological studies of the right brain to give a deeper understanding of a number of current societal and cultural problems, including anthropogenic trauma in wild elephants, gender differences between male and female social and emotional functions in development and the vulnerability of males to specific psychiatric disorders, the ubiquity of neurotoxic endocrine disruptors in the physical environment, dysregulated attachment dynamics and increasing violence here in the United States, and the lack of legislated maternal and paternal leave in America and entrance into early day care. I also discuss in some detail recent neuroscience and clinical research on the limitations of using online Zoom instead of face-to-face psychotherapy. In this section I offer warnings about left brain artificial intelligence, which, although it presents a façade of right brain functions, overlooks and cannot process human emotional intelligence, interactions of the social right brain, clinical intuition, implicit psychobiological attunement, and common sense. That said, I offer specific ideas about what we need to do to address each of these problems.

In the very last pages, I return to my opening paragraph of this introduction, where I described anxiety-inducing images of our present culture going through seemingly unpredictable changes, and asked how these ubiquitous stressful events in our everyday lives impact both our brains and bodies, our conscious minds and especially our unconscious minds. Integrating the information in these chapters, I offer thoughts on how current right brain social emotional stressors impact not only an individual unconscious but also the collective unconscious of the United States, the communal human psyche of American culture. I propose that the current polarized social context is increasing the imbalance of the left hemisphere's role in individuality, independence, power, and control, at the expense of the right hemisphere's seeking affiliation, warm relationships, and emotional connection with others, and thereby defensively altering our ways of being with other humans. With respect to the current multiple stressors on American culture, I suggest it is our right and not left brain that serves as the foundation for coping with the unpredictable, uncontrollable changes we are now experiencing. Recall Bob Dylan's "Forever Young": "May you have a strong foundation when the winds of changes shift."

Over the course of every chapter I discuss numerous recent discoveries of the adaptive functions of the emotional right brain, the psychobiological locus of the unconscious mind. A fundamental theme is that the right brain is dominant in what essentially makes us human, in what shapes the content of our character. Each chapter includes new information about the unique and essential functions of the cortical and subcortical areas of the right brain. Neuroscientists are now concluding that an expansion of the right frontal cortex relative to the left, the largest anatomical asymmetry in the human brain, is particularly responsible for greater right-sided neural plasticity, and that the right hemisphere generates the most complex and uniquely human functions of the cerebral cortex, the most highly evolved part of brain. As I mentioned earlier, only laterality research can uncover the deeper mechanisms of the human brain, ostensibly "the most complex object in the universe," including the left mind that creates this grandiose narcissistic illusion.

A central organizing principle running throughout this book is that the right brain unconscious system plays a central role in the early origin of human nature, defined by the *Oxford English Dictionary* (OED) as "the general characteristics and feelings attributed to human beings." This definition directly applies to the title of this book, *The Right Brain and the Origin of Human Nature*. In both the early attachment and psychotherapy relationships, the right brain illuminates the dark shadows of the terra incognita of the unconscious mind, the human psyche, and gives us direct access into what the deep unconscious emotional core of the human personality looks like, sounds like, and feels like. It is commonly accepted that *human psyche* refers to the parts of the human mind that affect the basic personality, which I identify in the right and not left mind. According to Freud, the psyche consists of the id, ego, and superego, and their functions at various levels, conscious, preconscious, and unconscious. The *OED* defines the psyche as "the soul, the spirit. The mind, especially in its spiritual, emotional, and motivational aspects. The collective, mental or psychological characteristics of a nation, people." The Greeks called Psyche the goddess of the soul—note the gender and the relation between the soul and "mother" nature.

A major theme of this book, like the others I've written, is that the origin of the human psyche is located in the unconscious emotional right mind and its connections to the peripheral autonomic nervous system and therefore the visceral body. One aspect of its subterranean psychic landscape was described by Carl Jung as the "shadow self"—the part of our psyche that we seek to hide and repress, which contains our darkest fantasies, negative emotions, and desires. The "shadow," Jung's personal unconscious, contains those areas of our mind/body that carry our forbidden feelings we project into others, that erupt in our relationships, and that can destroy intimacy. That said, recent neuroscience indicates that the right brain is also critically involved in the highest levels of human behavior performed by the subjective self, including empathy, intuition, creativity, imagery, symbolic thought, imagination, humor, music, poetry, dance, art, morality, altruism, compassion, spirituality, and love. Every one of these uniquely human higher cortical capacities sits atop an early-evolving right-lateralized subcortical foundation.

Running throughout these pages is the core principle that the human unconscious mind is always invisibly operating in everyday life, not only within us but between us, right brain to right brain. As these chapters show, communicating our emotions and making deep contact with close individuals we trust is an essential aspect of what fundamentally makes us human. In each chapter, I cite large bodies of brain laterality research indicating that at ultrarapid speed and thereby invisible levels beneath the awareness and control of the conscious mind, the empathic right brain subjective self can unconsciously intersubjectively communicate with another subjective self. A major intention in writing this book is that upon reading and pondering these chapters on the array of essential survival, emotional, and relational functions of the right brain, the reader may more readily recognize this unconscious system within his or her own subjectivity, especially in close relationships, and thereby experience an expansion of one's own emotional bodily-based subjective self-awareness. Toward that end, this book is about how we become who we are or, more fundamentally, how we become who we really are.

THE RIGHT BRAIN
AND THE ORIGIN OF
HUMAN NATURE

Chapter 1

Modern Attachment Theory: The Central Role of Affect Regulation in Early Human Development

Over the past three decades I have elaborated modern attachment theory, a neurobiologically informed update of John Bowlby's pioneering attempts to integrate Charles Darwin's biological explorations of the natural world and Sigmund Freud's psychoanalytic explorations of the human inner world in order to model the evolutionary origins of early human development. Beginning in 1994 in *Affect Regulation and the Origin of the Self* and continuing through that decade, I documented how attachment theory, informed and energized by ongoing neuroscience research, was experiencing a significant transformation and expansion, both scientifically and clinically. In 2000, writing a foreword to a reissue of Bowlby's seminal 1969 volume *Attachment and Loss, Volume 1*, I proposed, "In essence, a central goal of Bowlby's first book is to demonstrate that a mutually enriching dialogue can be organized between the biological and psychological realms" (Schore, 2000b).

Later that same year, I presented the Seventh Annual John Bowlby Memorial Lecture in London and offered recent findings from "the Decade of the Brain" to argue that modern attachment theory is essentially a regulation theory, and that Bowlby's (1969) first volume of *Attachment and Loss* refers specifically to the child's loss of interactive affect regulation that accompanies too frequent separations and dysregulating emotions. Soon after, I published an article in *Attachment and Human Development* identifying Bowlby's control system of attachment in the prefrontal areas of the right brain (Schore, 2000a). In a publication in the *British Journal of Psychotherapy* I then extrapolated this neuropsychoanalytic model of attachment to the clinical context, offering psychobiological models of attachment in the therapeutic alliance, and right-brain-to-right-brain communications in the transference-countertransference relationship between the patient and therapist (Schore, 2001a). Indeed, my groundbreaking integration of neuroscience with attachment theory led to my description as "the American Bowlby" and with emotional development as "the world's leading authority on how our right hemisphere regulates emotion and processes our sense of self" (see Dr. Allan N. Schore, https://www.allanschore.com).

Another major force that propelled the neurobiological transformation of attachment theory is the ongoing intense interest in the neuroscience of emotion and emotion regulation. At the dawn of modern neurology, Luys (1879) first suggested the existence of an "emotion" center in the right hemisphere, as opposed to the "intellectual" center in the left hemisphere. One hundred years later, in 1972 the neurologist Guido Gainotti proposed the "right hemisphere hypothesis," which posits a general dominance of the right hemisphere for all emotions, positive and negative. The current shift of attachment from its earlier focus on behavior and cognition into affect and affect regulation reflects the broader trend in the psychological sciences. In an editorial in the journal *Motivation and Emotion*, Ryan (2007) asserted, "After three decades of the dominance of cognitive approaches, motivational and emotional processes have roared back into the limelight. Both researchers and practitioners have come to appreciate the limits of exclusively cognitive approaches for understanding the initiation and regulation of human behavior."

In a more recent article, "Psychotherapy Beyond All the Words," in the *Journal of Psychotherapy Integration*, Fiskum (2019) cited my work on nonverbal affect regulation in attachment and psychotherapy (Schore & Schore, 2008) and asserted,

> There is reason to argue that the cognitive-verbal aspect is given overly much attention in psychotherapy and that an understanding of physiological and autonomic regulation needs further integration into clinical practice. . . . Other approaches are therefore needed that allow

the therapist to bypass the explicitly verbal or cognitive domains (p. 412). . . . Integrating . . . nonverbal interactions into psychotherapy can expand the patient's experience with and capacity for more complex states of self-organization and regulation. (p. 419)

In fact, a number of clinical and scientific disciplines are now experiencing a paradigm shift from the primacy of cognition to the primacy of affect, and this transition is expressed in a shift from cognitive to emotional and social theories of development.

Toward that end, modern attachment theory, grounded in developmental, affective, and social neuroscience, offers an early nonverbal right brain implicit and thereby unconscious emotional attachment model, in contrast to "classical," "academic" attachment theory that describes the explicit conscious behavioral-cognitive functions of the later-forming verbal left brain. The neuropsychoanalytic perspective of modern attachment theory highlights the critical importance of early unconscious forces that drive all human emotion, cognition, and behavior within an individual and sociocultural matrix. The outcomes of human attachment, the basic evolutionary system involved in the origin and development of human nature, are the product of the interactions of both nature and nurture, the strengths and weaknesses of the individual's genetically encoded biological predispositions (temperament), and the early dyadic relationships with caregivers embedded within a particular social environment (culture). From its beginnings, neurobiologically informed attachment theory, grounded in psychoanalysis and ethology (behavioral biology), has focused on how early emotional-relational implicit experiences directly impact the unconscious system.

One of the most common dimensions that is used by both clinicians and scientists is the distinction between implicit and explicit brain functions. In the recent neuroscience literature, Hart and his colleagues (2024) assert,

Both implicit (unconscious, automatic) and explicit (conscious, intentional) processes contribute to various kinds of learning. . . . There are two kinds of processes contributing to adaptation: those we are aware of and those we are not aware of. The processes we are aware of, which are usually intentional, involve a strategy, can be verbalized and are often effortful, are referred to as "explicit" adaptation. The processes we are not aware of are then not intentional but automatic, they cannot be verbalized and since they are automatic they usually require less effort, and these kinds of processes are often called "implicit" adaptation. A further distinction is that explicit processes can be voluntarily disengaged, as opposed to implicit processes. (p. 2)

Note the isomorphism of *implicit* and *unconscious*. Thus, when you read the word *implicit*, think *unconscious*.

The early-developing implicit right and later-developing explicit left hemispheres have different structural and functional properties, each of which are essential to optimal emotional and mental health (Schore, 1994/2016). One of the fundamental tenets of psychology asserts that there are two types of learning: implicit associative learning, also known as Pavlovian classical conditioning, and explicit instrumental learning. Instrumental learning involves voluntary behaviors or actions, followed by reinforcers that strengthen or weaken a motoric response and modify behavior by their consequences, while classical conditioning involves autonomic reflexes. As examples of the latter, a large body of studies have been done on the conditioned emotional response (Annau & Kamin, 1961), human Pavlovian heart-rate conditioning (Furedy & Riley, 1987), human autonomic conditioning (Furedy & Riley, 1987), and classical eyelid conditioning (Prokasy, 1965), all found soon after birth and across the first two years of human infancy.

Applying these dual learning principles to infant/child development, the pediatrician Martha Welch (2016, p. 1271) observes,

> It has been known for over 100 years that organisms learn and retain memory in two ways. They learn consciously in their brains, by way of operant conditioning, and they learn subconsciously in their bodies through Pavlovian or classical conditioning. . . . There have been notable theories and evidence presented that support the idea that emotions are primarily under the control of bodily mechanisms.

I suggest that the major process of learning in early human infancy is right brain classical conditioning associated with involuntary visceral/autonomic learning, and expressed in the attachment learning process of imprinting. Cloninger et al. (2019) refers to "the disposition of a person to learn how to behave, react emotionally, and form attachments automatically by associative conditioning."

Indeed, Pavlovian conditioning is responsible for the simultaneous nonconscious synchronous activation of multisensory limbic-autonomic responses. Furthermore, in imprinting face-to-face social encounters, this early evolutionary form of learning occurs in barely perceivable implicit facial, auditory, and gestural communications that result in rapid involuntary nonconscious fear responses to a sender that induces aversive emotional states in the receiver (Lundqvist & Ohman, 2005). This model is supported by Hugdahl's (1995) work, "Classical Conditioning and Implicit Learning: The Right Hemisphere Hypothesis," and Johnsen and Hugdahl's (1993) "Right Hemisphere Representation of Autonomic Conditioning to Facial Emotional Expressions."

Writing on the ongoing paradigm shift in psychiatry grounded in recent understandings of the functions of the imagistic, intuitive right hemisphere and linguistic, rational left hemispheres, the psychiatrist Paul Valent (2018), a brain laterality scholar, concludes that the emotional right hemisphere is associated with the activity of the unconscious involuntary nervous system while the cognitive left hemisphere is associated with the conscious voluntary nervous system. I suggest that the later-evolving voluntary conscious striatal motor learning generated in the left hemisphere is associated with instrumental learning, including behavioral reward and punishment. Indeed, the left brain is referred to as the instrumental brain.

Basic research indicates a superiority of the human left hemisphere during active (diurnal) daytime and the right hemisphere at more inactive (nocturnal) nighttime, including sleep and dreams (Casagrande & Bertini, 2008). Dreams, Freud's royal road to the unconscious (1900/1953), are a product of rapid eye movement (REM) sleep, which is associated with emotional homeostasis (Walker, 2009). Research demonstrates that the right hemisphere is activated during dreaming sleep (Bertini et al., 1984), and that human REM sleep is accompanied by intense activation of emotional and memory circuits (Maquet et al., 2005) involved in the consolidation of emotional memory formation (Wagner et al., 2001) and in the preservation of affective responses to social stress (Halonen et al., 2024).

Facilitation of emotional memory in REM sleep, particularly late-night sleep, which is rich in rapid eye movements, , shows right-dominant prefrontal activation (Nishida et al., 2008; Sopp et al., 2017). The longest REM periods usually happen at the end of the night, and so the dreams of this last REM period before wakening may thus be the major source of memories of emotional dreams brought to the psychoanalytic psychotherapist. According to Reitav and Thirlwell (2025), morning dreams contain more elements from much earlier life experiences, and are integrative of the dreamer's current emotional struggles. I suggest that these emotional experiences may include intense autobiographical memories activated in a "heightened affective moment" of a session, during transference-countertransference communications and reenactments of nonverbal attachment dynamics. Stimulation of the amygdala enhances REM sleep and induces highly emotional dreamlike images of autobiographical memory (Vignal et al., 2007).

Furthermore, the early right and later left lateralized dual systems use two different memory systems: a right brain implicit-procedural amygdalar memory that precedes a left brain explicit-semantic hippocampal memory system. The former is emotional and accessed instantaneously in implicit recognition memory. While left prefrontal areas process verbal episodic memory, the right prefrontal cortex contributes to the encoding and retrieval of nonverbal episodic memory (Wagner et al., 1998). Right prefrontal cortices are thus operating in the right brain critical period over the first two years, in the form of visuospatial working memory, while the later-forming declarative semantic working memory of the left hippocampal system does not mature until between the end of the second and third year and is associated with language encoding and retrieval. The right anterior temporal pole is associated with emotion and socially relevant memory and is the site of the recollection of personal, episodic memories, while the left anterior temporal lobe processes semantic memory (Olson et al., 2007).

The interdisciplinary perspective of interpersonal neurobiology posits that the synaptic wiring of the infant's early-developing right brain, which is dominant for the processing of emotional and social information, is imprinted in implicit, intersubjective, psychobiological transactions embedded in the child's attachment relationship with the mother. Throughout my work, I refer to *mother* interchangeably with *primary caregiver*, recognizing that the infant's primary attachment figure usually is but may not be the mother. The primary caregiver is the person who serves as the infant's right brain communicator and regulator, especially during moments of stress.

Over the course of the first two years of life, the length of the human brain growth spurt (Dobbing & Sands, 1973), this attachment relationship facilitates a state of rapid development of the infant's right brain and its array of adaptive emotional and relational survival functions. In one of the great classics of psychoanalytic theory, the pediatrician-psychoanalyst Donald Winnicott (1958b) moved beyond Freud's one-person intrapsychic ideas about early human development into a two-person interpersonal model. In his classic article "The Theory of the Parent-Infant Relationship," he boldly stated that "there is no such thing as an infant [apart from the maternal provision]" (1960b, p. 39). In this intersubjective context, the sensitive, responsive mother is providing, at levels beneath awareness, an emotional receptivity and regulation of her infant's emotional and bodily needs, giving rise to a state of mind in the child he called "going on being," a regulated, relaxed quiet alert state needed for the psyche to come to reside in the soma, the integration of mind and body. This maternal state of what McGilchrist (2016) calls "active passivity" is a state of sympathetic-parasympathetic balance of the mother's bodily-based autonomic nervous system. From early postnatal stages, the mother's and infant's right brain subjective self intersubjectively communicates their bodily-based emotional states nonverbally, right brain to right brain, with another human. In this manner the subjectivity of the self is cocreated in intersubjectivity.

A central focus of attachment dynamics is the primary caregiver's homeostatic regulation of the infant's developing brain/mind/body. Regulation theory also offers a conceptualization of the origins of both secure and insecure attachments, and of the etiology of resilience or vulnerability to later disorders of emotion dysregulation and relational deficits. Attachment is critical to more than just the development of overt behaviors and cognitive mental functions but more fundamentally to self-regulating emotional and social capacities that are essential for adaptive homeostatic organismic functioning. A study that I have been part of indicates secure attachment is the normative homeostatic state (Opie et al., 2020).

Modern attachment theory utilizes an interpersonal neurobiological perspective of development, one that describes how right brains align and synchronize their neural activities with other right brains in not only early but all later social interchanges, and how the structure and function of the brain and mind are shaped by social experiences, especially those embedded in emotional relationships. A large body of studies documents that the human infant's right brain begins a growth spurt in the last trimester of pregnancy and ends in the middle to end of the second year, when the left hemisphere begins its own, a period that also marks the end of the human brain growth spurt (Dobbing & Sands, 1973). Over the course of human infancy and toddlerhood, bodily-based attachment communications are interactively regulated between the right brains of the mother and infant, thus facilitating the relational experience-dependent maturation of the infant's rapidly developing right brain. In this manner, "the self-organization of the developing brain occurs in the context of a relationship with another self, another brain" (Schore, 1996, p. 60). With direct relevance to dyadic attachment communications, G. Benedetti (1987) asserts, "the birth of the self is composed of a mixture of interchangeable parts of oneself and others" (p. 194).

The Interpersonal Neurobiology of Optimal Attachment Dynamics

Over the last 30 years, my studies of attachment have utilized an interdisciplinary perspective to describe and integrate the developmental psychological, biological, neurochemical, and neuroendocrinological processes that underlie the formation of an attachment bond of emotional communication between the infant and primary caregiver (Schore, 1994/2016, 2003a, 2003b, 2012, 2019a, 2019b). Throughout my work I have offered a large body of research and clinical data that underscores the centrality of the evolutionary mechanism of early attachment bonding for all later aspects of human development, especially adaptive right brain functions essential for survival. Building upon and expanding John Bowlby's (1969) pioneering studies that integrated psychology, biology, and psychoanalysis, modern attachment theory incorporates current advances in developmental, affective, and social neuroscience in order to offer an overarching theoretical model of psychoneurobiological attachment dynamics.

A central principle of regulation theory dictates that attachment is the relational unfolding of an evolutionary mechanism, and that the essential developmental task of the first two years of human infancy is the cocreation of an attachment bond of emotional communication and regulation between the infant and the primary caregiver. Building upon prenatal physiological communications across the placenta between the mother and fetus, in ensuing perinatal and postnatal periods affective transactions are rapidly transmitted within the dyad, using more and more complex nonverbal sensoriaffective communications. In order to facilitate this relational-emotional mechanism, the mother must be psychobiologically attuned to the dynamic shifts in the infant's bodily-based internal states of central and autonomic arousal. Although initially these communications are mainly expressed in olfactory (Varendi et al., 2002) and tactile modalities (Conde-Agudelo et al., 2011), by the end of the second month the dyad utilizes more integrated visual and auditory channels of communications in mutual gaze interactions.

During synchronized, reciprocal right-brain-to-right-brain attachment transactions, the sensitive primary caregiver, at levels beneath conscious awareness, perceives (recognizes), appraises, and regulates nonverbal expressions of the infant's more and more intense states of positive and negative affective arousal. Via these communications, the mother regulates the infant's postnatally developing central (CNS) and autonomic (ANS) nervous systems. The attachment relationship thus mediates the interactive regulation of bodily-based emotional states. In this ongoing cocreated dialogue, the psychobiologically attuned mother and her infant coconstruct multiple cycles of both "affect synchrony" that upregulates positive affect in play states (e.g., joy-elation, interest-excitement) and "rupture and repair" that downregulates negative affect (e.g., fear-terror, sadness-depression, shame, disgust). These cycles of intersubjective attunement/misattunement/reattunement represent a preverbal psychobiological relational matrix that forms the core of the infant's emerging subjective self.

There is now agreement that emotion is initially regulated by others, but over the course of infancy it increasingly becomes self-regulated as a result of neurophysiological development and actual lived experience. These adaptive capacities are central to the emergence of self-regulation, the ability to flexibly regulate an expanding array of positive and negative affectively charged psychobiological states in various dynamic relational contexts, thereby allowing for the assimilation of a range of adaptive emotional-motivational states into a coherent and integrated self-system. Current attachment workers are now defining secure attachment as "flexibly integrated" (George & Aikins, 2023).

Optimal early emotional experiences that engender a secure attachment with the primary caregiver thus facilitate both types of self-regulation: interactive regulation of emotions accessed while subjectively engaged with other humans in interconnected contexts, and autoregulation of emotions activated while subjectively disengaged from other humans in autonomous contexts. Modern attachment theory describes emotional well-being as nonconscious yet efficient and resilient switching between these two modes (interconnectedness and autonomy), depending on the relational context. Internal working models of attachment encode both of these modes of coping strategies of affect regulation. At the most fundamental level, modern attachment theory is a regulation theory (Schore & Schore, 2008).

Synchronized, affectively charged relational attachment dynamics represent the biopsychosocial mechanism by which humans are sociophysiologically connected to others in order to coregulate their internal homeostatic affective states. The evolutionary mechanism of attachment fundamentally represents the regulation of biological synchronicity between and within organisms (Schore, 1994/2016). At all points of the lifespan, interactive psychobiological regulation supports the survival and growth functions of the right-lateralized human subjective self-system. This principle is echoed in developmental brain research, where Ovtscharoff and Braun (2001) reported, "The dyadic interaction between the newborn and the mother . . . serves as a regulator of the developing individual's internal homeostasis. The regulatory function of the newborn-mother interaction may be an essential promoter to ensure the normal development and maintenance of synaptic connections during the establishment of functional brain circuits" (p. 33). In this manner, dyadic attachment regulatory transactions impact the development of psychic structure, that is, they generate brain growth (Schore, 1994/2016).

In a number of contributions, I have elucidated how the maturation of the emotion-processing limbic-autonomic circuits of specifically the infant's developing right brain are influenced by implicit intersubjective affective transactions embedded in the attachment relationship (Schore, 1994/2016, 2003b, 2012, 2019a, 2019b). Over the first two years, more and more complex right-lateralized visual-facial, auditory-prosodic, and tactile-gestural nonverbal, implicit affective communications lie at the psychobiological core of the emotional attachment bond between the infant and primary caregiver. The very rapid implicit spontaneous processing of nonverbal affective cues in infancy is "repetitive, automatic, provides quick categorization and decision-making, and operates outside the realm of focal attention and verbalized experience" (Lyons-Ruth, 1999, p. 576).

The interpersonal synchronization of the mother's responses to the infant's signals is a key aspect of the mother's embodied and "pre-reflective sensitivity," expressed in the promptness of her timing to immediate moment-to-moment changes in the child's emotional states (Guedeney et al., 2011; Manini et al., 2013). The dictionary definition of sensitivity is "susceptible to the attitudes, feelings, or circumstances of others; registering very slight differences or changes of emotion" (*American Heritage Dictionary*). Sensitivity has been well studied in the developmental attachment literature, where researchers observe that maternal sensitivity cultivates synchronous, reciprocal, and jointly satisfying mother–infant interactions, which in turn foster the development of a secure attachment relationship.

From an interpersonal neurobiological perspective, the nonconscious joint processing of these attachment communications is the product of the synchronized operations of the infant's right brain interacting, connecting, coupling, uncoupling, and recoupling with the mother's right brain. Internal representations of attachment experiences are imprinted in right-lateralized implicit-procedural memory, including moments of mutual interactive regulation. The regulatory functions of mother–infant socioemotional interactions thereby impact the wiring of right brain circuits during a critical period of growth (Ammaniti & Trentini, 2009; Cozolino, 2010; Henry, 1993; Schore, 1994/2016, 2001a, 2003a, 2012; Siegel, 1999).

Lin and his colleagues (2013) published a near infrared spectroscopy study of newborn humans, reporting a higher blood flow in the right over left hemisphere at birth. They stated, "Our findings of right hemisphere dominance are in agreement with the 'Right-hemispheric conservation theory'" and concluded that "the right hemisphere develops earlier. . . . Moreover, in humans, as in animals, the right hemisphere sustains those functions necessary for the survival of the species, including visuospatial or emotional processes, which account for its earlier development" (p. 345). Note that this form of neuroimaging, which is low cost, portable, and easy to use with infants, can identify markers of typical and atypical right brain development at a far earlier age than behavioral assessments, which begin in the second year of life or later.

Describing the dynamic mother–infant nonverbal communication system, Walker-Andrews and Bahrick (2001) asserted, "From birth, an infant is plunged into a world of other human beings in which conversation, gestures, and faces are omnipresent during the infant's waking hours. Moreover, these harbingers of social information are dynamic, multimodal, and reciprocal" (p. 469). In these rapid attachment communications, the child uses the output of the mother's emotion-regulating right cortex as a template for imprinting the hard wiring of circuits in his right cortex that will come to mediate his expanding affective capacities that operate implicitly. All of this is occurring rapidly and spontaneously, as the intuitive mother's state of reverie is cocreating this emotional relationship unconsciously.

Via these face-to-face right-brain-to-right-brain nonverbal communications, the attachment relationship reflects a coordination, alignment, and synchronization between the mother's right brain unconscious and the infant's developing right brain, the psychobiological system of the human unconscious mind. In support of this model, neuroscientists document that the right hemisphere shows an earlier maturation than the left in prenatal and postnatal stages of human development (Gupta et al., 2005; Sun et al., 2005), that the strong and consistent predominance of the right hemisphere emerges postnatally (Allman et al., 2005), and that the mother's right hemisphere is centrally involved in emotional processing and mothering (Lenzi et al., 2009).

Relational attachment transactions thus shape the experience-dependent maturation of right subcortical-cortical systems, and in this manner they impact later personality development, especially of survival functions that act at ultrafast time frames, beneath conscious awareness. My work in developmental neuropsychoanalysis indicates that the implicit self-system of the right brain that evolves in preverbal stages of human life represents the early development of the psychobiological substrate of Freud's dynamic unconscious (Schore, 1997a, 2002b). Indeed, the relational attachment mechanism is generated by reciprocal bidirectional nonverbal communications between the mother's unconscious and the infant's unconscious (Schore, 2012). This right-brain-to-right-brain mechanism mediates the intergenerational transmission of unconscious structures and functions across the generations.

Consonant with this proposal, a body of studies documents that unconscious processing of emotional information is mainly subsumed by a right hemisphere subcortical route (Gainotti, 2012), that unconscious emotional memories are stored in the right hemisphere (Gainotti, 2005), and that this hemisphere is centrally involved in maintaining a coherent, continuous, and unified sense of self operating at levels beneath awareness (Schore, 1994/2016; Devinsky, 2000; McGilchrist, 2009). From infancy throughout all later stages of the lifespan, this right-lateralized system's rapidly acting emotional processes are centrally involved in the control of vital functions supporting survival, in enabling the organism to cope with stresses and challenges, and thus in emotional resilience and well-being.

A body of research now indicates that the right (and not left) lateralized orbital prefrontal system, the locus of Bowlby's control system of attachment, is responsible for the highest-level regulation of affect and stress in the brain (Cerqueira et al., 2008; Perez-Cruz et al., 2009; Schore, 1994/2016; Stevenson et al., 2008; Sullivan & Gratton, 2002; Wang et al., 2005). Indeed, there is now agreement that the human stress response is located in the right hemisphere (Schore, 1994/2016; Wittling, 1997). It is for this reason that "conscious thought processes are believed to only direct a weak influence on the stress-response system" (Fiskum, 2019, p. 417).

Furthermore, a central tenet of regulation theory dictates that early socioemotional experiences may be either predominantly regulated or dysregulated, imprinting secure or insecure attachments. Developmental neuroscience clearly demonstrates that all children are not "resilient" but "malleable," for better or worse. I refer the reader to my previous studies of the central role of organized and especially disorganized insecure attachments in the psychoneuropathogenesis of psychiatric disorders (Schore, 1996, 1997b, 2003a, 2012, 2013). During early critical periods, secure, insecure anxious, insecure avoidant, and disorganized attachment histories are "affectively burnt in" the infant's early developing right brain (Schore, 1994/2016, 2003a).

Less than optimal early dyadic experiences during a critical period of right brain development, including what I have termed relational trauma, are manifest in a form of chronic attachment trauma that results from repeated and prolonged exposure to highly stressful early social and emotional experiences without repair (Schore, 2001b). These intense interpersonal stressors are subjectively experienced by the infant as repeated minor "shocks" or cumulative miniature traumata associated with frequent highly stressful misattunements triggered by the dysregulating caregiver. The caregiver's responses are typically unpredictable, frightening, frightened, or unavailable to the child's attachment overtures, and they reflect "entrance into peculiar compartmentalized or even partially dissociated states of mind" (Hesse, 2010). Dyadic experiences of relational trauma of the early developing right brain are imprinted into right cortical-subcortical systems limbic-autonomic circuits, encoding disorganized-disoriented insecure internal working models of attachment that are nonconsciously accessed at later points of interpersonal emotional stress. For more on my work on relational trauma and its relation to disorganized-disoriented attachment and borderline personality disorder, I refer the reader to Schore (2001b, 2003a, 2009a 2012, 2019b). That said, in this book I focus on organized insecure avoidant and anxious attachments.

The right orbitofrontal system acts as the attachment control system. The first scientific research on the orbitofrontal cortex, the major emotional regulatory system in the brain, was published by my late colleague, the neurosurgeon Karl Pribram, in the *Journal of Neurophysiology* in 1950 (Pribram et al., 1950). This ventromedial cortex, which lies at the bottom part of the prefrontal cortex, is densely connected by the right uncinate fasciculus with the subcortical right amygdala deep in the temporal lobe and involved in the expression and control of emotional and instinctual behaviors. It is important to note that the right hemisphere cycles back into growth phases throughout the lifespan (Thatcher, 1994; Schore, 2001a) and that the orbitofrontal cortex, the executive regulator of the right brain, retains a capacity for plasticity in later life (Barbas, 1995). In light of the facts that the orbitofrontal areas are "critical to the experience of emotion" (Baker et al., 1997, p. 565) and fundamentally involved in "emotion-related learning" (Rolls et al., 1994) and "cognitive-emotional interactions" (Barbas, 1995), the therapeutic relationship can act as a growth-facilitating environment for this self-regulatory system.

Psychobiological Core of Attachment: Nonverbal Emotional Communication and Interactive Affect Regulation

The essential task of the first year of human life, the foundation of the human experience, is the cocreation of an attachment bond of emotional communication and interactive regulation between the infant and the primary caregiver. A central tenet of modern attachment theory dictates that attachment dynamics are expressed in the implicit or "subliminal" regulation of emotion (Koole & Jostmann, 2004). Bowlby (1969) suggested that attachment dynamics of a "reciprocal interchange" are associated with activity in the emotion-processing limbic system, and that in these interactions the mother appraises the infant's "state of arousal." There is now agreement that the regulation of arousal is the most basic level of regulatory processes (Tucker et al., 1995).

Within the emerging attachment relationship, the mother's "intuitive" interactive regulation of emotional arousal during episodes of psychobiological attunement, misattunement, and reattunement not only regulates the infant's internal state but also indelibly and permanently shapes the infant's developing right brain. Caregivers vary in terms of being able to appraise and regulate not only their infant's but their own emotional states, and this potently influences the quality of their attachment to the infant. Different styles of maternal synchronization and regulation of infantile affect and different patterns of regulation of emotions during separation and reunion have been observed in the various attachment typologies. The dynamic affective experiences in the caregiver–infant relationship are very different in securely and insecurely attached dyads.

The mother of the securely attached infant permits access to the child who seeks proximity at reunion and emotional reconnection after a separation. She shows a tendency to respond appropriately and promptly to the infant's spontaneous emotional communications, thereby engendering an implicit unconscious expectation in the secure infant that during times of stress the primary attachment object will remain relationally available and emotionally accessible. The psychobiologically attuned caregiver mutually regulates the child's arousal within a moderate range that is high enough to maintain interactions by stimulating the child up out of low arousal states, but not so intense as to cause distress by generating dysregulated high arousal states. This entails her actively initiating and participating in not only upregulating (arousal amplifying) and downregulating (arousal braking) transactions, but also in interactive repair (optimal arousal recovering) transactions after breaches of the attachment bond.

In these nonverbal communications, in order to "follow the affect," the mother must be psychobiologically attuned to the dynamic crescendos and decrescendos of the infant's bodily-based internal states of ANS and CNS arousal. In this manner the primary caregiver regulates a state of synchronous autonomic balance between the infant's energy-expending components of sympathetic arousal and energy-conserving parasympathetic arousal ("sympatho-vagal balance") and thereby a quiet alert state of safety. The brain/mind/body becomes alerted by sympathetic physiological activation or relaxed by parasympathetic activation. Underscoring the laterality of these ANS subsystems, Gainotti (2020) concludes that the sympathetic nervous system, which allows the organism to respond quickly and strongly to stressful emergency situations, is right lateralized.

On the other hand, my colleague Stephen Porges (2011) describes a "polyvagal" circuit of parasympathetic emotion regulation that emanates from the brainstem nucleus ambiguus and supports the functional dominance of the right side of the brain in regulating autonomic function. He suggests that "the right hemisphere—including the right cortical and subcortical structures—would promote the efficient regulation of autonomic functions via the source nuclei in the brainstem" (p. 139). In this "vagal circuit of emotional regulation" that supports a "social engagement system," right-lateralized structures exhibit greater control than the left of the autonomic physiological responses associated with emotion. Furthermore, he offers a model that "enables the individual to express complex voluntary levels of communication and movement via the left side of the brain, and more intense emotion-homeostatic processes via the right side of the brain" (p. 140).

Due to a stronger connection between the right hemisphere and stress regulatory systems in the sympathetic-adrenomedullary axis and the hypothalamic-pituitary-adrenocortical (HPA) axis, the right hemisphere is dominant for the human stress response (Henry, 1993; Wittling, 1997). Cortisol secretion is under the excitatory control of the right hemisphere (Lueken et al., 2009). During exposure to social stressors, cortisol increases in anticipation of the stressor onset and remains elevated for over an hour after stress exposure (Drevets et al., 2002). Functional magnetic resonance imaging (fMRI) research of HPA regulation of mothers with their infants reports that increased cortisol reactivity is associated with poor maternal functioning (Laurent et al., 2011). In a recent neuroimaging study, "The Orbitofrontal Cortex Modulates Parenting Stress in the Maternal Brain," Noriuchi's laboratory concludes, "Moderate levels of parenting stress. . . exert beneficial effects on maternal motivation. However, high levels of parenting stress often impair warm and responsive parenting, provoke harsh and reactive caregiving, and negatively influence the child-parent relationship, children's outcomes, and the well-being of the mother" (Noriuchi et al., 2019, p. 1). Within the mother–infant relationship, attachment stressors and their regulation are transmitted in rapid right-brain-to-right-brain communications.

Indeed, bodily-based attachment signals of both negative and positive states are bidirectionally transmitted in face-to-face emotional transactions. The right hemisphere is dominant for mutual gaze, "the process during which two persons have the feeling of a brief link between their two minds" (Wicker et al., 1998). Within episodes of eye-to-eye mutual gaze, the most intense form of human communication, the mother's and infant's right brains engage in synchronized, spontaneous facial, vocal, and gestural emotional communications, universal to all cultures (and thus essential to the origin of human nature). In these relational experiences, which the intuitive mother carries out "unknowingly and can hardly control consciously," she provides the infant with a large number of episodes, often around 20 per minute during parent-infant interactions (Papousek et al., 1991, p. 110). These researchers document that caregivers' intuitive contingent response to an infant vocalization occurs rapidly, within 800 milliseconds (Papousek & Papousek, 1987). In such unconscious right brain limbic-autonomic emotional transactions, the mother makes herself implicitly contingent, easily predictable, and manipulatable by the infant and thereby able to interpersonally synchronize her brain with her infant's developing brain. Such highly arousing, bodily-based, emotion-laden, face-to-face interactions allow the infant to be exposed to high levels of social and emotional information.

Thus, during these rapid bidirectional nonverbal affective communications, the mother intuitively synchronizes her bodily-based affective state with the infant's. The sensitive, responsive caregiver implicitly appraises changes in the nonverbal expressions of her infant's internal arousal, shares his or her affective states, and regulates them, all the while bidirectionally nonverbally communicating with the child. To accomplish this, the primary caregiver must successfully regulate nonoptimal high or excessively low levels of stimulation that would induce supraheightened or extremely low levels of arousal (hyperarousal or hypoarousal). These attachment events are occurring in a critical period of development of the infant's right brain. For the rest of the lifespan, attachment dynamics are expressed in right-brain-to-right-brain communications of affect and the interactive regulation of emotional arousal.

A large body of research and clinical studies clearly demonstrates that the primary caregiver is not always attuned and optimally mirroring, that there are frequent moments of stressful misattunement in the dyad, ruptures of their right brain attachment bond. Frequently the misattunement takes place because, in a heightened affective moment when the child's right brain is dysregulating and the caregiver remains in the left brain, they are asynchronized, in opposite hemispheres. The disruption of attachment transactions leads to a transient regulatory failure and an impaired autonomic homeostasis. In a pattern of rupture and interactive repair or disruption and repair, the good-enough caregiver who induces a stress response through misattunement will in a timely fashion shift out of the left and into the right and reinvoke a reattunement—an implicit right brain regulation of the infant's negatively charged arousal. In other words, a common form of misattunement and hemispheric asymmetry occurs when right brain implicit affect regulation is needed and a left brain explicit affect regulation is provided. This applies to both the mother–infant and patient–therapist dyads.

The repair process, common to secure but not insecure avoidant, insecure resistant, or especially insecure disorganized mother–infant dyads, allows the child to cope with stressful negatively charged affects and to gain self-regulatory skills in the form of maintaining persistent efforts to overcome interactive stress. The dyadic process of interactive repair that reestablishes safety also generates a sense of trust in the infant that the caregiver's right brain will be emotionally available at times of stress and in moments of mutual play. Modern attachment theory utilizes a two-person perspective of *interpersonal synchrony* to model right-brain-to-right-brain communications of interactive repair of negatively valenced states, and affect synchrony of positively valenced states. In the case of the latter there is also an *intrapersonal synchrony* between the mother's visual, tactile, and auditory sensory systems, as her eye contact, smiling face, caressing touch, and comforting voice all send signals of safety to the infant of the mother's positively valenced state.

Through right-brain-to-right-brain nonverbal visual-facial, tactile-gestural, and auditory-prosodic attachment communications, the caregiver and infant learn the rhythmic structure of the other and modify their behavior to fit that structure, thereby cocreating a moment-to-moment synchronized, specifically fitted interaction. According to Feldman and her colleagues (1999), "Synchrony in dynamic systems . . . reflects the degree to which interactants integrate into the flow of behavior the ongoing responses of their partner and the changing inputs of the environment." All of this is occurring rapidly and spontaneously, as the mother is intuitively cocreating this emotional relationship unconsciously, beneath levels of her awareness. Thus, the nonverbal communications embedded in the attachment relationship reflect a coordination, an interpersonal synchronization between the mother's right brain unconscious mind/body and the infant's developing right brain unconscious mind/body. Indeed, the mother is implicitly shaping her infant's unconscious mind, which, as Freud observed, develops before the emergence of the conscious mind.

In his seminal first volume, Bowlby (1969) cited Darwin's (1872/1965) observation that movement or expression in the face and body serve as the first means of communication between the mother and the infant. Bowlby proposed that mother–infant attachment communications are "accompanied by the strongest of feelings and emotions, and occur within a context of facial expression, posture, tone of voice" (1969, p. 120). In later classic studies on face-to-face intersubjective communications between mother and infant, Trevarthen (1990) described how synchronized, coordinated visual-facial eye-to-eye messages, tactile and involuntary body gestures, and prosodic vocalizations serve as channels of communicative signals in the earliest dialogues between the 2–3-month-old infant and mother, which induce instant positive emotional effects that are shared by both.

Cole asserted, "It is through the sharing of facial expressions that *mother and child become as one* [emphasis added]. It is crucial, in a more Darwinian context, for the infant to bond with her mother to ensure her own survival" (1998, p. 11). In fact, Darwin (1872/1965) asserted that dynamic changes in facial signals between two individuals ground emotion in homeostatic processes. Following these and other leads, in my first book I suggested that during attachment episodes of right brain visual-facial, auditory-prosodic, and tactile-gestural affective communications, the primary caregiver synchronizes and regulates the infant's internal homeostatic states of ANS peripheral and CNS central arousal (Schore, 1994/2016).

In this manner, the infant's early-maturing right hemisphere, which is dominant for the child's processing of visual emotional information, the infant's recognition of the mother's face, and the perception of arousal-inducing maternal facial expressions, is psychobiologically attuned to and imprinted by the output of the sensitive mother's right hemisphere, which is involved in the expression and processing of emotional information and in nonverbal communication. In order to process these nonverbal communications, the infant seeks not just physical but emotional proximity to the mother, who in an optimal context must be subjectively perceived as predictable, consistent, and emotionally available, and thereby an interpersonal source of safety and trust. Recall Erik Erikson's (1950) classic work demonstrated that the infant's basic trust develops in the first year of life in interaction with the primary caregiver, the mother.

It is now well established that the human female brain undergoes dramatic changes in reproductive hormones during pregnancy and early motherhood that allow her to become more sensitive to the visual, auditory, and olfactory signals from her infant (Kinsley & Lambert, 2006). Using near-infrared spectroscopy, Nishitani et al. (2011) investigated functional changes in a woman's brain when she becomes a mother. They find that compared to nonmothers, mothers discriminated happy, angry, sad, fearful, and surprised emotional facial expressions in their right and not left prefrontal cortex, specifically mentioning the right medial prefrontal cortex. These authors conclude that in social interaction with the infant, the mother's right hemispheric ability to respond appropriately to "nonverbal facial expression" with emotional empathy plays a key role not only in identifying her infant's emotions but also in her ability to bond with her infant. In this manner, the mother's right prefrontal cortex is preferentially involved in maternal behavior. Basic research indicates that the right ventromedial (orbitofrontal) cortex, as opposed to the left, is critically involved in empathy (Shamay-Tsoory et al., 2003) and emotional and social functions (Tranel et al., 2002).

On the other side of the mother–infant attachment relationship, early postnatal brain development in the infant is expressed in the massive outgrowth of dendrites and neurons, and synaptogenesis (Silbereis et al., 2016), especially in rapidly developing areas of the right brain. In the postnatal period, during dyadic attachment bond transactions the sensitive primary caregiver's right brain implicitly (unconsciously) attends to, perceives (perceptually recognizes), appraises, and regulates nonverbal expressions of the infant's more and more intense states of positive and negative emotional arousal. According to Trevarthen (1990), "The intrinsic regulators of human brain growth in a child are specifically adapted to be coupled by emotional communications to the regulators of adult brains."

In this manner infants express their attachment needs, not just through proximity-seeking explicit behaviors but through right-brain-to-right-brain implicit communications. The temporal dynamics of these right brain ultrarapid, spontaneous, bodily-based emotional states are bidirectionally expressed in intersubjective, implicit nonverbal facial, prosodic, and gestural communications, a connection of their right minds. In order to describe this interpersonal neurobiological inscription of attachment experiences within the mother–child relationship, I created the phrase "The infant is hardwired to connect." Neuroscience research documents that the right hemisphere is more deeply connected to the emotion-processing limbic system than the left, that it has more direct connections to both the sympathetic and parasympathetic branches of the involuntary ANS that relate to arousal and relaxation, respectively, and that it is dominant for the spontaneous processing and communication of unconscious emotionally salient attachment stimuli in everyday life.

Directly related to the cocreation of the limbic-autonomic attachment bond, Buck (1994) characterizes "spontaneous emotional communications":

> Spontaneous communication employs species-specific expressive displays in the sender that, given attention, activate emotional preattunements and are directly perceived by the receiver. . . . The "meaning" of the display is known directly by the receiver. . . . This spontaneous emotional communication constitutes *a conversation between limbic systems.* . . . It is a biologically-based communication system that involves individual organisms directly with one another: *the individuals in spontaneous communication constitute literally a biological unit* [emphasis added]. (p. 266)

Buck emphasizes the importance of the right limbic system in this interaction, and thereby describes a nonverbal conversation of two interacting emotionally communicating right brains. This directly applies to mother–infant and patient-therapist interactions.

As the right hemisphere is also dominant for the broader aspects of communication and for subjective emotional experiences, the face-to-face implicit communication of affective states between the right brains of the members of the infant-mother (and therapist-patient) dyad is best described as *intersubjectivity*. With respect to *visual-facial attachment communications*, research indicates that infants develop a preference for looking at the eyes over other regions of the face at two months (Maurer, 1985), and that by four months they can differentiate direct gaze from averted gaze (Vecera, 2006). A body of studies indicates that infants process faces holistically in the right and not left hemisphere, specifically in the right occipitotemporal cortex (de Heering & Rossion, 2015). Furthermore, researchers are documenting a developmental progression over the first year to more complex visual-affective functions. These data indicate that the future capacity to process the essential emotional information expressed in face-to-face communications, a central aspect of all later social relationships, is dependent on caregiver–infant attachment eye contact and visual gazing during early critical periods. Thus, how often and in what contexts the mother and infant spontaneously look (and not look) directly at each other is of key importance to an infant's development and the emotional health of the dyadic relationship.

Ongoing studies of *auditory-prosodic attachment communications* also highlight the role of the right brain. Neuroscience now supports the principle that the caregiver's use of infant-directed speech ("motherese") is critical for the development of the posterior areas of the right hemisphere that process prosodic-emotional functions. Independent of culture, infant-directed speech is preferred over adult-directed speech as early as a few weeks after birth. Compared to adult-directed speech, motherese, the vocal expression of emotion to infants, is higher in pitch, has a wider pitch range, and exhibits exaggerated pitch contours. These studies indicate the importance of not the verbal content but the affective melody of the mother's voice and whether or not she's using infant-directed versus adult-directed speech in her interactions with her child, especially in both calming soothing and exciting playful contexts. This use of infant-directed speech facilitates the development of the infant's right temporal areas and the burgeoning ability to read the emotional tone of the voice of others is an essential element of all later social relationships.

In terms of *tactile-gestural attachment communications* over the course of the first year, the attachment dyad uses interpersonal touch as a communication system, especially for the communication and regulation of emotional information. With respect to gestures, authors are now concluding that the early advantage of the right hemisphere in the first few months of life affects the lateralized appearance of the first imitative gestures. Thus, at all stages of the lifespan, "the neural substrates of the perception of voices, faces, gestures, smells and pheromones, as evidenced by modern neuroimaging techniques, are characterized by a general pattern of right-hemispheric functional asymmetry" (Brancucci et al., 2009, p. 895). This implicit perception of emotional stimuli takes place within the first attachment and all subsequent social contexts.

Supporting this model of the critical importance of right-brain-to-right-brain attachment communications in the progressive socioemotional experience-dependent lateralization of the right brain, hemispheric asymmetry studies now document that the right hemisphere is dominant in human infants. In classic laterality research on human brain development in the first two years, Fox et al. (1994) showed that typically developing infants display a resting relative right frontal asymmetry (higher activity in the right frontal lobe compared to the left) at 9 months that reverses at 14–24 months. Killeen and Teti found that "greater relative right frontal activation in response to seeing one's own infant is related to maternal negative affect matching during times of infant distress, and greater perceived intensity of infant joy during times of joy" (2012, p. 18).

Researchers are now agreeing that a significant measure of healthy infant development is lateralized behavior (Hall et al., 2008). A body of research indicates that attachment transactions influence "the early life programming of hemispheric lateralization and synchronization" (Stevenson et al., 2008) that underlies the dominance of the right hemisphere in the first and second years of life. It is now accepted that "expansion of the *right frontal cortex relative to the left, the largest anatomical asymmetry in the brain* [emphasis added] . . . is particularly responsible for greater right-sided neural plasticity" (McGilchrist, 2021a). Thus, the development of lateralization of the infant's right hemisphere, the emotional brain, the social brain, is dependent upon the emotional interactions embedded in the cocreated mother–infant attachment system. This is confirmed by a number of researchers, including Montirosso et al. (2012), who reported findings "consistent with Schore's (2005) hypotheses of hemispheric right-sided activation of emotions and their regulation during infant–mother interactions" (p. 826), and Minagawa and colleagues (2009), who observed at the end of the first year, "Our results are in agreement with that of Schore (2000b) who addressed the importance of the right hemi-sphere in the attachment system."

As the securely attached infant enters toddlerhood in the second year, his or her interactively regulated right-brain-to-right-brain visual-facial, auditory-prosodic, and tactile-gestural communications become more and more holistically integrated, allowing for the emergence of a coherent emotional right brain and subjective sense of self. This right-lateralized system stores a vocabulary of nonverbal affective facial expressions, prosody, and gestures—right brain signals used in implicit bodily-based attachment communications. Secure, interactively regulated attachment histories are imprinted into developing right cortical-subcortical circuits in implicit-procedural (and not semantic) memory, thus generating an internal working model of attachment that encodes strategies of affect regulation that non-consciously guide the individual through interpersonal contexts, especially in stressful, novel, and close intimate contexts.

Over the later stages of life, these adaptive capacities are central to the dual processes of a secure attachment and optimal regulation of the right brain subjective self: interactive regulation, the ability to flexibly regulate psychobiological states of emotions with other humans in interconnected contexts, and autoregulation, through the individual's own agency, which occurs apart from other humans in autonomous contexts. Furthermore, secure attachments are able not only to receive interactive regulation but to provide interactive regulation of others.

In a secure attachment, the right orbitofrontal cortex, operating beneath conscious awareness, generates an unconscious self-image, what I have termed a cohesive, continuous, and unified sense of self. The right orbitofrontal cortex enters a critical period of growth from 10–12 months to the end of the second year. Human self-awareness associated with self-recognition develops around the age of two years (Lewis et al., 1985). This exactly overlaps the end of a critical period of growth of the right hemispheric orbitofrontal growth spurt. A large body of brain laterality research demonstrates that self-related information, self-awareness, and the recognition of one's own face, voice, and body are processed in the frontal areas of the right hemisphere (e.g., Keenan et al., 2000, 2001; Kircher et al., 2001; Miller et al., 2001; Uddin et al., 2005; Platek et al., 2006; Morita et al., 2008; Rosa et al., 2008; Tsakiris et al., 2008).

Interestingly, the ventral tegmental area in the midbrain, a center of the reward pathway, exhibits greater activation to subliminal presentations of the self-face than those of other faces, while subliminal presentations of others' faces induced activation of the amygdala (Ota & Nakano, 2021). The right amygdala, the ventral anterior cingulate, and the anterior insula are all involved in the emotional processing of self-face recognition (Morita et al., 2014; Yoshimura et al., 2009). Medford and Critchley (2010) proposed that the anterior insular cortex and anterior cingulate, which have strong interconnections, represent the basis of self-awareness. The right insula's activity serves as a "topographic and dynamic glue or node for integrating different layers of self" (Scalabrini et al., 2021, p. 11) and functions as a "sentient self" (Craig, 2010).

Using self-report questionnaires on communication and emotion in social interaction, Anderson and Guerrero (1998) suggest that secure attachment in adulthood is expressed in an ability to form trusting relationships, have realistic expectations, acknowledge negative emotions, and turn to others for support. In the psychiatric literature on secure attachment, Maunder and Hunter (2009) cite a body of studies to show

> a person with secure attachment has developed sufficient self-confidence and confidence in the value of *close relationships* to allow flexibility in moving comfortably between autonomy and dependence in a way that is realistically and effectively responsive to circumstances. Relationships are valued. The give and take of close relationships are usually reciprocal and balanced. . . . The secure style is characterized by *resilience and effective collaboration* [emphasis added]. (p. 125)

According to these authors, secure individuals have a sense of positive self-esteem combined with sociability and enjoy being with others in interpersonal relationships. They experience others as being emotionally available, and when in contact with attachment figures experience increases in subjective comfort. They are not prone to anger but assertive, expressing anger that facilitates repair and resolution, and manage conflict effectively. Secure personalities are described as adaptable, warm, trusting, dependable, cooperative, understanding, playful, and loving. They use flexible strategies that activate or deactivate the attachment system and have a well-developed capacity for affect regulation, and can self-soothe using both internal resources and external support. That being the case, these individuals, like all human beings, at times experience conscious stressful insecurities that are felt in all their intensity, but without strong affect-repressing defenses.

For the rest of the lifespan, the right, and not left, lateralized prefrontal regions are responsible for the communication and regulation of affect and stress, especially the right orbitofrontal (ventromedial) cortex, the apex of the emotion-processing limbic autonomic system, which I have identified as Bowlby's attachment control system. The right orbital prefrontal cortex acts as the source of "hot" right hemisphere executive functions, as opposed to the left dorsolateral prefrontal cortex and "cool" left hemisphere executive functions. It is now thought that "the fronto-orbital part of the right hemisphere is responsible for the very complicated mental functions that characterize *only humans* [emphasis added]" (Rotenberg, 2021, p. 263). Note the direct involvement of this early-forming system in the origin of human nature, a central theme of these chapters. These complex functions include uniquely human maternal behavior. Noriuchi et al. (2019) now report that the right orbitofrontal cortex plays a central role in providing intrinsic maternal motivation and that its activation is critical for adaptation in daily parenting situations and the mother's sense of parenting competence.

The enduring legacy of a secure attachment with a psychobiologically attuned mother is an efficient right brain that can implicitly regulate positive and negative emotional experiences and thereby cope with the novelty and stress that is inherent in all human interactions. Over the lifespan, this more complex right brain is capable of regulating and maintaining an implicit subjective self: a cohesive, active mental structure that continuously appraises life's experiences and responds according to its scheme of interpretation (Schore, 2003a). My colleague Iain McGilchrist (2009) concludes an efficient right hemisphere is dominant for *integration*. In contrast to the left hemisphere,

> the right hemisphere has a greater degree of myelination, facilitating swift transfer of information between the cortex and the centres below the cortex, and greater connectivity in general. . . . At the experiential level it is also better able to *integrate* [emphasis added] perceptual processes, particularly binding together different kinds of information from different senses . . . this means in bringing together in consciousness

different elements, including information from the ears, eyes, and other sensory organs, and from memory, so as to generate the richly complex but coherent, world which we experience. (p. 42)

My fellow laterality researcher Russell Meares (2012) asserts that the brain's right side creates an "'inner,' emotionally laden experience" and a self-system that generates "*a background state of well-being.*" This hemispheric asymmetry model of a positive sense of self is supported by recent neuroimaging research showing that myelinated white matter tracts exclusively in the right hemisphere correlate with personality profiles predictive of subjective well-being and optimism (Kotikalapudi et al., 2022). These latter authors report

> The right hemisphere has been involved in a variety of integrative phenomena, including helping the implicit self maintain a positivity bias (Quirin et al., 2018). The implicit self is a highly integrative construct that processes vast amounts of self-relevant information. . . . Because personal experiences are inherently perceived as positive in healthy individuals, a functional implicit self is critical in maintaining a positivity bias by assimilating negative affective experiences within a network of predominantly positive experiences (Rotenberg, 2004; Schore, 1996). Due to this holistic nature, the implicit self is believed to be a function of the right hemisphere (Kuhl et al., 2015). . . . Our study thus supports previous findings that the right hemisphere is necessary for healthy individuals to express their positivity bias. (Kotikalapudi et al., 2022)

Furthermore, in the early critical period of right brain maturation from the last trimester of pregnancy through the second year, interactive emotional experiences within the mother–child relationship may be regulated or dysregulated, imprinting either secure or insecure attachments with a negatively biased self. Modern attachment theory explicates the interpersonal processes that shape, for better or worse, the survival functions of the right brain. Developmental neuroscience now clearly demonstrates that all children are not "resilient" but "malleable" (Leckman & March, 2011). In a 2011 editorial on an entire issue of the *Journal of Child Psychology and Psychiatry* titled "Developmental Neuroscience Comes of Age," these authors describe "the phenomenal progress of the past three decades of research" and assert that "a scientific consensus is emerging that the origins of adult disease are often found among developmental and biological disruptions occurring during the early years of life" (p. 333). Alluding to a paradigm shift, they confidently state,

> Over the past decade it has also become abundantly clear that in addition to the remarkable cascade of genetic, molecular and cellular events that ultimately lead to the formation of the billions of neurons that inhabit the human neocortex, the in utero and immediate postnatal environments and the dyadic relations between child and caregivers within the first years of life can have direct and enduring effects on the child's brain development and behavior. . . . *The enduring impact of early maternal care and the role of epigenetic modifications of the genome during critical periods in early brain development in health and disease is likely to be one of the most important discoveries in all of science that have major implications for our field* [emphasis added]. (Leckman & March, 2011, p. 334)

They further conclude, "our in utero and our early postnatal interpersonal worlds shape and mold the individuals (infants, children, adolescents, and adults and caregivers) we are to become" (p. 333).

Although the role of early expressed genetic factors continues to be an essential focus of current study, it has become clear that genes do not specify behavior absolutely; prenatal and postnatal environmental epigenetic factors play critical roles in early right brain attachment development. There is considerable interest across disciplines in the problem of specifically how genetic, hormonal, environmental, and social factors influence brain development, and how these act in the causal pathways that link early development with a predisposition to later resilience or psychopathologies and disease. All fields are now converging on the centrality of epigenetic mechanisms—heritable changes in gene expression that occur without a change in DNA sequence. Epigenetic DNA methylation determines gene expression and silencing during prenatal and postnatal critical periods (Novakovic et al., 2010).

According to Monk and her colleagues (2012) the in utero environment is regulated by placental function and is highly susceptible to maternal distress and a target of epigenetic dysregulation. In discussing gene regulation in the placenta and fetal development, they observe,

> This temporary endocrine structure regulates the transfer of nutrients to the developing fetus, buffers the fetus from toxins and maternal glucocorticoids, and by altering maternal hormone levels can also influence maternal mood and the priming of the maternal brain with consequences for the quality of postnatal mother–infant interactions. Thus gene regulation within the placenta can have functional consequences for both fetal and infant development.

The social environment, particularly the one created together by the mother and fetus/infant, directly affects gene-environment epigenetic interactions and thereby has long-enduring effects, for better or worse.

Indeed, during critical periods in utero and in infancy when the developing brain has heightened sensitivity to social environmental experiences, epigenetic programming that turn genes on or off by variations in maternal care imparts either a risk for or resilience to later psychopathology (Weaver et al., 2004; Roth & Sweatt, 2011). Research describes the detrimental effects of deficits of maternal care in the alteration of specifically the right and not left ventromedial cortex (Lyons et al., 2002) and the creation of a vulnerability to future psychopathologies (e.g., Schore, 1994/2016, 2003a, 2012, 2019a). Clinicians are concluding, "If children grow up with dominant experiences of separation, distress, fear and rage, then they will go down a bad pathogenic developmental pathway, and it's not just a bad psychological pathway but a bad neurological pathway" (Watt, 2003, p. 109). This is due to the fact that during early critical periods of rapid growth, organized insecure and disorganized insecure attachment histories of what I have termed "relational trauma" are "affectively burnt in" the infant's rapidly developing right brain (Schore, 2001b, 2003a). These stressful relational experiences are encoded in the nonverbal right brain as unconscious insecure internal working models of inflexible strategies of affect regulation and rigid ways of being in the social world.

Furthermore, in my 2017 article in the *Infant Mental Health Journal* "All Our Sons: The Developmental Neurobiology and Neuroendocrinology of Boys at Risk" (Schore, 2017a), I offered evidence to show that the developing right hemisphere stress system in male infants develops more slowly than in females, and that this maturational gender difference is expressed in more immature male infants being particularly negatively impacted by early development stress. This article has been multiply cited in various scientific and clinical literatures. As an example, in the journal *International Journal of Environmental Research and Public Health*, Pagani and her colleagues (2023) assert, on this gender variation in early stress,

> This is likely due to differences in sex hormones and differing rates of early right brain maturation processes favoring females (Schore, 2017). Neural circuitry targeted for stress regulation and socioemotional functioning develops more slowly in male than in female brains throughout the perinatal period. This delay may partly explain why boys might be more vulnerable to social stressors such as maternal depression (Schore, 2017). . . . Being a boy is a risk factor for difficult temperament in infants (Schore, 2017). Difficult temperament, which is a neurobiologically driven emotional self-regulatory problem in infants, increases risk of postnatal depression in women. (Letourneau et al., 2019)

In my earlier 2001 article in the *Infant Mental Health Journal*, "The Effects of a Secure Attachment Relationship on Right Brain Development, Affect Regulation, and Infant Mental Health," I concluded,

> Adaptive infant mental health can be fundamentally defined as the earliest expression of efficient and resilient strategies for coping with novelty, stress, and change, and maladaptive infant mental health as a deficit in these same coping mechanisms. The former is a resilience factor for coping with relational stressors at later stages of the life cycle, the latter is a risk factor for interruptions of developmental processes and a vulnerability to the emotional coping deficits that define later-forming psychopathologies. (Schore, 2001a)

Across disciplines there is now agreement that resilience involves the adaptive ability to bounce back from adversity, integrating emotional, social, and cognitive dimensions. It is thus a central factor in developmental change. This right brain perspective of resilience is consonant with Darwin's (1859/1958) principle that the ability of the brain to adapt to changing circumstances is the key to the survival and thriving of the human species.

The Role of the Father in Early Human Brain Development

The infant's right hemisphere ends its initial growth spurt in the middle to end of the second year, as the left hemisphere begins its own (Thatcher et al., 1987). Thirty years ago I provided extant developmental data which suggested that subsequent to the child's formation of an attachment to the mother in the first year, the child forms another, to the father in the second (Schore, 1994/2016). I also proposed that the mother's communications have a major impact on the baby's brain in the first year of right brain dominance, and the father's in the second year, when the infant's left brain enters a growth spurt. Indeed, classic developmental researchers observed that the formation of a second attachment system to the father emerges in the second year (Schaffer & Emerson, 1964), as the child now expresses a separation response to the absence of either parent and becomes involved in separation-individuation dynamics.

In classic developmental psychoanalytic studies, Margaret Mahler (1980) described the father's essential role in a rapprochement subphase of the separation-individuation phase of the practicing period at the end of the second year. Developmental psychological research demonstrated that the quality of the toddler's attachment to the father is independent of that to the mother (Main & Weston, 1981), and that at 18 months both a "mother attachment system" and a "father attachment system" are operational (Abelin, 1971). These two independent systems are respectively located in the child's right hemisphere, which is ending its growth spurt, and the left hemisphere, which is entering one. As opposed to the nonverbal right hemisphere, the left is dominant for not only verbal learning and emergent speech functions but for individuality, independence, and autonomy (Hecht, 2014). During a critical period of a left brain growth spurt, the secure father is thus shaping the child's emerging adaptive left brain abilities. That said, at any earlier time in the child's infancy, the secure father is capable of feeling and expressing tenderness in right-brain-to-right-brain communications. Though it may come as a surprise to some, we now have evidence that men do have right brains!

The role of the father in child development has been comprehensively summarized by, among others, Cabrera and Tamis-LeMonda (2013), Lamb

(2004), and Herzog (2001). The latter observed, "The biorhythmicity of man with infant and woman with infant" allows the infant to have "interactive, state-sharing, and state-attuning experiences with two different kinds of caregivers" (Herzog, 2001, p. 55). He further asserted that this paternal function is "entirely contingent on the presence of homeostatic-attuned caregiving by the mother." Herzog also pointed out that through the father's careful use of his own assertiveness, he helps the boy to modulate and integrate his own burgeoning aggression and states that his "stimulating, gear-shifting, disruptive, limit-setting play" mobilizes intense affect and facilitates "radical reorganization and further developmental progression" (p. 261).

A large body of studies indicate a difference between the mother's and father's play even in the first year, and that the father's is more arousing and energetic, while the mother's is more calming. Though the mother's soothing is essential to the child's attachment security, the father's arousing play is thought to be critical for the child's competent active exploration of the physical world. This physical exploration involves the striatal motor system operant instrumental reward learning, located in the instrumental left hemisphere. Expanding upon these ideas, I have suggested that although the mother is essential to the infant's capacity for fear regulation, in the second year the father is critically involved in male and female toddlers' aggression regulation (Schore, 2003a). I suggest the paternal attachment system of father-son interactions forges an androgenic neuroplastic imprint in the toddler's evolving left brain developing circuits, allowing for the father's regulation of the male toddler's testosterone-induced aggression ("terrible twos") and rough-and-tumble play.

Bowlby (1969) proposed that the child's experience with a supportive mother and "a little later father" (p. 378) indicates that the right-to-right transmission of attachment patterns between mother and infant precedes the subsequent left-to-left transmission between father and child. Building upon this, in *Affect Regulation and the Origin of the Self*, I offered the hypothesis that not only the infant's mother but also the father is impacting the growth of the baby's brain. In that work I argued that in the first year the mother is the major source of the environmental stimulation that facilitates (or inhibits) the experience-dependent maturation of the child's developing right brain neurobiological structures. In the second year, however, the father now becomes an important source of arousal induction and reduction, and his modulation of stimulation will influence the formation of those neural structures that are entering a critical period of growth of the toddler's left hemisphere.

In the last three decades, the vast majority of developmental neurobiological research has focused on the mechanisms by which specifically one particular adult, a mother, impacts the development of her offspring's brain. That said, a series of studies clearly demonstrates that paternal care affects synaptic development in the orbitofrontal cortex (Helmeke et al., 2009) and the anterior cingulate (Ovtscharoff et al., 2006). Interestingly, juvenile rough-and-tumble play, a behavior extensively investigated by Panksepp (1998), has been shown to be critically impacted by the father-child relationship (Flanders et al., 2010) and to depend upon orbitofrontal activity (Pellis & Pellis, 2007). This body of work shows that deprivation of a father or a father figure, especially in a critical period in toddlerhood, impacts the child's left hemisphere more than the right.

Anna Machin (2018) proposes that highly pleasurable rough-and-tumble play, which she describes as "the original and prototype father-child interaction," facilitates a rapid bond between the father and child. The author further posits that "paternal investment in the socialization of children" conferred "evolutionary advantages to humans." Note this evolutionary advance in both phylogeny and ontogeny of the human paternal function is initiated during the developmental growth spurt of the left brain and thereby on specifically left hemispheric functions, including uniquely human language, abstraction, verbal intelligence, social motivation, competition, and survival skills. Machin also discusses the paternal impact of rough-and-tumble play on the child: "Children of fathers involved in their education were more likely to develop the skills necessary for survival" (p. 152).

Flanders et al. (2013) describe the synchronized social learning and collaboration in joyful rough-and-tumble play between fathers and young children that involves both cooperation and competition:

> In playing aggressively with you, I am learning to modulate my behavior with respect to yours: I am allowing your motivational and emotional states to shape mine; and I am adopting a shared frame of reference. Over time, this embodied appreciation of other gives rise to more abstract, social cognitive abilities. (p. 375)

This social learning includes limits on aggressive behavior, as well as reciprocity (Barish, 2020). Citing my work (Schore, 1994/2016), this latter author observes that vigorous play with fathers in infancy and early childhood enhances a child's ability to recognize and express emotions. The father's physical play behavior at this time thus has different impacts on the dual cerebral hemispheres. Note the direct reference to right hemispheric cooperation and left hemispheric competition.

Indeed, in the middle of the second and into the third year, the structural development of the child's brain is shifting from a maternal experience-dependent maturation of the infant's postnatally developing right cortical system to a father or a father figure and a paternal experience-dependent maturation of an even later developing left cortical system. According to Bogels and Phares (2008),

> The father's role can be characterized by play, challenge, risk taking, *encouraging independence*, and, later in development, by helping the child make the transition to the outside world. Moreover, fathers are important in their role of supporting mothers and the family and through their marital relationship with the mother. Finally, fathers' unique role is not only important during childhood, but continues to be important in children's young adult years. (p. 544)

I suggest that in single-parent homes, the mother's left hemisphere (or a father figure's) is imprinting the child's left hemisphere.

In support of this hemispheric chronology, Meuwissen and Carlson (2015) offer research on the role of father parenting in the development of executive function of preschoolers in the third year, aged 35 to 41 months (early childhood, the exact time of a verbal left hemisphere growth spurt). These authors point out that executive functions show rapid development during the preschool years and that it is associated with higher levels of not only cognitive thinking but self-regulation skills. They observe that at this time the father's support of the child's autonomy, "the most important aspect of parenting for the development of independent action . . . facilitates self-regulation of behavior" (p. 2).

Other studies document that paternal autonomy support is important for the development of the child's left hemispheric emerging "cool" executive functions, which are involved in explicit self-regulation, conscious control, voluntary willpower, complex cognitive advances, psychological distancing, instrumental goal-related behavior, and reflective thinking (Giesbrecht et al., 2010; Mischel et al., 2011; Zelazo, 2004). From a neurobiological perspective, these emerging executive functions are located in the left hemisphere, specifically the left dorsolateral prefrontal cortex, which is involved in abstract thinking, cognitive control, and self-reflective consciousness (Andrews et al., 2011; Courtney et al., 1998; Dehaene & Naccache, 2001).

That said, in this left brain critical period, the father may be a source of authoritarian parenting, expressed in threats, harsh punishments, or shaming that induce externalizing behavior in the child. Reviewing the large literature on authoritarian parenting, Cramer (2011) states, "The Authoritarian/Autocratic parent tries to shape, control and evaluate the behavior of the child according to a set standard. Obedience to authority is stressed; orders are expected to be obeyed without explanation. Punitive measures are favored to bring about compliance" (p. 254). A large body of research shows a strong relation between harsh parental discipline and aggressive problems, especially in boys, as early as two and three years of age (Lyons-Ruth & Block, 1996), the same time frame as the accelerated growth in the child's left hemisphere. It is now well established that increased aggression is associated with elevated levels of testosterone (Rausch et al., 2015).

On the other hand, in my own studies in the *Infant Mental Health Journal* I have reported research documenting important hormonal changes in men associated with parenting (fatherhood) and marriage (Schore, 2017a). Testosterone levels are lower in married versus single men (Booth & Dabbs, 1993) and in fathers (Gray et al., 2006). Interestingly, fathers' testosterone levels drop during their partners' late pregnancy and early postpartum period (Perini et al., 2012; Storey et al., 2000), and men who provide more parental care have lower baseline testosterone levels than fathers who provide less care or fathers without children (Gettler et al., 2011). Lower levels of paternal testosterone have been linked not only with suppressing aggression toward infants but also with developing paternal nurturance expressed in tenderness and increasing empathy for the child.

Researchers are proposing that the reduction of testosterone in a committed romantic relationship is related to "pair bonding" (attachment) and that "affiliative interactions with a partner may decrease testosterone levels" (Burnham et al., 2003, p. 121). I suggest that these adaptive hormonal changes are a direct result of synchronized regulated right-brain-to-right-brain implicit, reciprocal, bodily-based affective attachment communications between the mother and the father, as well as in nontraditional relationships between two male parents, and they would be activated in paternal tenderness as well as father-child play. These interactions have organizational, programming effects on the growth of paternal circuits in the father's brain, paralleling documented increased growth in the mother's brain in the postpartum months (Kim et al., 2010).

Indeed, a functional MRI study reveals that the father's brain is sensitive to childcare experiences, and that while maternal caregiving involves an "evolutionarily ancient" brain-hormone-behavior subcortical-paralimbic network involved in emotional processing, paternal caregiving activates a later-developing brain-hormone-behavior cortical circuit involved in socio-cognitive understanding, mentalizing, and future planning (Abraham et al., 2014). In other words, this work characterizes two types of caregiving, right-brain-to-right-brain regulation of the infant's emotional brain, and later left-brain-to-left-brain regulation of the child's cognitive brain.

That said, to my mind there is one single primary caregiver that psychobiologically synchronizes with the infant's developing mind. A good definition of the primary caregiver is that, under stress, and when seeking interactive play, the baby moves toward this single person's right brain and not the secondary caregiver's in order to seek the external arousal regulation he or she needs at the moment. At the same time, the father, through his ongoing emotional interactions with the infant, is getting a good felt sense of who the baby is as well as emotionally supporting the mother. To my mind, the right-brain-to-right-brain primary bond in most cases is to the mother in the first two years of human infancy and toddlerhood. Many psychotherapists and family therapists are aware of the fact that in certain clinical histories the mother is the primary source of so much emotional stress that she cannot act as the primary affect regulator for the baby, and the father takes on the role of the right brain communicator and regulator for the infant.

There are extensive differences between females and males in terms of the ability to process emotional information. Females show an enhanced capacity to more effectively read nonverbal communications and to empathically resonate with emotional states than men. When it comes to reading facial expressions, tone of voice, and gestures, women are generally better than men. This is why in all human societies, the very young and the very old are mostly attended to by females. Furthermore, the orbitofrontal cortex, the control center of attachment and the brain's major system of affect regulation, is in general larger in females (Gur et al., 2002), although there is variation in size and complexity, dependent on early attachment experiences. Interestingly, magnetoencephalographic research reveals that the medial orbitofrontal cortex of both females and males rapidly and thereby implicitly responds to the image of an infant's face in 130 milliseconds (Kringelbach et al., 2008). These authors conclude the orbitofrontal cortex expresses a specific and rapid signature for not just maternal but parental instinct.

The question arises whether the gender distinction is a historic artifact from Bowlby's era. In contemporary society, there are now diverse family units, families with a mother and a father, two mothers or two fathers, and single-parent families. In those diverse situations, we are still looking at how the primary caregiver's right brain shapes the infant's right brain. There are differences in the wiring of the emotion-processing limbic system between males and females, influenced by individual attachment history. That being the case, in both males and females, there are different early internalizations around gender. Both developing males and females first internalize a maternal and then a paternal attachment. In the second year, in both sexes, psychological gender (the sense of maleness or femaleness) is not only genetically encoded but also epigenetically molded by early experiences with masculine and feminine caregivers. This allows access to affiliative and nurturant feminine aspects such as paternal tenderness and to pragmatic masculine aspects of power and independence in the evolving personality in developing females. We all have right brain feminine and left brain masculine internalizations.

Ultimately, what the infant needs for a secure attachment is direct access to a well-functioning adult right brain that can empathically synchronize, send, receive, share, and implicitly regulate the infant's positive and negative emotional communications. It's not just the gender but the attachment security and emotional health of the parent that is the key to who can best provide right brain primary caregiving in the first year. Indeed, securely attached males also have efficient right orbitofrontal systems. When you see families where there is a switch, where the father is the primary caregiver and nurturer, or where there are two fathers (or two mothers), I would suggest the couple has intuitively and rationally figured out together who's better at emotional-relational versus rational-analytic skills and have agreed to divide their roles accordingly. In terms of the best interest of the child, this important decision ensures that the developing infant has optimal access to the more efficient right-brain-to-right-brain communication system in that particular set of parents.

Chapter 2

Ongoing Neurobiological Updates of Freud's Unconscious Mind in Psychotherapy and Across Human Development

Within a short period of time following the publication of my *Affect Regulation* volume (Schore, 1994/2016), I was invited by the *Journal of the American Psychoanalytic Association* to publish an article, "A Century After Freud's Project: Is a Rapprochement Between Psychoanalysis and Neurobiology at Hand?" (Schore, 1997a). It is often forgotten that in his first professional career Freud was an internationally respected neurologist, who coined the term *agnosia* and offered important work on aphasia. And yet his early career as a scientist made an indelible impression upon his professional identity. In 1921 Freud wrote to a colleague, "If I had my life to live over again I should devote myself to psychical research rather than to psychoanalysis" (Jones, 1953, p. 392).

I began my 1997 article with Freud's description of his own mind at a point of significant changes in his career from neurology to the foundation of psychoanalysis. On April 27, 1895, Sigmund Freud wrote his friend and colleague Wilhelm Fliess that he was rapidly becoming preoccupied, indeed obsessed, with a problem which had now seized his mind. In what would turn out to be a creative spell, he was attempting to integrate his extensive knowledge of brain anatomy and physiology with his current experiences in psychology and psychopathology in order to construct a systematic model of the functioning of the human mind in terms of its underlying neurobiological mechanisms. In the preceding year, he had completed the final chapter on psychotherapy for *Studies on Hysteria*, and at this point in time, 20 years into his professional career, he had produced over 100 scientific works. Yet in his letter to Fliess he openly admitted, "I am so deeply immersed in the 'Psychology for Neurologists' as to be entirely absorbed until I have to break off, really exhausted by overwork. I have never experienced such intense preoccupation. I wonder if anything will come of it" (Jones, 1953, p. 380).

Throughout the summer, Freud continued to relay to Fliess messages of both his progress and frustration on the Project, describing his mood as alternately "proud and happy" or "ashamed and miserable." Freud's coauthor, Josef Breuer, wrote to Fliess in July 1895, "Freud's intellect is soaring at its highest" (Sulloway, 1979, p. 114). In September he feverishly began to write it out, and within one month he had filled two notebooks totaling 100 manuscript sheets, which he sent to Fliess in early October. In a letter of October 20, commenting on his ambitious attempt to work out the direct links between the operations of the brain and the functions of the mind, he wrote,

> One evening last week when I was hard at work, tormented with just that amount of pain that seems to be the best state to make my brain function, the barriers were suddenly lifted, the veil drawn aside, and I had a clear vision from the details of the neuroses to the conditions that make consciousness possible. Everything seemed to connect up, the whole worked well together, and one had the impression that the Thing was now really a machine and would soon go by itself. . . . Naturally I don't know how to contain myself for pleasure. (Jones, 1953, p. 382)

The state of elation and excitement would not last. A month later he admitted to Fliess, "I no longer understand the state of mind in which I hatched out the 'Psychology,' and I can't understand how I came to inflict it on you" (p. 383). In fact, he never asked for the return of the manuscript and never wanted to see it again. Fliess kept it, however, and after Freud's death it was finally published under the title "Project for a Scientific Psychology" (Freud, 1895/1966). Indeed, in his subsequent development of psychoanalytic theory, Freud attempted to expunge the neurophysiological and biological roots of his psychological model.

What was Freud attempting to accomplish, and why did the seeming possibility of achieving this goal create in him an exhilaration that he was hardly able to contain, yet his failure triggers a quick and apparently irreversible repudiation? What are the contents of this controversial document that appeared at the dawn of psychoanalysis, and how did they influence Freud's subsequent thinking? At the very outset of this short essay, Freud proclaims that the essential aim of the Project was to "furnish a psychology which shall be a natural science." He then presents, for the first time, a number of new elemental constructs that will literally serve as the foundation, the very bedrock of psychoanalytic theory.

In this remarkable document, Freud introduces the neurobiology of the unconscious, perception, and memory; preconscious psychic activity of primary and secondary processes; the principles of pleasure-unpleasure, constancy, and reality testing; the wish-fulfillment theory of dreams; and the theory of psychic regression. Importantly, this seminal work also contains Freud's earliest thoughts about the essential nature of three problems that he struggled with for the rest of his career: early development and the establishing of human contact, motivation, and affect. Thus Freud's earliest neurological formulations of the unconscious were first outlined in the Project and lie at the foundation of both theoretical and clinical psychoanalysis.

If it is true that Freud disavowed the Project, why are we so familiar with the concepts it introduced? Freud's biographer Ernest Jones provides us with the answer—it is contained in the seventh chapter of Freud's (1900/1953) masterwork, *The Interpretation of Dreams*. In 1896, Freud wrote Fleiss that he had revised the Project and formally renamed it "metapsychology." This was the same year that he would use the term *psychoanalysis* for the first time. In his essay "On the History of the Psycho-Analytic Movement," Freud (1914/1957) stated that *The Interpretation of Dreams*, though published in 1900, "was finished in all essentials at the beginning of 1896" (p. 22). For more on this first groundbreaking attempt to integrate neurology and psychology and Freud's creation of the field of psychoanalysis, I refer the reader to Chapter 6 of my 2003 volume *Affect Regulation and the Repair of the Self*.

In *The Claims of Psycho-analysis to Scientific Interest*, Freud (1914/1958) later asserted:

We have found it necessary to hold aloof from biological considerations during our psycho-analytic work and to refrain from using them for heuristic purposes, so that we may not be misled in our impartial judgement of the psycho-analytic facts before us. But after we have completed our psycho-analytic work *we shall have to find a point of contact with biology* [emphasis added]; and we may rightly feel glad if that contact is already assured at one important point or another. (pp. 181–182)

As *Affect Regulation and the Origin of the Self: The Neurobiology of Emotional Development* demonstrated, this contact point is emotion, which operates rapidly beneath levels of conscious awareness. In its last chapter, "A Proposed Rapprochement Between Psychoanalysis and Neurobiology," I offered a seminal articulation of the emergent field of neuropsychoanalysis, the neuroscience of psychoanalysis. Throughout the book I showed that although the bulk of Freud's writings describe an intrapsychic model of the unconscious, he laid the groundwork for, but never fully elaborated, a future two-person relational unconscious, an unconscious that communicates with another unconscious.

Toward that end, I cited his 1912 article where he stated, "The analyst must turn his unconscious like a receptor organ towards the transmitting unconscious of the patient . . . so the doctor's unconscious is able, from the derivatives of the unconscious which are communicated to him, to reconstruct that unconscious" (1912/1958, pp. 115–116). In that work Freud articulates the "fundamental rule of psychoanalysis" of how the clinician can receive these communications:

> He should withhold all conscious influences from his capacity to attend, and give himself over completely to his "unconscious memory." Or, to put it purely in terms of technique: "He should simply listen, and not bother about whether he is keeping anything in mind." What is achieved in this manner will be sufficient for all requirements during the treatment. (1912/1958, p. 112)

I have suggested that Freud's listening stance of "free floating," "wide ranging," "evenly suspended attention" is equated with a right brain quiet alert state that can receive and send right-brain-to-right-brain unconscious nonverbal communications.

Soon after, Freud observed, "Everyone possesses in his own uncon-scious an instrument with which he can interpret the utterances of the unconscious of other people" (1913/1958). In that same publication, Freud recommended,

> *The therapist must surrender himself to his own unconscious* mental
> activity, in a state of evenly suspended attention, to avoid so far as
> possible, reflection and the construction of conscious expectations,
> not try to fix anything that he hears particularly in his memory, and
> by these means *to catch the drift of the patient's unconscious with his
> own unconscious* [emphasis added]. (1913/1958)

In 1915, Freud continued to allude to an interpersonal model of the unconscious when he asserted, "It is a very remarkable thing that the unconscious of one human being can react upon that of another, with-out passing through the conscious" (1915/1957, p. 194). Following up on Freud, Carl Jung (1946), in *The Psychology of Transference*, proposed that unconscious-to-unconscious therapist–patient communication describes the affective nature of relationships. These psychoanalytic models alluded to a two-way, bidirectionally transmitting unconscious of emotional commu-nications within the coconstructed therapeutic relationship and in clinical models of unconscious transference and countertransference interactions.

Neuropsychoanalytic Advances of Freud's Clinical Model: Right-Brain-to-Right-Brain Emotional Communications in Transference-Countertransference Interactions

Current psychodynamic models of transference contend that "no appre-ciation of transference can do without emotion" and that "transference is distinctive in that it depends on early patterns of emotional attach-ment with caregivers" (Pincus, Freeman, & Modell, 2007). Transference involves a surrender to a regression, which Freud (1900/1953) defined as a return to an earlier unconscious stage of life and more "primitive methods of expression and representation." In his superb volume *The Neuroscience of Psychotherapy: Healing the Social Brain* my colleague Lou Cozolino asserts, "It is through transference that early relationships for which we have no conscious recollection are brought fully into therapy" (2024, p. 34).

Psychodynamic clinicians describe transference as "an established pattern of relating and emotional responding that is cued by something in the present, but oftentimes calls up both an affective state and thoughts that may have more to do with past experience than present ones" (Maroda, 2005, p. 134). This conception is echoed in neuroscience, where Shuren and Grafman (2002) assert, "The right hemisphere holds representations of the emotional states associated with events experienced by the individual. When that individual encounters a familiar scenario, representations of past emotional experiences are retrieved by the right hemisphere and are incorporated into the reasoning process" (p. 918). Indeed, autobiographical memory of one's own past is stored in the right temporal lobe (Markowitsch et al., 2000), specifically in the right inferior frontal gyrus, amygdala, and hippocampus, which are activated during autobiographical memory retrieval (Greenberg et al., 2005). The amygdala modulates the memory of salient emotionally arousing experiences (McGaugh, 2004) of both aversive and pleasant stimuli (Hamann et al., 1999). It is important to point out that these affective states can be negative or positive and thereby expressed in the positive or negative transference (in later chapters I discuss the often overlooked positive transference).

Transference has been characterized as "an expression of the patient's implicit perceptions and implicit memories" (Bornstein, 1999). According to Gainotti (2006), "The right hemisphere may be crucially involved in those emotional memories which must be reactivated and reworked during the psychoanalytical treatment" (p. 167). In discussing the role of the right hemisphere as "the seat of implicit memory," Mancia (2006) notes, "The discovery of the implicit memory has extended the concept of the unconscious and supports the hypothesis that this is where the emotional and affective—sometimes traumatic—presymbolic and preverbal experiences of the primary mother–infant relations are stored" (p. 83).

These transferential autobiographical memories of early attachment experiences emanate from both the patient's central and autonomic nervous systems, and are expressed in implicit-procedural right-brain-to-right-brain communications. In such bodily-based transmissions, facial indicators of transference are expressed in implicit visual and auditory affective cues quickly appraised from the patient's face, voice, and gestures.

Freud emphasized the fundamental role of transference in the origin of human nature: "A universal phenomenon of the human mind, it dominates the whole of each person's relationship to his human environment" (1927/1961, p. 42).

On the other hand, countertransference is defined as the therapist's "autonomic responses that are reactions on an unconscious level to nonverbal messages" (Jacobs, 1994). Nonverbal implicit bodily-based countertransferential processes are manifest in the capacity to interoceptively recognize and utilize the sensory (visual, auditory, tactile, kinesthetic, and olfactory) and affective responses and imagery that the patient generates in the psychotherapist. Countertransference dynamics are appraised by the therapist's interoceptive observations of his or her own bodily-based visceral reactions to the patient's unconscious emotional communications. As an example, Mucci (2023) observes that the clinician's "embodied witnessing" involves empathic attunement to the patient's stressful trauma that impacts the clinician's body and generates autonomic somatic sensations of nausea and pain, as well as headache, stomachache, and bowel movements. That said, there are also pleasurable physiological components of the positive transference.

In monitoring her somatic countertransferential responses, the empathic clinician's psychobiologically attuned right brain "follows the affect wherever it leads" and synchronizes with not only the arousal rhythms and flows of the patient's affective states, but also her own somatic interoceptive, bodily-based physiological responses to the patient's implicit facial, prosodic, and gestural nonverbal emotional communications of subjective self-states such as fear, aggression, sadness, and shame, as well as joy and excitement. The clinician's unconscious countertransferential responses to the patient's unconscious transferential nonverbal communications represent a synchronized right brain reciprocal interaction between the therapist's bodily-based autonomic and central nervous system and the patient's autonomic and central nervous system.

In 1915 Freud stated, "We have become aware of the countertransference which arises in [the analyst] as a result of the patient's influence on his unconscious feelings." Alluding to a relational two-person psychology, Racker (1968) asserted, "Every transference situation provokes a countertransference situation." Translating this into modern neuropsychoanalytic terms, transference-countertransference transactions are expressions of bidirectional, nonconscious, nonverbal, right brain/mind/body emotional communications between the patient and therapist. Right-brain-to-right-brain, nonverbal, transferential-countertransferential unconscious communications between the patient and therapist act as an essential relational matrix for the therapeutic expression of stressful unconscious negative emotion (Yang et al., 2011). Neuroscience documents "right hemispheric dominance in processing of unconscious negative emotion" (Sato & Aoki, 2006) and "cortical response to subjectively unconscious danger" (Carretie et al., 2005).

In all psychotherapy cases, transference-countertransference attachment dynamics play a fundamental role in the treatment. Cortina and Liotti (2007) describe the enduring impact of early relational stress on later attachment dynamics: "Experience encoded and stored in the implicit system is still alive and carried forward as negative expectations in regard to the availability and responsiveness of others, although this knowledge is unavailable for conscious recall" (p. 207). In this manner, an individual's unique past attachment history of strong right brain negatively valenced emotions without repair shapes the implicit self's unconscious negative expectations of the other's response to a transferential emotional communication of stressful affect dysregulation. This implicit negative expectation predicts the other will not take the negative transference communication and will not be emotionally available to provide interactive affect regulation.

In other words, throughout life, early right brain stressful, strong, and painful dysregulated attachments are the primal source of the unconscious negative transference. These stressful communications are transacted in implicit right brain/mind/body transactions within the therapeutic alliance. The clinician's capacity for intersubjective communication depends upon her "being open to intuitive sensing of what is happening in the back of the patient's words and, often, back of his conscious awareness" (Bugental, 1987, p. 11). Right brain bodily-based dialogues between the relational unconscious of the patient and the relational unconscious of the affectively sensitive therapist are activated in the "heightened affective moments" of transferential reenactments of early attachment dynamics. Enactments represent especially challenging moments for the clinician and may be decisive turning points in the therapy. These are times of both high risk and high gain for both patient and therapist (see Schore, 2012,

2019a, for an extensive interpersonal neurobiological model of working in clinical enactments).

These dyadic enactments are more common in severe psychopathologies that show histories of early attachment trauma. Borgogno and Vigna-Taglianti (2008) observed,

> In patients whose psychic suffering originates in . . . preverbal trauma . . . transference occurs mostly at a more primitive level of expression that involves in an unconscious way . . . not only the patient but also the [therapist]. . . . These more archaic forms of the transference-countertransference issue—which frequently set aside verbal contents—take shape in the [therapeutic] setting through actual mutual enactments.

In the treatment of such patients, Kalsched (2003) proposed,

> For our early trauma patients to get well again, they will have to suffer through a re-traumatization in their transferences. This repetition in the transference will be the person's way of remembering, and may actually lead to the potential of healing the trauma, provided that the therapist and patient can survive the *furor therapeuticus*, that such transformation requires.

There is now a consensus that despite the existence of a number of distinct theoretical perspectives in clinical work, the concepts of transference and countertransference have been incorporated into all forms of psychotherapy. Transference-countertransference affective transactions are currently seen as an essential relational element in the treatment of all patients, but especially in the early forming severe psychopathologies. It is important to note that transference-countertransference is now being seen as a central mechanism of not just psychodynamic but all forms of psychotherapy (e.g., Cartwright, 2011, "Transference, Countertransference, and Reflective Practice in Cognitive Therapy").

Freud, the creator of psychotherapy, referred to the two-person attachment process, the therapeutic relationship, and the central role of emotions in treatment. In his classic article "On Beginning the Treatment," he observed, "It remains the first aim of treatment to attach him [the patient] to it [the process of therapy] and to the person of the doctor" (1913/1958, p. 139). In subsequent work, he reported, "Even the most brilliant results were liable to be suddenly wiped away if my personal relation with the patient was disturbed. . . . The personal emotional relation between doctor and client was after all stronger than the whole cathartic process" (1927/1961, p. 42).

In my 1994 *Affect Regulation* volume, I used an interpersonal neurobiological perspective to show that the above observations of Freud's emotion-transmitting and -receiving unconscious transference-countertransference bidirectional attachment interactions were communicated right brain to right brain, and that the emotional core of the therapeutic relationship can be understood as an interpersonal context of early bodily-based nonverbal emotional communications from one relational unconscious to another. On the cover of the 1994 book was an image of a mother sharing a mutual loving gaze with her baby, a two-person interpersonal neurobiology. By the late 1990s, that book and my subsequent publications helped to establish the interdisciplinary field of neuropsychoanalysis, the scientific study of the unconscious mind, and thereby to promote a fundamental transformation in the study of the human unconscious mind and its relation to neuroscience.

The interdisciplinary fields of not only interpersonal neurobiology but relational psychoanalysis continue to describe the adaptive socioemotional functions of the right brain, the human unconscious mind, and how throughout the lifespan the generation and regulation of emotional states by the right-lateralized attachment mechanism are nonverbally communicated beneath awareness to other right brains via a "relational unconscious" or what Lyons-Ruth (1999) terms a "two-person unconscious." In my studies on the omnipresence of the unconscious in everyday life, I have described how one unconscious intersubjectively communicates, synchronizes, and interacts with another unconscious, right brain to right brain, right mind to right mind.

Over the last three decades, a paradigm shift has occurred within the concept of the unconscious. In its updated reformulation, this central construct of psychoanalysis has changed from an intrapsychic unconscious that expresses itself only in dreams at night to a relational unconscious, a "right mind" that, over the course of the day, emotionally communicates with the unconscious right mind of another. There is now widespread agreement that "unconscious communications can be apprehended through the particular tone of an expression, or an unexpected image or association, or a shift in body gesture; or even simply through a silence" (Tweedy, 2021, p. 11).

In light of the commonality of nonverbal, intersubjective, implicit right-brain-to-right-brain emotion-transacting and regulating mechanisms in the caregiver–infant relationship and the therapist–patient relationship, developmental attachment studies have direct relevance to the treatment process. As the right hemisphere is dominant for nonverbal communication (Benowitz et al., 1983), subjective emotional experiences (Wittling & Roschmann, 1993), and implicit learning (Hugdahl, 1995), the implicit communication of unconscious affective states between the right brains of the members of the therapist–patient dyad (as in the infant–mother dyad) is best described as intersubjectivity. As a result of dyadic right-lateralized interbrain synchronization, both the therapist and patient can cocreate a right-brain-to-right-brain system of nonverbal communication that can send and receive face-to-face unconscious emotional attachment communications (implicit face, voice, gesture) from one subjective self to another subjective self (intersubjectivity). By 2003, neuroscientists were underscoring the essential role of brain laterality studies on the origins of the self. Keenan, Gallup, and Falk (2003) concluded,

> By casting the right hemisphere in terms of self, we have a revolutionary way of thinking about the brain. A new model of the brain, therefore, must take into account the primary importance of the right hemisphere in establishing and maintaining our sense of awareness of ourselves and others. (p. 252)

These nonconscious right brain/mind/body intersubjective communications are reciprocal and thereby potentially valuable to not only the therapist's perception of emotional states but their communication to and from the patient. In describing the clinician's "therapeutic presence," the interpersonal mechanism by which the empathic therapist's social and emotional responses influence the client's physiological state, Geller and Porges (2014) observe, "This bidirectional communication between areas in the right hemisphere promotes adaptive interpersonal functioning between therapist and client (Allison & Rossouw, 2013; Schore, 2012;

Siegel, 2012)." Meares (1993) also observed the bidirectionality of these rapid communications:

> Not only is the therapist being unconsciously influenced by a series of slight and, in some cases, subliminal signals, so also is the patient. Details of the therapist's posture, gaze, tone of voice, even respiration, are recorded and processed. A sophisticated therapist may use this processing in a beneficial way, potentiating a change in the patient's state without, or in addition to, the use of words. (p. 124)

Neuroscience documents that pattern recognition and the comprehension of faces, complex pitch, graphic images, and voices is superior in the right hemisphere (van Lancker Sidtis, 2006). More than conscious left brain verbalizations, these subliminal visual-facial, auditory-prosodic, and tactile-gestural right-brain-to-right-brain communications reveal the deeper aspects of the personality of the patient, as well as the personality of the therapist (see Schore, 2003b). Intersubjective, relational affect-focused psychotherapy is not the "talking cure" but the "affect-communicating cure" between two unconscious minds.

Thus, in recent years the unconscious, the central theoretical construct of psychoanalytic and psychodynamic theory, has reappeared in a new form in both the scientific and clinical literatures. Psychoanalysis has been called the scientific study of the unconscious mind, clearly implying both that the unconscious is its definitional realm of study and that this realm is accessible to scientific analysis. Although originally closely tied to the psychoanalytic theory of repression, the construct of the unconscious is now being used across a number of psychological and neurobiological disciplines to describe essential implicit, spontaneous, rapid, and involuntary processes that act beneath levels of conscious awareness. Yet, despite current significant advances in brain laterality research, some clinicians and social scientists still continue to hold older and now unsupported ideas that the "primitive" nonverbal unconscious mind is a miniature version of the "more complex" verbal conscious mind, and that the "nondominant" right hemisphere is a lesser mirror of the "dominant" left hemisphere.

And yet, for over 30 years I have cited a large body of interdisciplinary research documenting the importance and universality of unconscious nonverbal emotional communications, not only in psychotherapy but in everyday life. For example, Mandal and Ambady (2004) assert,

> Human beings rely extensively on nonverbal channels of communication in their day-to-day emotional as well as interpersonal exchanges. The verbal channel, language, is a relatively poor medium for expressing the quality, intensity and nuancing of emotion and affect in different social situations. . . . The face is thought to have primacy in signaling affective information. (p. 23)

In the journal *Nature*, Buchanan (2009) describes "secret signals" rapidly transmitted between two individuals:

> A person's responses can often be explained by non-linguistic behaviors of other people and simple instincts for social display and response, without any recourse to conscious cognition. . . . This "second channel" of human communication acts in parallel with that based on rational thinking and verbal communication, and it is much more important in human affairs than most people like to think. . . . *It is incredibly naïve . . . to take conscious verbal communications as the primary way that people respond to each other* [emphasis added]. (pp. 528–529)

According to these authors, this channel of communication processes social signals that are expressed in intonation, fluctuating pace and amplitude of voice, upper-body movements, and "mirroring . . . which occurs when one participant subconsciously copies another's prosody and gesture" (p. 529). The outputs of this channel are an expression of "a more archaic brain system for non-linguistic social signals" (p. 529), clearly alluding to the early attachment system and rapid face-to-face right-brain-to-right-brain nonverbal communications. The *Oxford English Dictionary* defines *archaic* as "designating or belonging to an early or formative period." It is now held that the "non-verbal, prerational stream of expression that binds the infant to its parent continues throughout life to be a primary medium of intuitively felt affective-relational communication between persons" (Orlinsky & Howard, 1986).

Returning to the clinical context, in order to receive and monitor the patient's nonverbal bodily-based attachment communications, the affectively attuned clinician must shift from constricted left hemispheric attention that focuses on local detail to more widely expanded right hemispheric attention that focuses on global detail, a characterization that fits with Freud's (1912/1958) description of the importance of the clinician's "evenly suspended attention." Neuropsychologists confirm that the right hemisphere uses a broad, expansive attention mechanism that focuses on global features, while the left uses a narrow, restricted mode that focuses on local detail (Derryberry & Tucker, 1994). McGilchrist (2009) describes a broad attention that invites relationship and is open to the other, versus a narrowly focused and detailed form of attention aimed at analyzing and manipulating the world. Hill (2024) elegantly captures this duality of attention: "Global attention is like the diffuse light of a lantern illuminating the whole of a space. Focal attention is like the beam of a flashlight that puts a concentrated light on a part of the whole." A large body of classic studies shows a right hemisphere dominance for attention (e.g., Heilman & van den Abell, 1980; Deutsch et al., 1988; Whitehead, 1991; Sturm et al., 1999).

In the therapeutic alliance, as in the developmental attachment relationship, right-brain-to-right-brain auditory prosodic communications act as an essential vehicle of implicit communications between the patient and therapist. When listening to speech, we rely upon a range of cues on which to base our inference as to the communicative intent of others. To interpret the meaning of speech, how something is said is as important as what is actually said. Prosody, which Porges (2011) shows is due to autonomic involuntary changes in the right larynx, conveys different shades of meaning by means of variations in stress and pitch—irrespective of the words and grammatical construction. Research shows that musical pitch-based melodies of the human voice are processed by the right auditory and right temporal neocortices (Peretz & Zatorre, 2005) and that the emotional responses to music, like prosody, are generated by the right orbitofrontal and cingulate cortices (Blood et al., 1999).

It is now well established that the right hemisphere is dominant for prosodic communication (George et al., 1996; Ross & Monnot, 2008) for the affective melody of the human voice, for the holistic processing of prosodic and musical patterns (Nicholson et al., 2003), and for the emotional experience of listening to music (Satoh et al., 2011). Perani et al. (2010) documented that at birth infants show a right hemispheric specialization for processing Western tonal music. They assert that music modulates infants' attention and autonomic arousal level, and that the right-lateralized system plays a central role in the development of prosody. Lullabies, common among all cultures, have been described as regulatory "transferential transitional music" offered to the infant as a lulling comfort at the time of separation (Diaz de Chumaceiro, 1995). The psychobiological mechanism for this maternal comforting lies in the fact that music affects physiological autonomic regulation and emotional state (Ellis & Thayer, 2010) and that sedative music affects the human stress response by decreasing sympathetic and increasing parasympathetic autonomic activity of the HPA axis (Thoma et al., 2013). Thus, the prosodic affective melody of motherese can interactively regulate the infant's evolving right-lateralized limbic-autonomic circuits. Importantly, musical interaction is a potent context for creating physiological synchrony and intersubjective connections between two individuals (Fiskum, 2019), including the mother–infant and patient–therapist dyads.

These data support earlier psychodynamic suggestions that the preverbal elements of language—intonation, tone, force, and rhythm—stir up reactions derived from early mother–child relationships (Greenson, 1978). Andrade concludes, "It is the affective content of the analyst's voice—and not the semantic content—that has an impact on the patient's store of implicit memories" (2005, p. 683). Marcus (1997) observes, "The analyst, by means of reverie and intuition listens with the right brain directly to the analysand's right brain" (p. 238). The emotional right hemisphere, dominant for unconscious processes, is critical to the implicit processing of the "music" behind the patient's words. Intuition is defined as "the subjective experience associated with the use of knowledge gained through implicit learning" (Lieberman, 2000, p. 109).

It is certainly true that the clinician's left brain conscious mind is an important contributor to the treatment process. But perhaps more than other treatment modalities, psychodynamic psychotherapeutic models have focused upon the critical functions of the therapist's unconscious right mind. A neuropsychoanalytic right brain perspective of the treatment process allows for a deeper understanding of the critical factors that operate at implicit levels of the therapeutic alliance, beneath the exchanges of language and explicit cognitions. Clinical expertise, with all but especially more severely disturbed patients, taps into the nonconscious nonverbal emotional right brain rather than conscious verbal, rational left brain functions.

Sensitivity to different emotional states has been well studied in the developmental attachment literature, where researchers observe that maternal sensitivity cultivates synchronous, reciprocal, and jointly satisfying mother–infant interactions, which I have suggested foster the development of a secure attachment relationship and an efficient right brain. This attachment principle applies to the therapeutic relationship as well. The dictionary definition of sensitivity is, "susceptible to the attitudes, feelings, or circumstances of others; registering very slight differences or changes of emotion" (*American Heritage Dictionary*). I have described the operations of the therapist's right brain by which "the sensitive clinician's oscillating attentiveness is focused on barely perceptible cues that signal a change in state and on nonverbal behaviors and shifts in affects" (Schore, 2003b).

In classical writings on "the art of psychotherapy," Bugental (1987) stressed the importance of the sensitive clinician's ability to "learn to experience finer and finer distinctions or nuances." He stated, "The primary instrument brought to the support of the client's therapeutic efforts is the therapist's trained, practiced, and disciplined sensitivity. In many ways, this sensitivity is akin to a musical instrument which must be carefully prepared, maintained, tuned, and protected." The clinician's capacity for rapid intersubjective communication is expressed in her ability for right brain clinical intuition. According to Allman et al. (2005), "We experience the intuitive process at a visceral level. Intuitive decision-making enables us to react quickly in situations that involve a high degree of uncertainty which commonly involve social interactions" (p. 370). The "sixth sense" of intuition thus involves an autonomic "gut feeling." Carl Rogers (1989) describes his intuitive entry into this receptive state of the unconscious right brain: "As a therapist, I find that when I am closest to my inner, intuitive self, when I am somehow in touch with the unknown in me, when perhaps I am in a slightly altered state of consciousness in the relationship, then whatever I do seems full of meaning" (p. 137). Note the allusion to a left-right hemispheric shift.

Psychotherapeutic expertise is more than skills with different left hemispheric techniques. All technique sits atop these right brain implicit skills, which deepen and expand with experience: clinical sensitivity, the capacity to implicitly synchronize with a variety of patients; the ability to receive and express unconscious, nonverbal affective communications; and the use of intersubjectivity, affective empathy, clinical intuition, and implicit affect regulation. It is well established that the same technique can lead to different outcomes with different therapists. That said, "Technique, in general, should be invisible. The therapist should be viewed by the patient as engaging in a natural conversational dialog growing out of the patient's concerns; the therapist should not be perceived as applying a stilted, formal technique" (Valentine & Gabbard, 2014, p. 60). At the most essential level, the intersubjective work of psychotherapy is not defined by what the therapist does for the patient or says to the patient (left brain focus). Rather, the key mechanism is how to be with the patient, in both affectively stressful and joyful moments (right brain focus).

The Essential Role of Right Brain Interpersonal Neurobiological Processes in the Development of the Unconscious Mind

Despite the earlier devaluation of Freud's work in some academic circles, writers are concluding, "Freud's model of the unconscious as the primary guiding influence over everyday life, even today, is more specific and detailed than any to be found in contemporary cognitive or social psychology" (Bargh & Morsella, 2008, p. 73). These authors assert that only 5% of goal-directed actions are conscious and 95% unconscious. According to de Gelder (2005), "In the early days of scientific psychology, the notion of unconscious information processing was much debated and controversial. The idea that our thoughts result from deliberations we are not aware of is no longer provocative. . . . There is now growing consensus that facial expressions of emotion can be processed outside awareness" (p. 123). More recently Hoffmann (2021) concludes

> Conscious activity comprises 5% of all cognitive activities with 95% occurring non-consciously. . . . The overwhelming portion of incoming information is therefore processed subconsciously. Many survival aspects and important decisions occur without conscious awareness.

In *The Science of the Art of Psychotherapy*, I asserted that a deeper understanding of human development can never be attained by narrowly focusing infant studies on the precursors of language, voluntary behavior, and conscious thought (Schore, 2012). More recently, in *The Development of the Unconscious Mind* (Schore, 2019a), I offered evidence on the early-maturing yet long-enduring essential impact of the unconscious mind on all later aspects of human development. Freud's (1920/1953) assertion that "the unconscious is the infantile mental life" is supported by developmental neuroscience research that describes how the right brain unconscious system is activated in the earliest stages of human development.

Toward that end, I continue to present a large body of evidence indicating that the development of the unconscious right mind begins in the prenatal, perinatal, and postnatal stages of human infancy and continues across all later stages of the lifespan (Schore, 2019a). This model validates Freud's (1914–1916/1957) description of the human mind: "Every earlier stage of development persists alongside the later stage which has arisen from it. . . . *The primitive stages can always be re-established; the primitive mind is, in the fullest meaning of the word, imperishable*" (p. 286). I suggest that an integration of current findings in the neurobiological and developmental sciences can elucidate the fundamental origins and dynamic mechanisms of the system that represents the core of psychoanalysis, the right brain unconscious system. The construct of the unconscious has thus shifted from an intangible, immaterial, metapsychological abstraction of the mind to a psychoneurobiological heuristic function of a tangible brain that has material form. The direct relevance of this reformulation is a central theme of every book I've written, including my 2019 volumes *Right Brain Psychotherapy* and *The Development of the Unconscious Mind*.

Beginning in my inceptive 1994 volume, *Affect Regulation and the Origin of the Self*, I first integrated developmental psychology, developmental neuroscience, and developmental psychoanalysis to tie together the conceptual, clinical, and research links between early attachment, the experience-dependent maturation of the right brain, psychoanalytic object relational development, and the relational origins of the human unconscious, of all of which are unique to human beings. This first relationship, with the mother, acts as a template, as it permanently forges the individual's capacities to enter into all later emotional relationships. These early right brain experiences impact the origins of human nature and thereby shape the development of a unique personality, its adaptive capacities as well as its vulnerabilities to and resistances against particular forms of future psychopathologies. Indeed, the secure right brain attachment relationship between the mother and infant profoundly influences the emergent organization of an integrated system that is both stable and adaptable, and thereby the formation of the dynamic unconscious subjective self.

Over the past three decades, a huge body of interdisciplinary evidence across all mammalian species, including humans, documents the indelible, enduring impact of specifically the mother on the infant's prenatal and postnatal implicit subcortical and cortical brain development (Schore, 1994/2016, 2003a, 2003b, 2012, 2019a, 2019b). Thus I have continued to offer data supporting the organizing principle that the "first relationship" (Stern, 1977), "the earliest relationship" (Brazelton & Cramer, 1990) with another human is mediated by unconscious face-to-face right-brain-to-right-brain bodily-based attachment communications between the intuitive mother and infant, and that this primordial bond is mediated by rapid emotional interpersonal neurobiological communications between the mother's right brain unconscious and the infant's emerging right brain unconscious. In other words, early affective experiences during a critical period of right brain development from the last trimester through the end of the second year permanently influence the development of the right-lateralized psychic structures that process unconscious information. Indeed, researchers are now contending that "the right hemisphere develops first in the uterus and for the first three years" (Leisman et al., 2023, p. 66).

In 1924, Freud's disciple Otto Rank proposed, "The child and its physical representative, the Unconscious, knows only of the situation before birth" and that our unconscious strives "to establish nothing else than the already experienced condition before birth" (1924/2010, pp. 195–196). Modern developmental neuroscience now establishes that the early development of the unconscious begins in utero and continues to evolve after birth. Indeed, recent information suggests that even before birth, mother–infant interactions in the form of maternal–fetal placental transactions occurring in the last trimester in utero shape the primordial emergence of the deep unconscious (Schore, 2017a). As I discuss in a later chapter, authors are now concluding that "*in utero* the fetus is mostly in a state of 'unconsciousness'" (Lagercrantz & Changeux, 2009). In "The Emergence of Human Consciousness: From Fetal to Neonatal Life," these authors conclude the fetus is aware of its body as it perceives pain, reacts to smell, sound, and touch, and shows facial stimuli responding to external stimuli in the social world, in a state of unconsciousness. It should be pointed out that the fetus's right hemisphere is larger than the left (de Schonen and Deruelle, 1991).

The continuity of this right brain unconscious mechanism underscores Fischer and Pipp's observation, "A young infant functions in a fundamentally unconscious way, and unconscious processes in an older child or adult are to be traced back to the primitive functioning of the infant or young child" (1984, p. 88). These authors also conclude that unconscious thought does not remain static during childhood but undergoes subsequent systematic developments. Indeed, the right hemisphere enters into later growth spurts, including adolescence. Notice that the right brain unconscious mind continues to evolve over the lifespan.

Although a number of important developmental psychoanalysts such as Donald Winnicott studied the critical role of the unconscious in human infancy, John Bowlby integrated psychoanalysis and contemporary ethology and neuroscience to propose that in intimate emotional attachment contexts, human emotions are nonverbally unconsciously communicated through "facial expressions, posture, tone of voice, physiological changes, tempo of movement, and incipient action" (Bowlby, 1969, p. 120). As opposed to later-forming conscious left hemispheric secondary-process verbal communication, early right hemispheric nonverbal attachment communication has been described by Dorpat as unconscious "primary process communication" expressed in "both body movements (kinesics), posture, gesture, facial expression, voice inflection, and the sequence, rhythm, and pitch of the spoken words" (2001, p. 451). He concludes, "In normal awake adults, these two modes are integrated . . . although one or the other may predominate," clearly alluding to the right and left hemispheres.

In addition to psychoanalytic authors who have implicated the right brain in primary process functions, neuroscience researchers contend that "the right hemisphere operates in a more free-associative, primary process manner, typically observed in states such as dreaming or reverie" (Grabner et al., 2007, p. 228). A body of studies over the last 50 years demonstrates that the right hemisphere is dominant for primary process cognition (Galin, 1974; Joseph, 1996), for nonverbal communication (Benowitz et al., 1983), and for the perception of nonverbal emotional expressions embedded in facial and prosodic stimuli at unconscious levels (Blonder et al., 1991;

George et al., 1996; Wexler et al., 1992). In face-to-face as well as body-to-body transactions, the mother is implicitly yet indelibly shaping her infant's developing right-lateralized unconscious mind. The nonverbal socioemotional environment of the attachment relationship influences the developing patterns of neuronal connectivity that underlie implicit nonverbal communication and spontaneous emotional behavior (Schore, 2003a). The early-maturing, visuospatial, emotional, right cerebral cortex (as opposed to the later-developing lexical-semantic left cortex), which stores and processes self-and-object images, has been suggested to be responsible for the manifestations of unconscious processes (Galin, 1974). This data fits nicely with Bowlby's (1969) assertion that unconscious internal working models of the attachment relationship are located in the right hemisphere. These models are guides for future interactions, and the term *working* refers to the individual's unconscious use of the model to interpret and act on new experiences. They contain affective components and are unconsciously accessed and utilized in the generation of internal strategies of affect regulation, especially during times of stress and times of play. Recall, Bowlby (1988), who was psychoanalytically trained, asserted that the restoring into consciousness and the reworking of attachment internal working models is an essential task of psychotherapy.

Alluding to the differences between the hemispheres, Freud (1920/1953) described the unconscious as "a special realm, with its own desires and modes of expression and peculiar mental mechanisms not elsewhere operative." In *The Ego and the Id*, Freud proposed that "thinking in pictures . . . approximates more closely to unconscious processes than does thinking in words, and it is unquestionably older than the latter both ontogenetically and phylogenetically" (1923/1961, p. 21).

These proposals are echoed in brain laterality research, where Howard and Reggia (2007) conclude, "The right hemisphere develops a specialization for cognitive functions of a more ancient origin and the left for a specialization for functions of more modern origin" (p. 121). This speculation about the origin of human nature is confirmed by a body of data suggesting that the right hemisphere matures before the left (e.g., Geschwind & Galaburda, 1985; Gupta et al., 2005; Mento et al., 2010; Saugstad, 1998; Sun et al., 2005) and is dominant in human infancy (Chiron et al., 1997; Schore, 1994/2016). Neurobiological data thus support Freud's suggestion that highly visual, nonverbal, implicit primary-process cognition, dominant in infancy, ontogenetically precedes later-forming semantic, verbal, explicit secondary-process cognition.

Mirroring Freud's idea that early unconscious processes precede later conscious processes, Buklina (2005) describes the general dynamic bottom-up principle:

> The right hemisphere performs simultaneous analysis of stimuli. . . . The more "diffuse" organization of the *right* hemisphere has the effect that it responds to any stimulus, even speech stimuli, *more quickly and thus earlier.* The *left* hemisphere is activated *after* this and performs the *slower semantic* analysis [emphasis added]. . . . The arrival of an individual signal initially in the right hemisphere and then in the left is more "physiological." (p. 479)

Due to its central role in unconscious functions and primary-process activities, psychoanalysis has been intrigued with the unique operations of the implicit right brain since the last quarter of the 20th century. In 1981, Roger Sperry's split-brain research won the Nobel Prize for his discoveries of the specializations of each hemisphere, including his work showing that many of the higher functions of human beings are centered in the right hemisphere. Advances in brain laterality, especially on implicit functions, have been linked to recent reformulations of Freud's unconscious. Neuroscience authors are concluding that "the right hemisphere has been linked to implicit information processing, as opposed to the more explicit and more conscious processing tied to the left hemisphere" (Happaney et al., 2004, p. 7). It is important to note that this lateralization includes subcortical areas—research shows that a subcortical pathway to the right amygdala mediates "unseen fear" (Morris et al., 1999), and that the right amygdala plays a central role in unconscious emotional learning, as opposed to the left amygdala in conscious emotional learning (Morris et al., 1998; Davidson, 2008).

Writing in the psychological literature on the implicit functional abilities of the human unconscious, Hassin (2013) cited studies indicating,

> The function of extracting patterns from our environment, also known as implicit learning, has been repeatedly demonstrated; maintaining

evidence from past experience, also known as memory, can happen outside of conscious awareness; people can extract information about emotion and gender from subliminally presented facial expressions; comparing oneself with others, a central social function, occurs non-consciously and even with subliminally presented others; and physical sensations affect perception and social perception. . . . A review of the literature through functional glasses quickly reveals that *many functions that were historically associated with conscious awareness can occur nonconsciously* [emphasis added]. (p. 200)

Over the last three decades, I have continued to offer a large body of research implicating right brain structural systems in implicit, rapid, and spontaneous anticipation, recognition, expression, communication, and subliminal affect regulation of bodily-based emotional states beneath levels of awareness (see Schore, 2012, 2019a, b). Consonant with these ideas, the neuropsychologists Tucker and Moller concluded, "The right hemisphere's specialization for emotional communication through nonverbal channels seems to suggest a domain of the mind that is close to the motivationally charged psychoanalytic unconscious" (2007, p. 91).

Indeed, recent research is now validating this central tenet of my evidence-based neuropsychoanalytic model: The right brain is the psychobiological substrate of Sigmund Freud's unconscious. Researchers are reporting a "right hemisphere dominance for unconscious emotionally salient stimuli" (Ladavas & Bertini, 2021). Authors are documenting that voice processing is associated with "right-lateralized unconscious, but not conscious, processing of affective environmental sounds" (Schepman et al., 2016). In work on "the unconscious guidance of attention," Chelazzi and colleagues (2018) show that the right hemisphere temporoparietal junction plays an essential role in implicit attentional functions that operate outside conscious awareness. According to Kahneman (2011), unconscious processing occurs hundredths of seconds quicker than conscious awareness. fMRI tracking of the unconscious generation of free decisions in the human brain showed that when a subject's decision reached conscious awareness it had been influenced by unconscious brain processes for up to 10 seconds (Bode et al., 2011). The processing of effortless willpower occurring beneath levels of awareness is associated with right brain activation, as opposed to left brain effortful willpower (Quirin et al., 2021).

Functional Relationships Between and Within the Right and Left Hemispheres

A central theme of both my ongoing clinical and developmental studies dictates that the human brain and mind are in actuality a dual right brain–left brain system. Across all my writings I have been offering a continuous stream of clinical data and experimental research to show that the conscious mind resides in the "top-down" explicit left hemisphere, while the unconscious mind resides in the "bottom-up" implicit right hemisphere (Schore, 1994/2016, 2003a, 2003b, 2012). This hierarchical model of multiple levels of brain organization traces back to the foundations of brain laterality research in the 19th century and to the origins of psychoanalysis in the early 20th century. It not only emphasizes the functional differences between the hemispheres but also models the relationships between the cerebral hemispheres, as well as the relationships between the conscious and unconscious minds.

Figure 2.1 represents the hierarchical organization of the cerebral hemispheres: unconscious implicit processing of the "lower" early-developing right brain and its subsequent connections to the "higher" later-developing left brain conscious explicit system, and then back into the right. In the figure, note the lower position of the autonomic nervous system, what the neurologist John Hughlings Jackson (1931) termed "the physiological bottom of the mind." The peripheral autonomic nervous system is thus centrally involved in what Freud termed drives, the energetic determinants of our motivational force and behavior linked to our bodily constitution.

With respect to the right, left, right sequence, McGilchrist (2009) observes, "The right hemisphere . . . underwrites and 'delivers' our experience to the world, which the left brain then 'unpacks' and processes, before returning it to the right hemisphere, to be reintegrated into the wider picture" (pp. 38–39). This right-left-right sequence thus involves holistic experiencing by the right brain; logical examination and categorization by the left; then a return to the right for a final synthesis with the abstract analysis, in order to generate an integrated and transformed whole. In this manner, "the rationality of the left hemisphere must be resubmitted to, and subject to, the broader contextualizing influence of the right hemisphere, with all its emotional complexity" (p. 203). He concludes,

The representation of the two hemispheres is not equal, and that while both contribute to our knowledge of the world, which therefore needs to be synthesized, one hemisphere, the right hemisphere, has precedence, in that it understands the knowledge that the other comes to have, and is alone able to synthesize what both know into a usable whole. (p. 176)

This formulation, like my own, clearly implies that the affective and relational functions of the right hemisphere are a defining marker of the human experience.

FIGURE 2.1
Hierarchical organization of the left and right cerebral hemispheres

Note the vertical axis of the unconscious right brain processing on the right side of the figure, as well as the sequence of efficient transfers between the hemispheres, right, left, and then back right, and downward, which allows for a securely attached, flexible, reversible dominance of the balanced hemispheres.

Illustration by Beth Schore

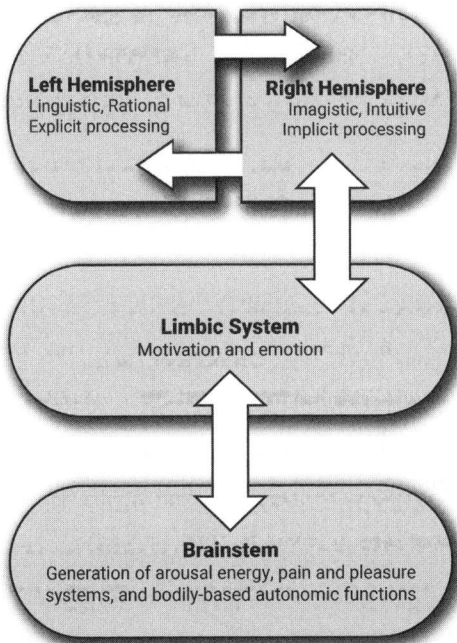

Left Hemisphere
Linguistic, Rational
Explicit processing

Right Hemisphere
Imagistic, Intuitive
Implicit processing

Limbic System
Motivation and emotion

Brainstem
Generation of arousal energy, pain and pleasure systems, and bodily-based autonomic functions

In addition, McGilchrist states that each hemisphere is capable of sustaining a different form of consciousness. In agreement, I suggest that while the early-maturing right hemisphere generates an enduring unconscious self, the left hemisphere is associated with the conscious self. In classic writings, Poincaré underscored the complexity and efficiency of the unconscious self:

> A first hypothesis presents itself: the subliminal self is in no way inferior to the conscious self; it is not purely automatic; it is capable of discernment, it has tact, delicacy; it knows how to choose, to divine. . . . It knows better how to divine than the conscious self, since it succeeds where that has failed. (quoted in Hadamard, 1945, p. 23)

The current expanding bodies of knowledge of neuroscience and neuropsychoanalysis now support a major alteration in Freud's conceptualization of a dynamic unconscious, a central construct of psychoanalysis, the science of unconscious processes. For most of the past century, the contents of the dynamic unconscious were thought to be the products of repression. And yet, in classic writings Freud emphasized, "Everything that is repressed must remain unconscious; but let us state that at the very outset that the repressed does not cover everything that is unconscious. The unconscious has the wider compass: the repressed is a part of the unconscious" (1915/1957, p. 166).

In my earlier neuropsychoanalytic studies, I offered the following update of this "wider compass": Freud's seminal model of a dynamic, continually active unconscious self describes the moment-to-moment operations of a hierarchical, self-organizing implicit-procedural regulatory system that is located in the emotional, social right brain (Schore, 2003b). The dynamic unconscious processing, organization, communication, and regulation of emotional and relational stimuli are specifically associated with activation of the right and not left hemisphere. This contemporary reformulation of Freud's theories indicates that not only thoughts but also affects can be unconscious (Schore, 2012). Furthermore, due to the incorporation of neuroscience and neurophysiology, psychoanalytic theory is now being transformed from a theory of the unconscious mind into a theory of brain/mind/body: unconscious systems operating at unconscious levels are inextricably linked to the visceral body.

The relationship of the conscious to the unconscious mind was initially discussed by Freud (1900/1953) in his topographical model of stratified unconscious, preconscious, and unconscious systems, and later in his structural model (1923/1961) of "higher" superego and ego functions that sit astride the id, the most primitive part of the unconscious mind. My own neuropsychoanalytic conceptualization of an integration of Freud's topographical and structural models describes a hierarchical organization of the conscious, preconscious, and unconscious minds. The neuroscientist Joseph LeDoux concludes, "[that] explicit and implicit aspects of the self exist is not a particularly novel idea. It is closely related to Freud's partition of the mind into conscious, preconscious (accessible but not currently accessed), and unconscious (inaccessible) levels" (2002, p. 28).

In terms of the fixed sequence of neurobiological maturation, the right brain evolves before the left brain in a bottom-up, caudal to rostral, subcortical to cortical, posterior to anterior direction, with the brain stem autonomic and arousal structures maturing earliest, then the right hemisphere and the emotion-processing limbic system, and last the verbal functions of the left hemisphere (see Figure 2.1). This translates into an early evolution of the deep unconscious, then to the unconscious, then preconscious, and finally the higher levels of the conscious mind in the left hemisphere. In earlier work I suggested that the deep unconscious represents activity of the early-developing subcortical right amygdala and the right insula, the unconscious and the later-developing right anterior cingulate medial frontal system, and the preconscious, the last-developing right orbitofrontal corticolimbic system (Schore, 1994/2016, 2003a, 2003b, 2012; see Figure 2.2). In addition to reciprocal connections with the right amygdala, insula, cingulate, and temporal pole, this higher level of the orbitofrontal right mind, located in the ventromedial areas of the right brain, also vertically connects to lower levels of the subcortical unconscious–deep unconscious right mind and the bodily-based autonomic nervous system.

As I explained in *Right Brain Psychotherapy*, reversing the sequence of this hierarchy of regulatory systems in Figure 2.1, Freud's construct of regression was drawn from the English neurologist John Hughlings Jackson's description of a dissolution: "The higher nervous arrangements inhibit (or control) the lower, and thus, when the higher are suddenly rendered functionless, the lower rise in activity" (Jackson, 1931). Note that as the "higher" conscious mind is taken offline, the more "primitive,"

FIGURE 2.2
Neuroanatomy of the right-lateralized socioemotional
brain and the hierarchical limbic system

Note the amygdala (blue), the anterior cingulate (yellow), and the orbitofrontal
(ventromedial) prefrontal cortex (red), as well as the posterior somatosensory
cortex (green) in the right hemisphere. The right insula is located deep within the
lateral sulcus, which is the large fissure that separates the frontal and parietal lobes
from the right temporal lobe. See figure in color on insert after page 190.

Reprinted from *Current Opinion in Neurobiology*, Vol 11, Issue 2, Ralph Adolphs, "The neurobiology
of social cognition," pages 231–239, Copyright 2001, with permission from Elsevier.

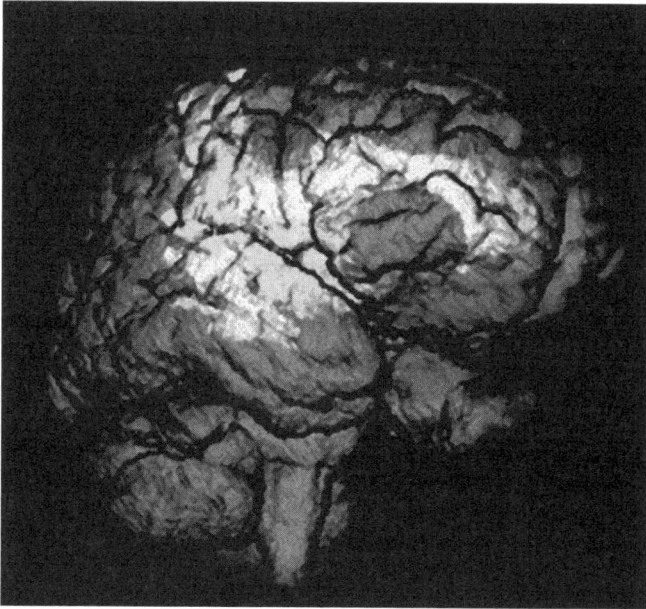

"lower" unconscious mind now increases activity and dominates awareness. According to Giovacchini (1990), "Regression implies that there are
various levels and layers that are contained within the psychic apparatus.
The regressive movements proceed from higher or later psychic levels, to
earlier . . . more primitive ones" (p. 228). In his clinical writings, Freud
asserted, "Unconscious processes only become cognizable . . . when processes of the higher preconscious system are set back to an earlier stage
by being lowered (by regression). In themselves they cannot be cognized"
(1915/1957, p. 186).

Recall in "Project for a Scientific Psychology" Freud (1895/1966) offered a "theory of psychical regression." Building upon that groundbreaking attempt to create a psychology as a natural science, I have offered a reformulation of Freud's concept of regression. I propose two types of adaptive neurobiological regressions: an interhemispheric topographical form (a horizontal state switch from a conscious left prefrontal cortical to a preconscious right prefrontal cortical system), and an intrahemispheric structural regression (a vertical hierarchical state switch from higher to lower right brain), downward cortical to subcortical, from preconscious to deeper unconscious levels of the right brain (see Figure 2.1 horizontal and vertical arrows).

A topographical regression thus involves an intrapsychic shift from the later-developing conscious left mind to the earlier-developing unconscious right mind. In order to directly enter into this right hemispheric realm, the emotionally focused therapist rapidly instantiates, at levels beneath awareness of the conscious left mind, an inversion of hemispheric dominance, a left-right callosal shift that takes place in 50 to 100 milliseconds. On the other hand, a structural regression is expressed in a shift from higher right to lower right levels of the unconscious mind.

For three decades I have been offering a neuropsychoanalytic conceptualization of the hierarchical organization of the conscious, preconscious, and unconscious minds. This neurobiological update of Freud's metaphor of an iceberg floating in the sea is presented in Figure 2.3 as a psychocartography of the depths of the human mind. Over nine-tenths of its mass is submerged below the surface, with most of it hidden below, allowing it to follow the deeper and more constant oceanic currents. Recall research indicates that 95% of goal-directed actions are unconscious and 5% conscious. In the figure note that the sequence of a top-down horizontal topographical regression from the left conscious mind into the right and then a vertical structural regression from the right preconscious downward allows direct access to unconscious repressed emotional memories and then to dissociated memories of the deep unconscious. This neurobiological conception underlies my clinical model of working with clinical regressions. For more on mutual regressions, see the chapters and case material discussions in *The Science of the Art of Psychotherapy* (2012) and *Right Brain Psychotherapy* (2019b), and again in upcoming chapters.

Note the bottom-up ontogenetic organization of the early evolving deep unconscious right amygdala and right insula, then the unconscious right

FIGURE 2.3
Revised update of Freud's iceberg metaphor

Illustration by Beth Schore

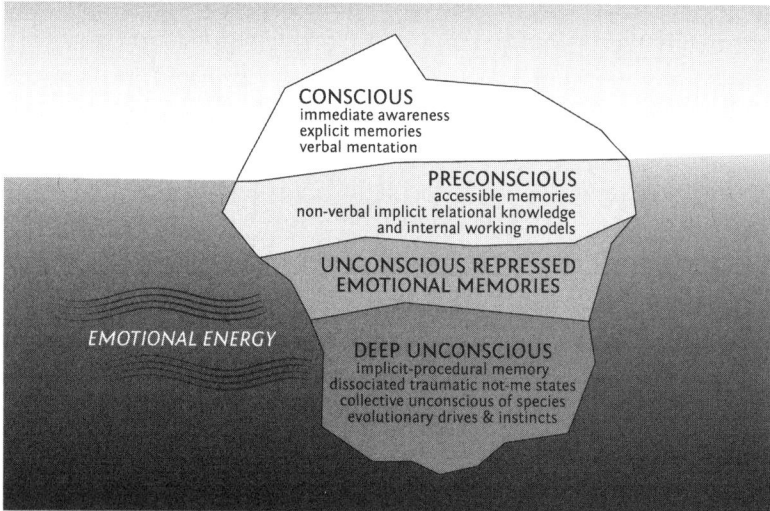

CONSCIOUS
immediate awareness
explicit memories
verbal mentation

PRECONSCIOUS
accessible memories
non-verbal implicit relational knowledge
and internal working models

UNCONSCIOUS REPRESSED
EMOTIONAL MEMORIES

EMOTIONAL ENERGY

DEEP UNCONSCIOUS
implicit-procedural memory
dissociated traumatic not-me states
collective unconscious of species
evolutionary drives & instincts

anterior cingulate, followed by the preconscious right orbitofrontal cortex, and the lastly developing "tip of the iceberg," the left dorsolateral cortex of the conscious mind. The iceberg image also appears on the cover of this book, where the top of the figure contains an embedded horizontal image of a face that is sleeping and dreaming, what Freud called the royal road to the deeper unconscious strata below, the right brain origin of human nature.

With respect to the three-tiered, right-lateralized unconscious system, the right orbitofrontal cortex, the preconscious mind, operating beneath conscious awareness, generates a cohesive, continuous, and unified sense of self. This right brain subjective self implicitly performs not only intra-psychic functions within the organism but also interpersonal functions between organisms. In this manner, the moment-to-moment bodily-based operations of the right-lateralized subjective self that is centrally involved in nonverbal emotional communications, interpersonal connections, and empathic relationships intersubjectively interacts with other subjective self-systems.

McGilchrist (2021a) now asserts that the "experiential self, the self in the present moment, the self sensing what is occurring in one's feelings and body state and noticing how things are from one moment to the next is associated with widespread right hemisphere activations" and that "the self as empathically inseparable from the world in which it stands in relation to others, and the continuous sense of self, enduring over time, are more dependent on the right hemisphere" (p. 117). In earlier work he asserted that the "emotional" right hemisphere "has the most sophisticated and extensive, and quite possibly most lately evolved representation in the prefrontal cortex, the most highly evolved part of the brain" (McGilchrist, 2009, p. 437). Over the lifespan, the right orbitofrontal system and its subcortical connections, shaped by optimal early attachment dynamics, act as an implicit executive regulator of the entire right brain.

Since the early 1990s I have continued to offer new research on the adaptive functions of the right brain, the psychobiological substrate of the human unconscious mind. The essential implicit, perceptual, relational, communicational, and empathic functions of the imagistic emotional right hemisphere were described by the neuroanatomist Jill Bolte Taylor, after she suffered a left hemispheric stroke:

> Our right hemisphere is designed to remember things as they relate to one another. Borders between specific entities are softened, and complex mental collages can be recalled in their entirety as combinations of images, kinesthesia and physiology. To the right mind, no time exists other than the present moment, and each moment is vibrant with sensation. . . . The moment of now is timeless and abundant. . . . The present moment is a time when everything and everyone are connected together as one. As a result, our right mind perceives each of us as equal members of the human family. . . . It identifies our similarities and recognizes our relationship with this marvelous planet, which sustains our life. It perceives the big picture, how everything is related, and how we all join together to make up the whole. Our ability to be empathic, to walk in the shoes of another and feel their feelings, is a product of our right frontal cortex. (2008, pp. 30–31)

In addition to these adaptive functions of the human right mind, I would add recent discoveries of other adaptive states of the right brain and their central role in the origins of the highest levels of human nature, including empathy, intuition, imagery, creativity, metaphor, imagination, humor, music, poetry, art, morality, compassion, spirituality, and love. Modern neuroscience confirms Freud's top-down description: "The conscious mind may be compared to a fountain playing in the sun and falling back into the *great subterranean pool of the unconscious from which it rises*," and Jung's bottom-up observation, "Man's task is . . . to become conscious of the *contents that process upward from the unconscious*. . . . His destiny is to create more and more consciousness."

That said, even in the present time a common bias still exists across the sciences that favors the "higher" left brain rational conscious mind over the "lower" right brain emotional unconscious mind. Music (2023) observes, "Western culture, including our academic institutions, and also some psychotherapies, can overly privilege the cognitive and thinking over nonverbal realms such as body-awareness and emotional states" (p. 2). Echoing the respective differences between the "nondominant" right and "dominant" left hemispheres, Aron and Bushra (1998) point out that "regression, the body, the woman, the child, the playful, the passionate, and the fantastic have often been positioned unfavorably behind/below progression, the mind, the man, the adult, the industrious, the cerebral, and the realistic" (p. 390). Note the clear implication of this duality for the right and left hemispheres, respectively. I suggest that this devaluation also includes an implicit bias currently shared by science and psychology, expressed in a blind spot to the unconscious processes not only in current research and clinical models, but also in overlooking the central role of the right brain unconscious in everyday life.

I end this chapter with some more thoughts about psychotherapeutic regressions. Clinical regressions transiently reverse the left hemispheric overriding of the right hemispheric unconscious mind, allowing us to enter into awareness of our own intersubjective mind, not through controlled voluntary action but by letting go of the left hemisphere, which is dominant for control. In the words of John Lennon and Paul McCartney, in these moments we need to "let it be" so that we are not doing to, but empathically being with, the patient. This is especially so during both the creation and the rupture and repair of the attachment bond with a variety of different types of patients.

That said, the ability to work with adaptive regressions is an advanced therapeutic skill gained by clinical experience, especially in long-term deep psychotherapy, as well as knowledge of hemispheric laterality and right brain interpersonal neurobiology. Toward that end, over time the clinician learns how to implicitly use his or her unconscious bodily-based subjective self in order to synchronize with a variety of different attachment styles, personalities, and defensive organizations. I believe much of this psychodynamic capacity to intuitively access right-brain-to-right-brain communications is taught to the clinician by the patient, if he or she is open to the patient's feedback. Of course, one's own psychotherapy, clinical case supervision, and ongoing reflective self-awareness are other sources of working more effectively in the depths of the right brain.

Although Sigmund Freud initially articulated the psychoanalytic theory of regression in 1900, Carl Jung was the first early clinical explorer of regressions. In 1912 he asserted, "With the concept of regression, psychoanalysis made probably one of the most important discoveries in the [psychological] field." In that work he described the importance of supporting the patient's therapeutic regressions back to the earliest stages of life in order to make contact with a vital generative core of the self that was hidden in the unconscious. In other words, deep psychotherapy, a mutual journey inward into the early roots of the right brain core self, can allow for a direct bottom-up access to the regenerative depths of human nature. The renowned pediatrician-psychoanalyst Donald Winnicott wisely offered advice about the important role of regression in the service of the ego in everyday life: "Let down your taproot to the center of your soul. Suck up the sap from the infinite source of your consciousness and be evergreen." Our unconscious right brain continues to grow over the lifespan and is central to our lifelong ongoing search for meaning, especially the deeper meaning of our own human nature.

Chapter 3

Relational Trauma, Insecure Disorganized Attachment, and Development of the Dissociative Defense

As mentioned earlier, the mother–infant attachment relationship can either facilitate a healthy resilience to stress or create a vulnerability to characterological affect dysregulation and deficits in social relationships, and thereby later psychopathology. As opposed to a secure attachment, in an early right brain context of insecure attachment the primary caregiver frequently misattunes and fails to coordinate, synchronize, and repair their infant's dysregulated emotional states. In my work I have focused on the contrast between the interpersonal neurobiology of a secure attachment and an insecure disorganized attachment. In the latter, what I have termed relational trauma, chronic attachment trauma that results from repeated and prolonged exposure to highly dysregulated early relational and emotional experiences without repair induces disorganized insecure attachments that imprint a physiological reactivity and susceptibility to early-developing disorders of affect regulation (Schore, 2001b, 2002b, 2003a, 2003b, 2012, 2019a, 2019b). This highly stressful attachment context in a critical period of right brain development also generates the unconscious defense of dissociation, a survival strategy associated with an energetic weakening of the right brain, which is thereby inefficient in adaptively regulating relational stress and novel information.

Insecure Disorganized Attachment and the Growth-Inhibiting Energy Dynamics of Relational Trauma

In marked contrast to the previously described optimal psychobiologically attuned attachment scenario of Chapter 1, in a relational growth-inhibiting early environment of relational trauma of abuse and/or neglect, the primary caregiver of an insecure disorganized-disoriented infant habitually misattunes and induces traumatic states of enduring negative affect in the early postnatal period. This caregiver is too frequently emotionally inaccessible and reacts to her infant's expressions of stressful affects inconsistently and inappropriately (massive intrusiveness or massive disengagement) and therefore shows minimal or unpredictable participation in the various types of relational arousal-regulating processes. Instead of regulating, she induces extreme levels of stressful stimulation and arousal, very high in abuse or very low in neglect. Due to the fact that too frequently she provides no interactive repair, the infant's intense negative affective states last for long periods of time.

Beatrice Beebe and her colleagues (2012) describe the disorganized infant-mother attachment pair as cocreating "mutually escalating overarousal" that amplifies the infant's hyperarousal. This results from a sudden increase of ANS sympathetic nervous system energy-expending activity that generates a significantly elevated heart rate, blood pressure, and respiration in the traumatized infant. With respect to the response of disorganized mothers during these moments of relational trauma, Beebe observes, "They may shut down their own emotional processing and be unable to use the infant's distress behaviors as communications, in a momentary dissociative process."

If early trauma is experienced as psychic catastrophe, then the survival defense of dissociation is detachment from an unbearable situation, the escape when there is no escape, a last-resort defensive strategy. That last resort is the right brain survival strategy of the dissociative defense. I have offered evidence to show that the dissociative metabolic defense represents a sudden shift in dominance from sympathetic autonomic hyperarousal to parasympathetic hypoarousal, from high-energy aerobic ventral vagal to low-energy dorsal vagal anaerobic metabolism. Recall, the right-lateralized autonomic nervous system consists of the energy-expending sympathetic and energy-conserving parasympathetic branches. The emotional right hemisphere, as opposed to the left, is known to operate not only at increased but reduced arousal levels (Dimond & Beaumont, 1974).

Over the lifespan, all emotion is composed of two dimensions: valence (positive-negative, pleasant-unpleasant, approach-avoidance of discrete emotions) and arousal (energy, intensity, calm-excited). In 1994 I suggested that right brain emotional arousal is associated with changes in mitochondrial metabolic energy, that supports the high aerobic energy metabolism of the brain (Wong-Riley, 1989). At all points of the lifespan, the metabolic defense of characterological pathological dissociation represents a sudden shutdown of right brain emotional energy, but this is especially problematic during the critical period of attachment when brain mitochondria must increase and shift from anaerobic to aerobic metabolism in order to provide energy that is essential to synaptogenesis. The transformation of energy production in various developing brain regions represents the physiological basis of critical period phenomena, as during optimal developmental contexts of accelerated growth increases in energy production occur in expanding numbers of infant brain mitochondria. The following discussion of energy dynamics bears directly upon my colleague Dan Siegel's (1999, 2012) important work on the role of energy in attachment dynamics.

For three decades I have discussed the importance of energy in both optimal and less than optimal early brain development (Schore, 1994). The mitochondrion, the powerhouse of the cell, generates cellular and thereby organismic metabolic energy in the process of oxidative phosphorylation by cytochrome oxidase, the generator of adenosine triphosphate (ATP), the principal donor of free energy in biological systems. It contains "the other human genome," and its circular DNA, unique from nuclear DNA, utilizes its own genetic code, is maternally inherited, is governed by non-Mendelian mechanisms, and has a mutagenicity rate 10 times that of nuclear DNA (Schore, 1994). Although mitochondrial DNA represents less than 1% of total cellular DNA, its gene products are essential for normal cell function. It is now well established that maternal–infant social and emotional experiences epigenetically impact the nuclear DNA genome, that mitochondria control epigenetics (Naviaux, 2008), and that epigenetic changes in the nucleus are regulated by mitochondrial DNA (Smiraglia et al., 2008; Castenega et al., 2015).

Thus, mitochondrial DNA, like nucleic DNA, can be epigenetically modified by the social environment for better, or for worse, as in stressful relational attachment trauma, thereby impacting changes in the bioenergetics of developing attachment circuits. The fundamental principle of allostasis, "stability through change," dictates that all bodily functions need to be dynamically adjusted in response to continuously changing environmental conditions in order to sustain optimal arousal and fitness for long-term survival (Sterling & Eyer, 1988). The relational trauma of disorganized attachment acts as an extreme stressor of the infant brain, increasing allostatic load and arousal dysregulation during a right brain critical period of energy-dependent brain development. Energy-producing mitochondria act as key components of the stress response (Manoli et al., 2007). Receptors for the glucocorticoid stress hormone cortisol located in mitochondria of human cells are activated during stress (Scheller et al., 2000), allowing corticosteroids to regulate mitochondrial DNA expression (Psarra & Sekeris, 2011; Hunter et al., 2016). Research now reveals bidirectional connections between these glucocorticoids and changes in the physiology and functions of mitochondria (Picard et al., 2014; Lapp et al., 2019).

The stressors of attachment trauma that challenge homeostasis induce important alterations in mitochondrial function that reduce their ability to sense environmental changes in the internal milieu and adjust their bioenergetic and oxidative responses to reestablish homeostasis (Manoli et al., 2007). As an example, Manoli and his colleagues suggest that mitochondria are responsible for the enormous energy demands of the flight-or-fight response (which is highly activated in disorganized attachment). To cover the increased energy demand of allostasis, glucocorticoids induce the mobilization of energy substrates into the bloodstream by the energy-expending sympathetic nervous system. But chronic levels of corticosteroid stress hormones impair energy synthesis in mitochondria of the developing brain, and this energy deficit has been suggested to be the cause of subsequent impaired brain development (Katyare et al., 2003). Every metabolic, gene expression, neuroendocrine, and inflammatory change triggered by stress is regulated by mitochondria (Andrieux et al., 2021; Picard et al., 2015), which coordinate the stress response systems that are activated by allostatic load (Naviaux, 2019).

Mitochondrial activation is centrally involved in apoptosis (Newmeyer & Ferguson-Miller, 2003), an adaptive process of programmed cell death that plays a crucial role in the early development and growth of living systems (Schore, 1994/2016). Mitochondria provide not only the cellular energy for stress and immunity (Mills et al., 2017) but also the main source of oxidative stress and act as the "sovereign of inflammation" (Tschopp, 2011). Indeed, the mitochondrial genome is vulnerable to oxidative damage (Capaldi, 2000). I have suggested that the dysregulating events of abuse and neglect during a critical period of right brain growth create chaotic, severe alterations of metabolic energy in the developing infant brain, causing allostatic overload and excessive wear and tear on the ANS, HPA axis, immune, and cardiovascular systems (McEwen & Wingfield, 2003). These homeostatic stressors intensify the normal process of apoptotic oxidative programmed cell death and thereby alter the developmental trajectory of the right brain (see Schore, 1994, 2003a, 2012, 2019a, 2019b).

During this early critical period of rapid growth there is a significant increase in energy metabolism in developing areas of the infant's right brain (Schore, 1994/2016, 2012, 2019a, 2019b), but the stress of relational trauma of disorganized attachment interferes with this upshift in energy needed for myelination and synaptogenesis. This disruption of energy resources for the biosynthesis of right-lateralized limbic-autonomic synaptic connections is expressed in a developmental overpruning of the corticolimbic system, especially one that contains a genetically encoded underproduction of synapses. The early stress of childhood maltreatment is known to be associated with alterations in the control system of attachment, the orbitofrontal (ventromedial) frontolimbic cortex and its connection with the amygdala (Hanson et al., 2010). With respect to lateralization, deficits in maternal care specifically alter the infant's right and not left ventromedial cortex (Lyons et al., 2002) and the right amygdala, which is more greatly affected by early rearing experiences than the left (Joseph, 1992).

There is now agreement that individuals who experience stressful early adversity such as childhood maltreatment and attachment trauma are at a heightened risk for a wide range of psychiatric disorders including posttraumatic stress disorder, depression, and substance and alcohol abuse (Nemeroff, 2016). Chronic childhood maltreatment, including abuse and neglect, evokes a complex dysregulation of the HPA axis (Tarullo & Gunnar, 2006). Recent research shows that the long-lasting biological and psychological changes associated with a history of childhood maltreatment in women are related to persistent alterations in psychobiological reactivity to stress and dysregulation of the HPA axis, and an alteration of the function and density of mitochondria. Gumpp et al. (2022) conclude that childhood maltreatment affects the energy production of cells in the developing brain by "altering the function and density of mitochondria, i.e., the body's main energy suppliers" (p. 3793).

Chronic unrepaired stress in postpartum periods induces mitochondrial alterations in the mother that reflect allostatic load of her brain mitochondria, expressed in an amplified release of proinflammatory cytokines that interferes with her epigenetic maternal functions (Maes et al., 2001). In a study of mitochondrial oxygen consumption in postpartum women with childhood maltreatment, Boeck et al. (2018) concluded,

> According to the mitochondrial allostatic load model, mitochondrial functioning might set the limits for an individual's capacity to adapt to external stressors, whereby a higher mitochondrial content and function is associated with an increased potential for adaptability and biological resilience, while reduced mitochondrial functioning limits the adaptive capacity and opens the way for the development of stress-related pathologies. (p. 75)

In my earlier writings I suggested that chronic allostatic overload induced by disorganized attachment trauma results in later health risk and disease, and the creation of a vulnerability to future psychopathologies (e.g., Schore, 2003a). This model is supported by recent studies showing the central role of excess apoptosis, developmental cell death, and oxidative stress in the epigenetics of neurotrauma (Dagra et al., 2022). It is also confirmed by Naviaux's (2019) essential work on the fundamental role of metabolic energy-generating mitochondria in "the cell danger response." In later chapters I further discuss the fundamental role of energy-generating mitochondria in critical periods of maladaptive neurotoxic endocrine disruptors that impair the growth of the limbic system and generate negative emotional states, as well as in the adaptive facilitation of biosynthetic activities of synaptogenesis which generate positive emotional states that optimize right brain development.

Further Thoughts on Disorganized Attachment and the Defense of Pathological Dissociation

With respect to chronic relational trauma, frequent highly stressful interactions between the chronically misattuned mother and her infant inscribe an indelible energy deficit and reduced synaptogenesis in the child's developing cortical, limbic, and autonomic regions of the right-lateralized implicit regulation system. The chaotic and dysregulated alterations of state induced by attachment trauma thus become imprinted into the child's right brain. This developmental trauma of disorganized attachment has enduring effects in later stages of childhood, adolescence, adulthood, and parenthood: an immature and metabolically limited right brain capacity to regulate later-life stressors that generate high levels of negative and low levels of positive affective states (Schore, 2003b). Regulation theory offers an interpersonal neurobiological model of the intergenerational transmission of both trauma and the dissociative defense against overwhelming and dysregulating affective states.

At the most fundamental level, over the lifespan the characterological use of pathological dissociation engenders an inability of the right brain cortical-subcortical implicit self-system to adaptively recognize and process external stimuli (exteroceptive information coming from the relational environment) and on a moment-to-moment basis integrate them with internal stimuli (interoceptive information from the body, somatic markers, the felt experience). This failure of integration of the higher right hemisphere with the lower right brain induces an instant collapse of both subjectivity within a mind and intersubjectivity between minds. Stressful affects, especially those associated with emotional pain, are thus not experienced in consciousness, but the physiological dysregulation continues.

For over 20 years I have offered a large body of neurobiological research and clinical studies that support this right-lateralized model (see Schore 2003a, 2003b, 2012, 2019b). Enriquez and Bernabeu (2008) offered research showing that "dissociation is associated with dysfunctional changes in the right hemisphere which impair its characteristic dominance over emotional processing" (pp. 272–273). Helton et al. (2011) reported that high dissociators have difficulty in specifically coordinating activity within the right hemisphere, and that such deficits become evident when this hemisphere is "loaded with the combined effects of a sustained attention task and negative emotional stimuli. . . . Thus, the integration of experiences, which rely heavily on right hemispheric activation (e.g., negative emotion, sense of self with reference to the experience) may be compromised in high dissociators" (p. 700).

In fMRI research on PTSD and its dissociative subtype, my colleagues and I demonstrated that the periaqueductal gray in the midbrain involved in defensive autonomic blunting when confronting threatening stimuli shows strong connectivity with areas of the right hemisphere, namely the right anterior insula, right fusiform gyrus, right temporoparietal junction, and right postcentral gyrus (Harricharan et al., 2016). Subsequently, my coresearcher Ruth Lanius in the same laboratory published a resting-state neuroimaging study of the dissociative subtype of posttraumatic disorder, characterized by "overmodulation with associated emotional numbing, hypoarousal, and feelings of detachment from one's body and surrounding" and thereby "a psychological escape from intolerable affect" (Rabellino et al., 2018). Observing "a strong laterality effect" and "a right dominance of functional connectivity alterations," they assert,

> In addition to its key role in the human stress response (Schore, 2002), the right hemisphere is thought critical for processing emotional experience and for the development of emotion regulatory capacities (Schore, 2000; Schore, 2001; Tanaka et al., 2012) appearing significantly affected by early-life stress. Our results support these observations by revealing aberrant function connectivity of right cortical regions . . . thus providing further evidence of trauma-related right hemispheric dysfunction involving multisensory integration and bodily consciousness. (p. 3368)

Furthermore, in agreement with earlier studies (Heilman & Van den Abell, 1979; Levy et al., 1983) and my own work (Schore, 1994, 2003a, b), Hartikainen (2021) now presents data showing that the right brain plays a central role in the arousal of both hemispheres. Citing my studies on the early organization of the right hemisphere (Schore, 1997b), S. Othmer and S. F. Othmer (2020) offer evidence to show that in normal contexts, "a reciprocal relationship exists in which the right hemisphere bears the primary burden of organizing our resting states, and that in this capacity also governs the left hemisphere. The left hemisphere, in turn, supervises our engagement with the outside world, and in that role also governs right hemisphere function" (p. 19).

I suggest, however, that in a prolonged traumatic state of low-energy dissociative hypoarousal, this reciprocal capacity is impaired and results in a pattern of imbalanced hemispheres. It is thus important to note that relational trauma and defensive dissociation involve not just the underactivated right but also the overactivated left hemisphere. Joseph (1992) states, "Sometimes the conscious self-image is fashioned in reactions to unconscious feelings, traumas, and feared inadequacies that the person does not want to possess, but that nevertheless, are unconsciously maintained."

Spitzer and his colleagues (2004) report that dissociation is associated with a right hemisphere dysfunction in the form of lack of integration in the presence of emotionally distressing or threatening stimuli. But they also pointed out that "dissociation may involve a functional superiority of the left hemisphere over the right hemisphere or, alternatively, a lack of an integration in the right hemisphere. This corresponds with the idea that the right hemisphere has a distinct role in establishing, maintaining, and processing personally relevant aspects of an individual's world" (p. 167). Similarly, McGilchrist (2009) concludes that the defense of dissociation represents "a disconnection from the right hemisphere, and an interhemispheric imbalance in favor of the left. . . . In dissociation, the hemispheres are more than usually disengaged, with an effective 'functional commissurotomy,' or disruption of functioning in the corpus callosum" (p. 236). He observes, "Activation of the left hemisphere in subjects especially prone to dissociation results in faster than usual inhibition of the right hemisphere, whereas those not prone to dissociation exhibit a balanced inhibition, corroborating the idea that dissociation involves a functional superiority of the left hemisphere over the right hemisphere" (p. 236). Note the maladaptive hemispheric asymmetry of a strong left hemisphere over a weak right hemisphere in pathological dissociation.

As Phillip Bromberg (2011) observes, "Dissociation as a defense is responsive to trauma—the chaotic, convulsive flooding by unregulatable affect that takes over the mind, threatening the stability of selfhood and sometimes sanity." He offers the important clinical observation that the function of pathological dissociation is to act as an early warning system that anticipates potential affect dysregulation by trauma before it arrives. That said, the characterological use of dissociation comes at a considerable

cost. Dissociation represents a deficit in the right hemispheric corporeal self
and thereby in maintaining a coherent, continuous, and unified sense of
self. This defensive process disrupts the integration of affective, sensorial,
perceptual, conceptual, and behavioral information and is characterized by
a depleted awareness of one's internal state and external environment (Spiegel & Cardena, 1991). McGilchrist (2009) asserts, "Dissociation is . . . the
fragmentation of what should be experienced as a whole—the mental separation of components of experience that would ordinarily be processed
together . . . suggesting a right hemisphere problem" (p. 236).

The ensuing emotional deficit in right brain subjectivity is accompanied
by a relational deficit in interpersonal intersubjectivity, the loss of the ability to engage in right-brain-to-right-brain communications in stressful contexts. Relational trauma-triggered dissociation thus induces an emotional
disconnection within the self, as well as between self and other. These
fragile personalities use the affect-deadening defense of dissociation that
defends against an anticipated pathological regression of affect dysregulation. This brittle defensive structure too frequently fragments under stress,
leading to a reexperiencing of the affective and interpersonal deficits of a
pathological, malignant regression, a reenactment of attachment trauma.
Donald Winnicott (1974) offered a classic article, "Fear of Breakdown,"
where he suggested that the breakdown is one that has already happened,
a long time ago, but is still being defended against. I have described an
enduring pathological object relation, an internal representation of a dysregulated self affectively interacting with a misattuning object, which is
reactivated in a mutual enactment.

According to Donnel Stern (2009),

> It is by now a clinical truism that experience dissociated in the
> strong sense—dissociated with unconscious defensive purpose—does
> not simply disappear into some untended part of the mind, but is
> instead repetitively externalized, unconsciously enacted in relation-
> ship. . . . Enactments are more or less stereotyped, rigid, constricted,
> and highly selective ways of behaving and experiencing. (p. 661)

Due to their right brain maturational deficits of implicit affect regulation
under stress, these patients show a periodic loss of reality testing. In recent
work, McGilchrist (2021a) states that the right hemisphere–dominated grip

on reality becomes increasingly tenuous the more impaired these functions become. Being susceptible to pathological regressions, these personalities are vulnerable to periodic losses of their right brain subjective self. He offers an evocative portrait of this dis-integration:

> Loss of self may be experienced in a number of ways: a loss of bound-aries between the self and other; as the self breaking apart; as alteration in the form of the face or body, in a lack of the sense of ownership of the body and of its actions, as well as in an alienation of the self from empathic connection with the world and with others, from which in normal circumstances the self draws its life. We are experiencing a rise in so-called dissociative disorders, such as borderline personality disorders, conditions in which the sense of one's identity is weakened or lost altogether. (p. 334)

This breakdown of the self is associated with a weakness and failure of the borderline's capacity for right orbitofrontal affect regulation (Meares, Schore, & Melkonian, 2011). Due to an early history of relational trauma and disorganized attachment without repair, the borderline's right orbi-tofrontal cortex is unable to regulate the right amygdala under times of stress. In fact, the emotional regulatory dysfunction of borderline person-ality disorders is associated with amygdala hyperactivity to fearful and to neutral stimuli that represent the most ambiguous threat (Donegan et al., 2003). This enhanced amygdala activation reflects the intense negative emotions triggered in response to relational stressors in borderline person-ality disorders (Herpetz et al., 2001). Neuroimaging research documents a fronto-limbic dysfunction (Salavert et al., 2011) and right amygdala–right orbitofrontal disconnection (New et al., 2007) in borderline personal-ity disorder.

In neurophysiological studies of psychoanalytic defense mechanisms, Northoff and his colleagues (2007) reported,

> The orbitofrontal cortex plays a crucial role in constituting more mature and cognitively guided defense. . . . Dysfunction in this region . . . might make the constitution of cognitively guided defense mechanisms impos-sible. This, in turn, might induce regressive processes with the consecu-tive predominance of rather immature and emotionally guided defense

mechanisms like splitting, projective identification, denial and psychotic introjection/projection. For example, one would suspect dysfunction in the orbitofrontal cortex in patients with a borderline personality, where projective identification predominates. (p. 148)

The interpersonal neurobiological mechanism of projective identification used by borderlines represents a form of primitive communication (Bion, 1957), a "silent dialogue" of rapid nonverbal communication (Rigas, 2008) that plays an important role in human interactive behavior in which people affect each other, through relationships, by altering the feeling state and self-representation of another person. Note the reference to a dysregulated right-brain-to-right-brain communication between self and other, and an unconscious internal object relational dialogue being reenacted, especially as it is affectively played out in transferential-countertransferential communications of the therapeutic alliance. As such, projective identifications into an other are a universal feature of the externalization of an internal object relation (see Chapter 3, "Clinical Implications of a Psychobiological Model of Projective Identification," in Schore, 2003b).

The right brain defense of projective identification occurs when the emotions and unconscious memories associated with early attachment trauma are expected to be subjectively intolerable. The patient unconsciously projects into the other member of the therapeutic alliance the state of traumatic affect dysregulation in rapid nonverbal right brain channels but immediately dissociates so that he or she is no longer subjectively experiencing nor overtly expressing the projected distress, but the empathic therapist is.

Furthermore, the borderline splitting defense acts as an unconscious process that fails to integrate both the positive and negative qualities of the self or others into a cohesive whole and splits the mental representation of self and other into two opposing realities (e.g., good mother and bad mother; good self and bad self). Merced (2015) offers the clinical observation,

The predominant borderline personality defense is splitting, which "splits" contradictory thoughts and feelings and results in people and events being perceived in one dimensional ways. Clinically splitting typically manifests as a dramatic and unpleasant rupture in the therapeutic alliance. When a borderline patient "splits," it can occur with a speed and intensity that leaves the clinician startled, disoriented, and frightened. It may seem to come "out of the blue" but is most likely to happen around the clinician's physical absences, or failures in empathy or attunement.

When used characterologically, splitting typically results in great distress and unstable, tumultuous relationships.

Indeed, those with borderline personality disorder, which is 12% in out patient and 10–20% in patients who present in psychiatry units (Widiger & Frances, 1989), show difficulties in maintaining close attachment relationships, characterized by oscillations between opposing fears of abandonment and dependency, neediness and withdrawal (Melges & Swartz, 1989). These "oscillations in attachment" reflect dysregulating emotional instability, expressed in alterations between states of undercontrolled intrusive hyperarousal and overcontrolled disengaged hypoarousal. The former is associated with anger-related impulsive aggression and elevated levels of testosterone (Rausch et al., 2015), while the latter is associated with dissociation. According to Stiglmayr et al. (2001), this emotional instability results in strong negatively valenced dysregulated affective states, including terror, panic, pain, anger, and shame. Rusch et al. (2007) note that implicit shame is prominent in borderline women with low self-esteem and greater anger-hostility, as well as implicit disgust (Rusch et al., 2010).

Meares (2012) describes the borderline state as "painful incoherence." These personalities lack internal affect regulatory mechanisms—self-soothing introjects that perform self-consoling and regulatory functions during emotional upheaval. In addition, borderline personality disorders fail to develop a "reflective self," a metacognitive "thinking about thinking" that can take into account one's own and others' mental states (Diamond et al., 2014), as well as affective empathy, achievements that are essential steps in emotional development.

In *Borderline Bodies: Affect Regulation Theory for Personality Disorders*, Mucci (2018) describes the impact of relational trauma on the borderline's body. For Mucci the body is an essential go-between in the relationship between the bodily-based self and the other. The major clinical expression of personality disorders is not only relational impairments but also their stressful dysregulation of the bodily-based autonomic nervous system. The body is the depository of intergenerational transmissions that are responsible for a kind of traumatic graft into the body derived from early relational trauma and subsequent affect dysregulation. These enduring deficits of early-forming borderline disorders are expressed in altered right-lateralized limbic-autonomic circuits, poor connectivity between the orbitofrontal cortex and the amygdala, and an enduring prevalence, under stress, of dissociative defensive reactions, all manifestations of functional deficits of the early-developing right brain/mind/body.

In the early history of borderlines, the body becomes a critical site where subjective experiences of the massive misattunements of relational trauma are painfully inscribed. In addition to chronic affective dysregulation without repair over the first year, by the second year the body can also become the target of nonverbal and verbal negative parental introjects, a receptacle of persecutory parts and feelings projected onto the body as a disgusting and hated other, a cause of maladaptive bodily sensations, and ultimately the target of self-destructive attacks felt as a foreign dissociated "not-me" state. Mucci demonstrates how in personality disorders the body becomes the place, almost detached from "me," where unrecognized or disavowed affects are evacuated, resulting in forms of self-persecution and self-abuse, which are ways of externalizing the negative affects projected onto the body.

Early chronic relational trauma is imprinted as a right brain internalized victim-persecutor dyad, where the individual oscillates between these two opposing hypoaroused and hyperaroused self-states, expressed in different transferential-countertransferential communications in enactments. In *Borderline Bodies*, Mucci (2018) states,

> These enactments occur in a continual sequence that alternates between affects linked to *victim* position that have been internalized (depression, self-loathing, and low self-esteem) and affects linked to the *persecutor* position that has been internalized (aggressiveness, hate, violence, envy, rage), with the persecutor affects externalized onto another or onto one's body for regulatory reasons. (Schore, 2003)

These dual self and other representations of victim-persecutor interactions in unconscious memory become a way of being that operates without the conscious awareness of the patient. Furthermore, these unconscious dissociated states may be overtly expressed when the fragile regulatory system fails, in the form of aggression being directed inwardly in an agitated depression, or outwardly in the form of an attack on the other.

Dissociation is a key feature of not only borderline personality disorder but all disorders associated with a disorganized attachment history: PTSD, autism spectrum disorders, psychotic disorders, eating disorders, substance abuse, and alcoholism. The painful dysregulation associated with the loss of the self may bring the individual into psychotherapy. In the clinical context, these patients frequently access dissociation, a state of mind characterized by a break in the continuity of conscious experience, one associated with detachment, loss of ability for self-monitoring, and emotional blunting. In the adult literature, this disorganized attachment is known as *fearful avoidance*. On the Adult Attachment Inventory, the disorganized unresolved adult shows a drastic collapse in the monitoring of left hemispheric discourse or reasoning on specific questions related to childhood loss and abuse, involving "entrance into peculiar compartmentalized or even partially dissociated states of mind" (Hesse, 2010, p. 570). This self-disorganization occurs as a sudden emotional disengagement and rupture of the fragile attachment bond within their relationships.

The enduring negative impacts of early relational trauma affect the right-lateralized subjective self's capacity for communicating with other minds, that is, intersubjectivity, as well as attachment, the interactive regulation of emotion. Psychotherapy with such insecure-disorganized-disoriented patients needs to attend to the severe dysregulation of affect that characterizes the developmental self-pathologies associated with histories of relational trauma, as well as with the dissociative defense. My colleague and coauthor Russell Meares (2017) observes that in the developmental histories of various personality disorders, including borderline personality disorder who subjectively experience "painful incoherence,"

> the self has been damaged, distorted, and stunted by trauma. In the case of relational trauma, at least, it must be the primary concern of the therapist. Such trauma is not approached by strategies, techniques, interpretations, and so forth, dictated by the agenda of a particular theory. Rather, it is through the establishment of a specific kind of relationship, which is not artificially imposed or manipulated but is allowed to emerge in conversational interplay. (p. 138)

In these cases of early right brain maturational failures, implicit interactive affect regulation acts as a central mechanism of right brain change processes, in both short-term symptom-reducing and long-term growth-promoting psychotherapy. The hallmark of trauma is damage to the relational life, and thus the repair and resolution of relational trauma must occur in a therapeutic relational context. My colleague Clara Mucci (2023) articulates the clinical principle, "What has been damaged in a relationship needs to be repaired in a relationship." Bromberg (2017) points out that in the treatment, "accessing early trauma is, at heart, personally relational: It does not free patients from what was done to them in the past, but from what they have had to do to themselves and to others in order to live with what was done to them in the past" (p. 32). What they have done to themselves is to overrely on the affect-numbing autoregulating dissociative defense. In this challenging work, more than left brain cognitive understanding, right brain relational factors lie at the core of the change mechanism.

The cocreation of a therapeutic alliance may take longer in patients with disorganized rather than organized attachments and in patients who under relational stress characterologically access the early-forming primitive defense of dissociation (Schore, 2012, 2019a). In these cases, a central focus of the therapy is on building a relatively stable therapeutic relationship of emotional engagement with a patient who has had a long history of relationships that provided low levels of predictability, sensitivity, safety, and trust. In such cases of deep psychotherapy, over time, due to the strengthening attachment bond of interactive regulation within the therapeutic alliance, the patient's safety and trust, at implicit levels, begin to increase. In classic writings, Bordin described a fundamental therapeutic principle, especially in patients using primitive defenses: "Some basic level of trust surely marks all varieties of therapeutic relationships, but when attention is directed toward the more protected recesses of inner experience, deeper bonds of trust and attachment are required and developed" (1979, p. 254).

This adaptive change in the patient's right brain facilitates an ability to momentarily suspend, reduce, and alter the affect-blocking defense of right brain dissociation. In long-term treatment, the stronger therapeutic alliance enables the patient to begin to confront dissociated inner states associated with frightening or shamed aspects of the self. This occurs in adaptive therapeutic reenactments of attachment trauma in regulated mutual regressions. Enactments represent the most stressful moments of the treatment, yet these mutual regressions also offer opportunities for interactive regulation and progressions in the treatment.

In her article "Progressing While Regressing in Relationships," Levine (2011) asserts, "Regression may be a necessary means of accessing and addressing the inaccessible parts of the self. Regressions move to different emotionally vulnerable and unformulated points of trauma, developmental and structural weaknesses, and unresolved conflict" (p. 625). She concludes, "More primitive interpersonal interactions . . . can sometimes provide opportunities for the development both of a more integrated self and more mature relating" (p. 621). I suggest that as a result of the evolving therapeutic alliance, the patient's dissociative defenses against affect are transiently lessened, thereby allowing attachment trauma to be more easily activated, communicated, and interactively regulated, including "unconsciously strong or even overwhelming affect" and states of "subjectively unconscious danger" embedded in the patient's right brain traumatic memory. The patient can now shift into bringing more intense negative affect and ultimately traumatic experiences into the session, including reenacted attachment trauma that is shared between the patient and the therapist.

As I have discussed in *The Science of the Art of Psychotherapy* and *Right Brain Psychotherapy* (Schore, 2012, 2019b), the general interpersonal neurobiological principle of working with relational trauma in an adaptive mutual reenactment and indeed with any disturbance of affect regulation dictates that the psychobiologically attuned empathic therapist facilitates the patient reexperiencing overwhelming affects in incrementally titrated, increasing affectively tolerable doses in the context of a safe and trusting environment, so that dissociated overwhelming traumatic feelings can be communicated and shared, regulated, come into consciousness, and be adaptively integrated into the patient's emotional life.

Therapeutic enactments (reenactments of early two-person attachment dynamics) are now seen as an emergent property of an evolving therapeutic relationship that provides an intersubjective context of effective communication and regulation of strong affects. The therapeutic resolution of a mutual regression embedded in an enactment is not a cognitive insight but an affectively charged corrective emotional experience and an intersubjective negotiation. Creative, adaptive regressions within sponta-neous mutual enactments thus represent an optimal intersubjective context of implicit therapeutic change mechanisms, including new ways of being with self and other. The key to an adaptive mutual regression in an enact-ment is a synchronized shift from the patient's and the therapist's rational, linear, verbal left minds into their nonlinear, nonverbal emotional right minds, and thereby the coconstruction of a working relationship between their unconscious minds.

Clinical expertise, especially with severely disturbed patients, taps into nonconscious, nonverbal right brain rather than conscious, verbal left brain functions. In this challenging work, more than cognitive understanding, relational factors lie at the core of the change mechanism. Disorganized-disoriented attachments, difficult as they may be, represent valuable learn-ing experiences for the therapist, as they provide for the learning and mastery of expert skills with more severe disorders of affect regulation. Neurobiologically oriented affectively focused psychotherapeutic treatment of such patients can facilitate neuroplastic changes in the right brain, which is dominant for attachment functions throughout the lifespan.

Ultimately, effective long-term psychotherapeutic treatment of early-evolving self-pathologies and personality disorders can alter insecure inter-nal working models of early relational trauma by facilitating neuroplastic changes in the right brain, which is dominant for emotional and social functions of attachment over the lifespan. Over time, these therapeutic changes occur in the patient's synaptic connections between the right orbitofrontal cortex and subcortical right amygdala. There is now agree-ment that therapeutic change in trauma patients ultimately requires con-nection to bodily experience that has been dissociated (Schore, 2012). It is important to note that I am referring not just to adult and adolescent psychotherapy but to early-intervention infant and child psychotherapy, as well as prevention in the prenatal and postnatal periods that are provided by the culture.

For clinical examples of working with insecure disorganized attach-ment, early relational trauma, and the dissociative defense, I refer the reader to my regulation model and analyses of Kalsched's case of Mike in *Right Brain Psychotherapy* (Schore, 2019b) and the Sands case of Lillian in *The Science of the Art of Psychotherapy* (Schore, 2012). For assessing child-hood trauma history in the relational-socioecological context in which childhood maltreatment occurs, I refer the reader to my involvement in the development of an online Childhood Attachment and Relational Trauma Screen (CARTS), which includes the relationship of the abused child to abused persons, the emotional availability or inability of caregivers, and the respondent's feelings, thoughts, and actions in response to maltreatment (Frewen et al., 2013, 2015). In 2013 I received the Distinguished Practice Award from the American Psychological Association Division of Trauma Psychology for Outstanding Contributions to the Practice of Trauma Psychology.

Chapter 4

Development of the Repression Defense and Its Relation to Insecure Avoidant Attachments

I now shift my focus from the early-forming dissociative defense of disorganized, disoriented, insecure attachment to the later-forming repression defense accessed in organized insecure and secure attachments. The first blocks affect from reaching conscious awareness in the emotional right brain, and the latter blocks right brain affect from reaching consciousness in the rational left brain (Schore, 1994/2016, 2003b, 2012, 2019b). Solms and Turnbull assert what is blocked from left brain consciousness in repression is specifically right hemispheric affect: "Thus we seem to have rediscovered, from a neuroscientific standpoint, the obvious fact that what we feel about our experience is what renders them susceptible to 'repression'" (2002, p. 162).

In his 1900 inaugural volume, *The Interpretation of Dreams*, Freud (1900/1953) placed the defensive construct of repression at the central core of the new field of psychoanalysis, the study of the unconscious mind. Freud (1935/1953) stated that the essence of the defense of repression lies in keeping something out of the conscious mind. More specifically, he contended,

> We remain on the surface so long as we treat only memories and ideas. The only valuable things in psychic life are, rather, the emotions. All psychic forces are significant only through their aptitude to arouse

emotions. Ideas are repressed only because they are bound up with releases of emotions, which do not come about; it would be more correct to say that repression deals with the emotions, but these are comprehensible to us only in their tie-up with ideas.

At the end of the 20th century, the neuropsychologist Rhawn Joseph (1992) asserted, "A defense mechanism is a protective strategy most often used by the conscious mind and left brain. Defense mechanisms serve to protect conscious recognition of information that is in some manner threatening to the conscious self-image" (p. 304). In earlier work, I asserted that defense mechanisms, which can be adaptive or maladaptive, are in essence forms of right brain unconscious, implicit emotion regulation strategies for avoiding, minimizing, or projecting out affects that are too difficult to tolerate (Schore, 2003b). Freud (1915/1961) asserted that projection is an unconscious emotional response, and clinicians now observe, "It is often extremely difficult to recognize in ourselves the tendency to project unwanted emotions onto others" (Chodorow, 1991). Vaillant (1994) concludes, "Rarely can we identify our own defenses, and we often fail to recognize them in others or even project our own." He underscores the importance of adaptive involuntary unconscious defenses to mental health, and of the fundamental clinical task of transforming maladaptive defenses into more adaptive defenses, by increasing social supports, interpersonal safety, and intactness of the CNS. Clinicians are describing the clinical importance of "making conscious the organizing patterns of affect" (Mohaupt et al., 2006).

Beneath conscious awareness, the dual affective defenses of left hemisphere repression and right hemisphere dissociation act as self-protective systems to hide from not only others but our own true self, the core of the personality (Winnicott, 1960a). They represent major counterforces to the emotional-motivational aspects of the change process in psychotherapy, and thus a graded lowering of these defenses and a release of negative affect during mutual regressions provide a valuable opportunity for intense painful affects beneath the surface to be subjectively experienced, communicated, and interactively regulated within the coconstructed therapeutic alliance, thereby increasing the patient's affect tolerance. Changes in the patient's characterological unconscious defenses only take place in the long-term, growth-promoting treatment of deep psychotherapy. Long-term psychodynamic therapy has been shown to be effective in reducing maladaptive defenses (e.g., Bond & Perry, 2004).

The patient brings not only her stressful symptoms and painful memories but also her failing unconscious defenses into psychotherapy. Operating at levels beneath conscious awareness, an overuse of the passive defense of dissociation and the active defense of repression are potential major contributors to the patient's unconscious resistance to psychotherapeutic change and thereby have major restraining intrapsychic impacts on the processes that underlie the psychotherapeutic repair of the self. These unconscious defenses determine the rate of development if not the resistance to the establishment of the therapeutic alliance. They also play a significant causal role in the patient's sudden discontinuance of treatment and in the high drop-out rate of experimental subjects in clinical research (see Gnaulati, 2019).

Authors have differentiated the defense of dissociation from the defense of repression:

> As a defense mechanism, dissociation has been described as a phenomenon quite different from repression. Repression has been considered an unconscious mechanism, placing unwanted feelings away from the conscious mind because of shame, guilt, or fear. . . . However, in order to repress, you must to some degree have processed the feelings. Dissociation is about not having processed the inputs at all. (Diseth, 2005)

Similarly, Bromberg (2011) offers a distinction between these defenses:

> Repression as a defense is responsive to anxiety—a negative but regulatable affect that signals the potential emergence into consciousness of mental contents that may create unpleasant, but bearable intrapsychic conflict. Dissociation as a defense is responsive to trauma—the chaotic, convulsive flooding by unregulatable affect that takes over the mind, threatening the stability of selfhood and sometimes sanity.

As opposed to dissociation's role in regulating strong negative emotion and traumatic affect, repression, aside from its interhemispheric actions regulating uncomfortable right brain emotion, also controls left brain anxiety. The duality in hemispheric functions of these defenses is seen in the differences of the two hemispheres that regulate strong and even traumatic affect versus anxiety. Engels and her colleagues (2007) offered an fMRI study that differentiates left hemispheric verbal anxious apprehension, expressed in worry, verbal rumination, and unpleasant thoughts, from right hemispheric physiological hyperarousal. Repression represents a top-down left lateralized defense for regulating left hemispheric conscious anxiety (anxious apprehension), while dissociation describes a bottom-up right-lateralized defense for regulating early-appearing right hemispheric traumatic physiological autonomic sympathetic hyperarousal.

Expanding upon my own earlier work on defenses, a central function of repression is to act as a strategy used by the higher left brain conscious mind to cope with potentially dysregulating painful emotional states that emerge in the lower subcortical right brain, the depths of the unconscious mind (Schore, 1994, 2003b, 2012, 2019a, 2019b). The hierarchical bottom-up relationship of the right to the left cerebral hemispheres was previously described by Buklina (2005) in Chapter 2, and visually represented in Figure 2.1 as ascending vertical arrows. Note the deep right brain source of the rhythmic crescendos and decrescendos of bioaminergic autonomic-emotional arousal, energy oscillations which then arise from the right into the left hemisphere. Recall the autonomic nervous system acts as "the physiological bottom of the mind" (Jackson, 1931).

Repression represents a top-down left lateralized defense inhibiting right brain affect, a left hemispheric control of the surface conscious mind over the deeper right hemisphere unconscious mind. According to Winnicott, "An instinct repressed along abnormal paths is liable to be shoved down deep into the subconscious and there act as a foreign body . . . for a whole lifetime" (in Rodman, 2003; see Figure 2.3). That said, in a rigid, maladaptive repression defense, there is a chronic imbalanced strong left over a weak right hemisphere.

The Hemispheric Asymmetry and Neuropsychoanalysis of the Repression Defense

Thus the repression defense, like the dissociative defense, generates a superiority of the left over the right hemisphere. The right brain unconscious system contains not just repressed but also dissociated "not-me" states of self (see Figure 2.3). In both cases, an energetically inefficient right hemispheric unconscious mind is compensated by a hyperactivation of the left hemispheric conscious mind. Notice the imbalanced hemispheric asymmetry. According to Rotenberg (2021),

> The functional insufficiency of the right hemisphere mode of thinking can lead to the hyperactivation of the brain during task solutions in an attempt to compensate for this insufficiency using those skills that they already have. Subjects with such insufficiency of image thinking adopt the long-lasting experience of exploiting their left hemisphere mechanisms during the engagement on any difficult task. (p. 268)

According to Nemiah (1989), "Dissociation resulted from the *passive* falling away of mental contents from an ego that was too *weak* to retain them in consciousness, whereas, for Freud, repression was characterized as the result of the *active* repression of undesirable and emotionally painful mental contents by an ego that was *strong* enough to banish them from conscious awareness." Spiegel and Cardena (1991) define repression as "a pushing (or pulling) of ideas *deep into the unconscious* where they cannot be accessed." Northoff et al. (2007) refer to repression as "moving thoughts unacceptable to the ego into the unconscious, where they cannot be easily accessed." Watt (1986) describes the left hemisphere disconnecting itself from stressful primitive, dystonic, and threatening affect-laden self-and-object images processed in the right hemisphere, which become the split-off repressed parts of the self.

More recently, Tweedy (2021) concludes,

> Repression does not emanate from the (right brain) unconscious, but from the "conscious" left brain system. The conscious mind is not however aware of doing this, hence the rather curious situation in which the apparently conscious mind generates the (repressed) unconscious due to its own unconsciousness. . . . Freud repeatedly notes . . . how deeply resistant the conscious, explicit self is to both change and self-knowledge. (p. 17)

Freud's "dynamic unconscious" still remains a central construct of psychoanalysis, "the science of unconscious processes." In classic writings, Freud (1915/1957) emphasized, "Everything that is repressed must remain unconscious; but let us state at the very outset that the repressed does not cover everything that is unconscious. The unconscious has the wider compass: the repressed is a part of the unconscious" (p. 166). As mentioned, the right brain unconscious is composed of both repressed and dissociated "not-me" states of self (see Mucci, 2021). Bromberg (2011) offered the important observation that we all have a multiplicity of conscious and unconscious self states associated with different affects and motivations, including unconscious "not-me" states hidden beneath the dissociative defense. Although these not-me states originate in a fear of annihilation, the dissociative state remains as "a vaguely defined organization of experience; a primitive, global, nonideational affective state" (D. B. Stern, 1997, p. 119). In contrast to the survival strategy of dissociation that represents a loss of vertical connectivity within cortical and subcortical limbic-autonomic areas of the right brain, the later-developing repression defense represents decreased horizontal lateral shifts in interhemispheric processing and cortical disconnectivity between higher left and right frontal structures (see Figure 2.1).

As I previously discussed in *Right Brain Psychotherapy*, Freud proposed,

> We have learned from psychoanalysis that the essence of the process of *repression* lies, not in putting an end to, in annihilating, the idea that represents an instinct, but in *preventing it from becoming conscious*. When this happens we say of the idea that it is in a state of being "unconscious," and we can produce good evidence to show that *even when it is unconscious it can produce effects, even including some which finally reach consciousness* [emphasis added]. Repression has to do with an active removal from consciousness of material or contents that have undergone a process of repression by a subject. (Freud, 1915/1957, p. 166)

Citing Brenner's (1957) classic definition of repression proper, the hallmark of the dynamic unconscious, Jones (1993) asserted that

> events, feelings, or wishes which were unquestionably at one time in conscious awareness and accessible to verbal representation came to be excluded from consciousness or memory. As Freud pointed out, this exclusion of memories from conscious recall appears to be due to the mobilization of guilt, shame or disgust which are aroused by the event, feeling, or wish in question.

Furthermore, I have offered developmental neurobiological research indicating that dissociation, the right brain defense against overwhelming trauma, appears in the prenatal and postnatal periods, in the hypoxic human fetus (Reed et al., 1999) and soon after birth (Bergman et al., 2004), and in what was previously referred to as the preoedipal stage of development. On the other hand, Freud showed that repression appears later in early childhood, previously described as the oedipal stage.

In Chapter 1, I cited developmental neurobiological data indicating that although the right hemisphere's growth spurt precedes that of the left, at the middle to end of the second year when it ends, the left enters its own critical period growth spurt. Note that initial left hemispheric verbal communication skills appear between 18 and 24 months, when the right hemisphere still dominates. Thatcher's (1996) EEG coherence research shows that this left hemispheric growth spurt continues through the third year, early childhood. In *Right Brain Psychotherapy*, I cited Levin's (1991) classical research indicating that left-to-right interhemispheric commissural transmission is clearly operative at three and a half years, a time period of intense interest to Freud's masculine oedipal sexual and aggression dynamics. Levin observed, "The beginning of the oedipal phase, a psychological and neuroanatomical watershed in development, coincides with the onset of the ability (or inability) of the hemispheres to integrate their activities" (p. 21).

In classic writings in neuropsychoanalysis, Levin (1991) proposed that in this time frame of human childhood,

> a system of two properly functioning cerebral hemispheres with a high level of interhemispheric (i.e., left-right and right-left) connectedness comes into being. . . . The resulting integrative tendency of affective-cognitive processing that results from the integration of the two hemispheres makes a further contribution to the cohesiveness and to the early formation of the repression barrier. . . . The remainder of the development of this defensive function, which Freud called the *repression barrier*, is accomplished by the increasing and *reversible dominance* of the left over the right hemisphere, which is known to occur during brain maturation. That is, the assumption of left-hemispheric dominance provides us with improved control over sexual and aggressive impulses. (p. 194)

Basch (1983) suggested "in repression it is the path from episodic to semantic memory, from right to left brain, that is blocked" (see Figure 2.1, arrows from right to left hemisphere). Research indicates the left hemisphere is dominant for control (Schore, 2012). But defensive overcontrol leads to an imbalance of the two hemispheres: a strong left regulation system over a weak right regulation system. Repression can thus be either adaptive and fluid, or maladaptive, rigid, and pathological as in Figure 4.1.

A large body of studies indicates that individuals with a heavily repressive personality style, who habitually inhibit negative affects, are at risk for both psychological and physical disorders. Heavily defensive or repressive coping styles that block transmission from the right into the left hemisphere block interoceptive awareness of right brain autonomic stress signals from the body. Indeed, Gainotti (2020) confirms that "the main function of sympathetic activation is to allow the organism to respond quickly and strongly to emergency situations" and that this energy-expending system is lateralized to the right hemisphere. The highly repressed individual is thus not subjectively conscious of this ongoing physiological dysregulation and thereby unaware that they are in an enduring state of chronic right brain autonomic hyperarousal. I suggest this hemispheric asymmetry mechanism underlies research on highly repressed personalities that document increased cardiovascular autonomic activity, higher blood pressure, and worse outcomes for cardiovascular disease (e.g., King et al., 1990; Miller, 1993), as expressed in Type A personalities (Williams et al., 1980). Classic research reveals that repressors show decreases in immunological functions (Esterling et al., 1993; Jamner et al., 1988). Repression is also associated with psychosomatic disorders, somatic representations, and somatic delusions (Galin, 1974).

In a classic article in the *American Journal of Psychiatry* on hemispheric asymmetry, "Implications for Psychiatry of Left and Right Cerebral Specialization," Galin (1974) cited then-pioneering split-brain research to propose,

In normal intact people mental events in the right hemisphere can become disconnected functionally from the left hemisphere (by inhibition of neural transmission across the cerebral hemispheres), and *can continue a life of their own.* This . . . suggests a neuro-physiological mechanism for . . . repression and an anatomical locus for the unconscious mental contents (p. 572). . . . According to Freud's early "topographic" model of the mind, repressed mental contents functioned in a separate realm that was inaccessible to conscious recall or verbal interrogation, functioning according to its own rules, developing and pursuing its own goals, affecting the viscera, and *insinuating itself in the stream of ongoing consciously directed behavior* [emphasis added]. (p. 574)

FIGURE 4.1

Bihemispheric model of rigid, inflexible, pathological repression, a top-down left-lateralized defense inhibiting right brain affect, a left hemispheric control of the surface conscious mind over the deeper right hemisphere unconscious mind

As opposed to Figure 2.1, note the vertical axis weak connections between the lower and higher levels of the right brain, as well as the repression barrier in the upper part of the top figure and the heavy horizontal inhibitory blockade of the left over the right hemisphere and reduced right-to-left transmission, and the imbalance between a strong left and weak right hemisphere.

Illustration by Beth Schore

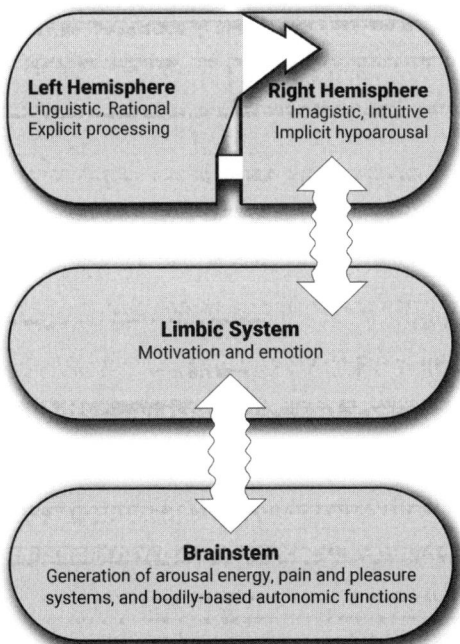

Galin suggested this research demonstrated not only the neurophysiological mechanism for repression but also an anatomical locus for the unconscious mental contents: the right hemisphere. Galin's proposal that the right hemisphere is the locus of unconscious processes is supported by a large body of research I've previously cited, including the recent work of Ladavas and Bertini (2021), "Right Hemisphere Dominance for Unconscious Emotionally Salient Stimuli," where they describe the "specialization of the right hemisphere in the processing of emotional stimuli occurring outside the focus of awareness" (p. 6). Confirming these ideas, EEG research on the human frontal lobes by Davidson (1985) reported that repressors demonstrated deficits in the interhemispheric transfer of negative affective stimuli from the right to left hemisphere. Subsequent studies documented that the defensive repressive coping style is associated with left hemispheric activity in both men and women (Kline et al., 1998). For example, Sander and colleagues (2003) report left (not right) lateralized activity in high-repressive women in the identification of sad prosodic tones of voice.

Freud's concept of the dynamic unconscious is classically understood to refer to the self-regulatory capacities of an unconscious system that operates via the process of repression in order to bar access of sexual and aggressive wishes to consciousness. In the clinical literature, Wolberg (1977) updated and expanded this, stating that not ideas but the emotions related to them are repressed:

> Among repressed and repudiated aspects of psychic activity are fears and fantasies . . . and sexuality. There are hostile and destructive impulses directed toward other persons and the self. . . . There are incestuous desires and other unresolved oedipal elements. . . . There are such normal strivings as desire for love, companionship, recognition, self-esteem, independence of self-fulfillment, which have developed incompletely, or, for anxiety reasons, been abandoned. There are, in addition, rejected neurotic drives for affection, dependence, superiority, dominance, ambition, power and detachment as well as conflicts that these drives initiate. (pp. 574–575)

Each of these repressed aspects of the patient's personality may appear as a focus of the treatment.

Importantly, Wolberg stated that repression has its limits, and that under stress there is a *"constant failing of repressive barriers with a breakthrough and release of repressed material* [emphasis added]" (1977, p. 413). In other words, this left hemispheric callosal inhibition has its limitations, and at time results in "a return of the repressed" in stressful clinical reenactments of dysregulated early right brain attachment dynamics. Returning to Figure 4.1, when the individual's fragile higher vertical right brain stress-regulating capacities are continuously overwhelmed, the repression barrier in the upper part of the top figure fails, and the horizontal callosal transfer of the lower dysregulated negative arousal associated with painful past experiences into the left significantly increases, disrupting left brain consciousness and producing symptomatic behavior.

Relational therapeutic work with defended repressed affect is a central theme of psychodynamic long-term deep psychotherapy, and it involves synchronized mutual regressions from the patient's and therapist's later-forming left brain conscious minds into both of their early-developing right brain unconscious minds, and therefore a joint exploration into the early-appearing depths of human nature. According to the *Oxford English Dictionary, regression* is defined as "a reversion to an earlier or less developed psychological state, either as a defensive response to circumstances, or as a result of hypnosis, psychoanalysis, or psychotherapy." These reenactments of transferential dysregulated attachment dynamics illuminate the dark shadows of the terra incognita of the unconscious mind and give us a glimpse into what the depths of human nature look and feel like.

This subterranean psychic landscape was described by Carl Jung as the "shadow self"—the part of our psyche that we seek to hide and repress, which contains our darkest fantasies and desires. The shadow is an essential quality that we prefer not to have, a powerful unconscious dynamic and defense in our everyday life that is projected onto some other person. Jung (1959) states, "It is not the conscious subject but the unconscious that does the projecting. Hence one meets the projections, one does not make them. The effect of the projection is to isolate the subject from the environment, since instead of a real relationship to it there is now an illusory one."

Not infrequently, a failing of the repression defense is associated with sudden self-exposure and conscious painful shame and early attachment dynamics. Such a return of the repressed leads to an increase of symptom-atology and a potential entrance into psychotherapy. And yet this expe-rienced painful affective dysregulation allows for interactively regulated mutual regressions in which the psychobiologically attuned empathic ther-apist enters into, monitors, and regulates the patient's nonverbally commu-nicated unconscious states below the repression defense. This means that in working with the left-over-right repression defense, both must "mistrust sweet reason" (Reik, 1956) and surrender out of the left and into the right. This relational approach involves joint excursions directly into both the patient's and therapist's right brains. Thus, the mutual synchronized psy-chotherapy relationship and interactive affect regulation are at the core of the change of defensive mechanisms of neurobiologically informed psycho-dynamic psychotherapy.

Recall, at the beginning of this chapter I suggested that the patient brings not only stressful symptoms and painful memories but also failing maladaptive unconscious defenses into psychotherapy. Due to the increased intensity, negativity, and frequency of a personally salient social stressor, emotionally dysregulating subjective experiences of shame affect are gen-erated in the right brain subjective self. This highly negatively charged emotional state is then callosally transmitted from the right to the left mind, overwhelming the patient's left brain repression defense. In these stressful moments, the left brain is inadequate in coping with the altered levels of dysregulated arousal, and thereby the patient's symptomatology increases. In other words, the patient's presenting symptomatology reflects a failure of his or her usual unconscious repression defense to block affect and maintain a familiar secure or insecure attachment regulatory orga-nization. It also reflects the experiencing of elevated levels of anxiety and "neuroticism." The left hemispheric defensive signal of anxiety continu-ously anticipates expected upcoming high levels of right hemispheric sym-pathetic arousal intruding into the left.

In contrast to those with severe personality disorders, who access dis-sociation under even mild stress, what was previously termed *neurotic* patients, who access repression in general, present with an attachment his-tory of more efficient regulation and repairs of relational ruptures. Echoing early emotional development, interpersonal synchrony is more frequent, alliance ruptures are not as severe, and therapeutic misattunements are not responded to with extremely intense dysregulated negative affect, projective identification, nor chronic dissociative disengagement. These personalities include organized insecure attachments.

The Hemispheric Asymmetry of Insecure Avoidant Attachment

I now present a clinical model for working long term with more stable personality organizations and more complex character structures than insecure disorganized attachments, especially those who characterologically use not dissociation but excessive repression as a major source of defensive inhibition of affect, cognition, and behavior. As I have suggested, an inefficient right frontal system is centrally involved in pathological repression dynamics, and an insecure attachment and weak right hemisphere underlie maladaptive strong left over weak right repression dynamics. This rigid, inflexible repression defense is specifically associated with an organized insecure attachment. The relational deficits of insecure attachments are described by Feinberg and Keenan (2005):

> The right hemisphere, particularly the right frontal region, under normal circumstances plays a crucial role in establishing the appropriate relationship between the self and the world. . . . Dysfunction results in a two-way disturbance of personal relatedness between the self and the environment that can lead to disorders of both under and over relatedness between the self and the world. (p. 15)

Right-lateralized insecure avoidant dismissive attachments are characterized by a disturbance between the self and the social environment, specifically an underrelatedness between the self and the world (as opposed to insecure anxious attachment and an overrelatedness to the world).

In order to understand the structural outcomes of mother–infant relationships that generate insecure avoidant attachments, the maternal and infant patterns of affective exchanges of this interpersonal system must be understood. In the first two years of life, the mother of an insecure avoidant infant exhibits very low levels of affect expression (emotional hypoarousal) and presents a maternal pattern of interaction manifested in emotional withdrawal, hesitancy, and reluctance to organize the infant's attention or affect. She has problems surrendering out of the left brain, can't read the affective melody of the infant's voice, and is tone deaf to sadness. The avoidant caregiver typically experiences contact and interaction with her baby to be aversive and actively blocks access to proximity-seeking (attachment) behavior. In the Strange Situation, Main and Weston (1982) observed that this mother manifests a general aversion to physical contact and at times expresses an unverbalizable physical response of withdrawing or pushing the child away.

This caregiver, when she rebuffs her infant, represents an assault from his haven of safety, and further, due to her aversion to physical contact, will not permit access to help him regulate attachment stress, nor the painful emotions aroused by her behavior. Infant-initiated contacts thus elicit not empathic care but parental aversion, behaviorally expressed not only in the caregiver wincing and arching away from the infant's approach but also in keeping her head at a different level from the infant's, thereby blocking right-brain-to-right-brain communication and precluding mutual gaze transactions. Joseph (1992, p. 256) states, "This feeling of aversion is communicated via the right half of the brain. The child responds accordingly because of its own right brain perceptions."

With respect to the other member of the dyad, the insecure avoidant infant shows no interest in an adult who is attempting to attract his attention and exhibits little motivation to maintain contact. This infant characteristically does not appear distressed by the mother's departure nor happy at her return; at reunion, the child does not express distress or anger openly. However, there is evidence that it does experience anger during reunion episodes. The insecure avoidant infant, unlike the securely attached infant, does not stop experiencing anger once reunited with the mother but, unlike the insecure anxious child, does stop expressing it. This suppressed anger may represent a muffled protest response accompanying the infant's frustrated proximity need as he encounters the irritation, resentment, and sometimes outright anger and subsequent active blockade of the contact-aversive mother.

In return, he actively avoids the mother, or in her presence ignores her by extensive use of gaze aversion, rather than seeking comfort from the interaction. Thus, this avoidance reflects an expectation of an unsatisfying and rejecting dyadic contact. Reunited with the mother, he actively turns away, looks away, and seems deaf and blind to her efforts to establish communication (Main & Stadtman, 1981). These authors interpret avoidance as a mechanism to "modulate the painful and vacillating emotion aroused by the historically rejecting mother" (p. 293).

As a result of the deprivation of maternal right brain attachment functions such as mutual gaze to interactively regulate internal physiological disruptions that accompany separation, the insecure avoidant infant habitually autoregulates by breaking eye contact and utilizing averted gaze, generating a downregulation of arousal. What is avoided is a negatively valenced emotional communication expected to emanate from the mother's face and body. Gaze aversion and avoidance of (withdrawal from) the mother who herself withdraws from her infant is proposed to reflect a hypoaroused state of parasympathetic conservation-withdrawal, a primary regulatory process for organismic homeostasis. The infant thus develops a bias toward this parasympathetic-dominant state, one characterized by heart rate deceleration and low levels of activity.

Indeed, Izard (1991) verified that the insecure avoidant infant has a relatively high level of parasympathetic tone. Its autonomic balance is parasympathetically dominated and geared to respond maximally to low levels of socioemotional stimulation. Psychophysiologically, the overcontrolled and restrained nature of insecure avoidant attachment reflects a parasympathetically biased, inhibitory affective core that has a problem shifting out of parasympathetic low arousal and in regulating sympathetic, high-arousal states, such joy. This attachment organization shows a pattern of "minimizing emotion expression" (Cassidy, 1994), a limited capacity to experience intense negative or positive affect, and a susceptibility to overregulation disturbances and overcontrolled psychopathologies. Thus, avoidant individuals are implicitly biased to autoregulate and not interactively regulate the right brain attachment system. For the rest of the lifespan, when relationally stressed, the avoidant personality will convey an unconscious, nonverbal message that says, "Stay away. I don't need you. Don't connect."

As I have discussed, the stage of human infancy-toddlerhood, grounded in the rapid development of the unconscious, nonverbal right brain, closes at the end of the second year. With the onset of a critical period of maturation of the verbal left brain at the end of the second and beginning of the third year, the infant enters into the stage of early childhood, where the later-evolving left can now interact with the earlier developing nonverbal emotional right brain. I suggest that in this overlap period the bidirectional callosal growth which was previously right-to-left changes left-to-right over the course of the third year. The third year begins a rapid expansion of verbal and cognitive skills that are accessed in behavioral assessments and conscious verbal self-reports of both the child and parent, the realm of classical attachment theory. That said, the unconscious insecure avoidant attachment associated with a blocking of right brain emotion into the left continues as an insecure dismissive attachment.

George and Aikins (2023) observe that later in childhood, the dismissing avoidant parent discourages attachment and deactivates the child's attachment needs by minimizing, neglecting, and ignoring them, seeing them as signs of weakness.

> Parent-child activities have a quality of pseudo-togetherness where interactions lack emotional sharing, intimacy, and enjoyment. Problem-solving efforts are limited to the facts needed to achieve a rational solution. Emotions are unwelcome and discouraged, especially anger and sadness. There is a strong emphasis on avoiding conflict and rejecting people and situations at the source. This posture helps parents maintain an authoritarian position. . . . Dismissing parents quickly notice misbehavior and transgressions, the source of fault, and punish. This approach to parenting undermines the development of empathy. . . . Discouraging attachment is also accompanied by shifting away from relationship closeness to stress independence, achievement, and success for social status and material gain.

These authors further conclude that over time this parental distancing and rejection associated with the child's attachment deactivation also results in "a fractured agency, synchrony, and connectedness." This in turn shifts the developmental context away from right brain relationship closeness to stress left brain independence, achievement, and success for social status and material gain. They conclude that the defining quality of dismissing attachment is "defensive deactivation." I propose that this refers specifically to excessive use of the defense of strong repression and that it represents a bias to emotional hypoarousal. This bihemispheric pattern of deactivation of the right hemisphere and overactivation of the left generates a strong tendency to left hemispheric autoregulation over right hemispheric interactive regulation, especially under relational stress. I also suggest that these insecure avoidant psychodynamics underlie the overregulation psychopathogenesis of a personality with a rigid repression defense, as well as an underrelatedness between the self and the world. Berant and colleagues (2005) similarly showed that the implicit unconscious processing of an insecure avoidant style in an adult is expressed in a deactivation of attachment, an inhibition of support seeking, a compulsive self-reliance and handling stress alone, a discomfort with intimacy and dependence, and difficulties in implicit emotion regulation. They further suggest that avoidant attachment reflects "denial and *repression* [emphasis added] of basic needs for proximity and security" (p. 73). Their description of an attachment-deactivating strategy applies directly to the insecure avoidant, heavily repressed patient who enters psychotherapy:

> The goal of deactivating strategies is to keep the attachment system down regulated to avoid the frustration and pain associated with attachment-figure unavailability. Pursuing this goal leads to denial of attachment needs; avoidance of intimacy and dependence in close relationships; maximization of cognitive, emotional, and physical distance from others; and striving for self-reliance and independence. In addition, deactivating strategies foster personal disengagement and detachment from challenging and demanding social interaction, which are viewed as potential sources of threat that can reactivate the attachment system. (Berant et al., 2005, p. 72)

In parallel writings, Sonnby-Borgström and Jönsson (2004) observed,

> Dismissing-avoidant attachment individuals are . . . characterized by a partly deactivated attachment behavioral system and *repression* of anxiety-provoking negative information. . . . Dismissing avoidant individuals are, in addition, assumed to have *incompatible internal working models operating at different levels of awareness* [emphasis added]. A model-of-self, assumed to operate out of awareness at an earlier, automatic level of information processing is . . . associated with . . . more negative affect than the more conscious, positive model-of-self, operating at later stages of information processing. (p. 111)

The authors conclude that in this manner these two different attachment models operate at different levels of consciousness. Note the direct allusion to hemispheric asymmetry of the early-developing right and later-developing left hemispheres (see Figure 4.2).

Indeed, hemispheric asymmetry research shows that these personalities use a left-dominant inhibition of their right hemisphere that underlies excessive repression. Neuroscientists refer to "early emotional learning occurring in the right hemisphere unbeknownst to the left; learning and associated emotional responding may later be completely inaccessible to

FIGURE 4.2
Bihemispheric model of insecure avoidant attachment

As opposed to Figure 2.1, note the left-to-right top-down deactivation of the right brain attachment system, vertical bias toward restrained and diminished emotional hypoarousal, underactivation of the right hemisphere and overactivation of the left, and imbalance between a strong left and weak right hemisphere. Under stress, avoidant personalities show a bias for left hemispheric autoregulation over right hemispheric interactive regulation and a susceptibility to overregulation disturbances.

Illustration by Beth Schore

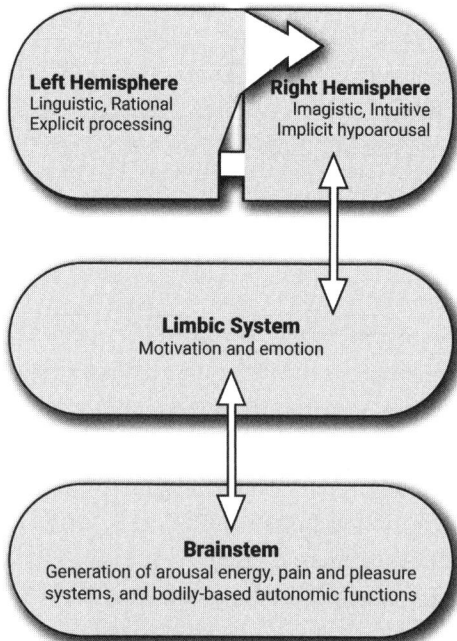

the language centers of the brain, even when extensive interhemispheric transfer is possible" (Joseph, 1982, p. 243). Laterality studies demonstrate that the verbal and nonverbal cortical hemispheres contain separate, dissociable memory systems. The right anterior temporal pole is associated with emotion and socially relevant memory and centrally involved in the recollection of personal, autobiographical memories, while the left anterior temporal lobe processes semantic memory (Olson et al., 2007). Left-dominant insecure avoidant personalities are known to have diminished access to their autobiographical memories.

Directly relevant to psychotherapy, research establishes that individuals with a repressive coping style are less able to remember autobiographical memories associated with negative affect states such as fear, anger, and sadness (Newman & Hedberg, 1999). They have difficulty not only in recalling distressing experiences from the past but also in seeing connections to current life situations. They are averse to surrendering or letting go of the left into the right brain. They talk about emotion, rather than experiencing it, and are unconsciously threatened by uncertainty and change. Due to this lack of access to right-lateralized autobiographical memory, "well-kept secrets of the right hemisphere" may not be accessible to the left (Risse & Gazzaniga, 1978)—a good definition of a defensive, highly repressed personality, who essentially attempts to live his or her life in the left brain. Joseph (1992) asserts, "If the left brain maintains functional dominance at all times and relegates the right brain to second-class status, the personality may be put at a tremendous disadvantage, as the right brain is so emotionally and socially astute whereas the left brain is not" (p. 63).

Joseph (1992) also offers a neuropsychological model of a right brain unconscious self-image and a left brain conscious self-image. This parallels Winnicott's (1960a) differentiation of a "true self" which is at the core of the personality, expressed in spontaneous gestures, and a trauma-induced "false self," a "pseudo adult self" designed to protect it. He described the true self as a bodily self, a source of authenticity, psychic aliveness, creativity, and a continuity of being. The compensatory false self or "social self" protects the authenticity of the true self by social compliance in order to shield it from traumatic exploitation, nonacceptance, and annihilation. I have offered evidence to show that the true self is right-lateralized, while the false self is left-lateralized (Schore, 2002a, 2010, 2019a, 2019b).

Commenting on Winnicott's model, Flanagan (2022) asserts,

> The True Self is the repository of individuality, uniqueness, difference. In relationships characterized by genuine attachment, the separate individuality of both persons is seen, respected, and encouraged to flourish. But if the child's striving for separateness is thwarted, the holding environment can become a prison, a limiting rather than an expansive force. . . . The highly individuated . . . True Self cannot emerge when the environment fails to be genuinely attuned to the child's uniqueness. What happens instead is that the child may develop a *False Self*, one that seeks to suppress individuality and molds itself to the needs and rules of others. . . . This False Self, unconsciously trying so hard to please and placate and pacify others, ultimately becomes rigid and overtly compliant. Uniqueness, vibrancy, idiosyncrasy, and difference are all submerged. In this debilitating, constricting process, the energy, the power, the "wildness" of the True Self is lost. (p. 101)

Meares (1993) put forth a model of a weakened attachment bond and the development of the false self of the conscious mind: "The child will do anything to maintain the bond [with the parent], even to the extent of sacrificing his or her reality. . . . The child searches for an indication of what the mother wants. He or she learns to emit certain behaviors in order to keep some link with the mother" (p. 115).

In neuropsychoanalytic terms, early dysregulated-insecure attachment dynamics generate an underlying weakness of the bodily-based right brain true self that is masked by a left brain pseudo-adult false self. This caretaker self usually becomes identified with the conscious mind, leaving the true self languishing in the body. In light of the fact that the nonverbal right hemisphere matures before the verbal left hemisphere starts, this clearly implies that the true self evolves before the false self, one associated with a developmental shift in dominance in early childhood from the right to left hemisphere. This occurs in humans at the end of the second and into the third year, early childhood, when the right brain ends a critical period, and the left begins one. This dynamic is seen in all personalities but is greatly overexpressed in highly repressed personalities with a history of an early stressed insecure right brain true self that is compensated by a left hemispheric idealized positively valenced false self.

In classic clinical writings, Thomas Ogden (1994b) described the defensive function of the false self in certain personalities:

> The false self is . . . a caretaker self that energetically "manages" life so that an inner self might not experience the threat of annihilation resulting from excessive pressure on it to develop according to the internal logic of another person. . . . The dread of annihilation experienced by the true self results in a feeling of utter dependence on the false self personality organization. This makes it extremely difficult for a person to diminish his reliance on this false self mode of functioning despite an awareness of the emptiness of life that devolves from such functioning. Functioning in this mode can frequently lead to academic, vocational, and social success, but over time, the person increasingly experiences himself as bored, "going through the motions," detached, mechanical and lacking spontaneity. (p. 96)

This bilateral configuration of an energetically strong left hemisphere overcompensating an energetically weak right hemisphere underlies the hemispheric asymmetry of highly repressed personalities. Mikulincer and Shaver (2003) documented that insecure avoidant (dismissive) attachment reflects denial and repression of basic needs for proximity and security, and personal disengagement from challenging and demanding person-environment interactions, as well as a self-facade (a false self). Characterologically, they dismiss and detach from their feelings, which frequently are expressed in unrecognized somatic symptoms. They avoid negative information and feedback and inhibit subjectively experiencing negative affect.

It is often overlooked that avoidant personalities detach from both negative and positive feelings, and are unable to experience, share, and amplify spontaneous joy and excitement with another self. These personalities thus show an inability to integrate positive interpersonal experiences into an enduring positive sense of self. With respect to relational functions, avoidant personalities show high levels of gaze aversion and tolerate little direct eye-to-eye emotional contact, thereby blocking cocreated right-brain-to-right-brain intimate connection and interactive affect regulation. As a result, they can only autoregulate and not interactively regulate emotional stress.

In the psychiatric literature on attachment, Maunder and Hunter (2009) give a brief snapshot of an insecure avoidant personality:

> Dismissing attachment is characterized by high levels of self-reliance and greater interpersonal distance. Others may be approached with mistrust, and situations that require dependence, intimacy or vulnerability may be aversive. The dismissing patient is characterized by *deactivation of the attachment system*; proximity seeking is reduced, attachment figures are considered unimportant and signs of personal distress or vulnerability are suppressed. (pp. 125–126)

These authors cite research indicating that dismissing avoidant adults explicitly see themselves as self-reliant and independent and devalue interpersonal relationships. Relational interactions are not reciprocal because of mistrust, where they expect others to be unresponsive, exploitative, controlling, or hostile. Because they do not experience emotional closeness as soothing or desirable, intimacy is aversive, and they resist depending on others, giving the impression that they are aloof, cool, and distant. Importantly, they do not seek social support when stressed, and their social behavior appears ungenuine or scripted. Communications that have their origin within the false self do not feel real. In conversation, their expressions of emotion are muted and vague, and they use verbal expressions to control dialogue rather than expressing interest in the other's experience. Anger is used to increase interpersonal distance. They are described as ambitious, autonomous, competitive, individualistic, rational, sarcastic, and unemotional. With respect to affect regulation, insecure dismissing personalities cope with stress by cognitive distancing from emotions and emotional disengagement.

According to Berant and colleagues (2005), avoidant adults frequently feel distant and bored in their daily interactions with friends and romantic partners, and are impervious to the induction of negative or positive affect. Unable to share the joys of an intimate relationship that enhances a positive sense of self, avoidant personalities use "defensive self-enhancement," characterized by self-praise and/or denial of weakness, a behavior associated with overt grandiose narcissism. They observe,

> Avoidant individuals' perception of themselves as confident and powerful was a *defensive façade* that helped them handle distress and convince others that they do not need help or support. . . . Avoidant

individuals reacted to threatening situations by *inflating their positive self-views* [emphasis added]. . . . This defensive response was a means for convincing others of their self-reliance. (Berant et al., 2005, p. 79)

Furthermore, they typically show "an arrogant face," hold a negative view and lack of trust in others' good intentions, and present with an exaggerated sense of self and the use of narcissistic defenses. Research shows high rates of avoidant dismissive attachment among grandiose narcissists (Dickinson & Pincus, 2003).

Notice that these data on the insecure avoidantly attached individual's strong left over weak right hemispheric asymmetry, a false self that defensively inflates an illusory positive view of the self, negates and refutes a common clinical and research misperception that avoidant personalities have a negative view of others but a positive view of the self. As I have previously stated, these insecure individuals are unable to integrate positive interpersonal experiences into an enduring positive sense of self.

This bihemispheric model of avoidant personalities and their bias for left hemispheric autoregulation over right hemispheric interactive regulation of relational stress has direct implications for working with dismissive patients. The clinical focus, as with all patients, is not on the compensatory conscious left hemisphere but on the unconscious affect dysregulation of the right hemisphere, the domain of attachment dynamics, beneath the words of the false self. In clinical research on both psychodynamic and cognitive psychotherapy, Håvås and her colleagues (2015) offer an article, "Attuning to the Unspoken: The Relationship Between Therapist Nonverbal Attunement and Attachment Security in Adult Psychotherapy." They documented that higher levels of nonverbal attunement and matching of affect (synchrony) in the initial stages of the treatment were associated with a decrease of avoidant attachment at termination. Citing my work on the central role of right brain nonverbal regulatory mechanisms in generating positive therapeutic outcomes (Schore & Schore, 2008), these authors suggest that for avoidant attachments, nonverbal (and not verbal) attunement renders interactive regulation less threatening and more feasible: "As a consequence, for these patients steady nonverbal matching may have expanded on and improved the repertoire, functionality and effectiveness of their overall regulatory activity, in particular interactive regulation, thereby leading to greater attachment security and treatment termination" (Håvås et al., 2015, p. 14).

Chapter 5

Clinical Applications of Hemispheric Asymmetry: Working with Grandiose and Vulnerable Narcissism and Repressed Shame

A similar left-over-right hemispheric dynamic is also expressed in the psychopathogenesis of narcissistic personality disorders (Schore, 1994/2016, 2012). In 1979, Christopher Lasch's book *The Culture of Narcissism*, published by Norton, argued that American culture had become more narcissistic and self-focused during the 1970s. As I will show, recent research indicates this trend continues to increase even more today. In terms of hemispheric asymmetry, McGilchrist (2009) observes, "The left hemisphere's world is ultimately narcissistic, in the sense that it sees the world 'out there' as no more than a reflection of itself" (p. 438). Narcissistic personality disorders present with a left hemisphere conscious grandiose false self and a right hemisphere unconscious insecure vulnerable true self.

Note the marked discrepancy between Joseph's (1992) left hemispheric superficial positive grandiose conscious self-image and a deeper split-off right hemispheric negative unconscious bodily-based insecure self-image. Clinical researchers have argued that narcissists are high in explicit but low in implicit self-esteem (Morf & Rhodewalt, 2001) and that an imbalanced self occurs at both explicit and implicit levels (Campbell et al., 2007). The former authors suggest that a repression mechanism disconnects the slow-acting positive explicit self-esteem system based on logic, reason, and effortful processing (left hemisphere) from the faster negative implicit self-images that are affect based and automatic (right hemisphere).

It is important to point out that narcissism, first introduced by Freud (1914/1957), may be adaptive or maladaptive. Both Heinz Kohut (1971) and Otto Kernberg (1984) understood narcissism as a normal aspect of development that evolves as the individual matures, expressed in self-cohesion and a realistic sense of self-esteem. There is now agreement that all individuals have normal narcissistic needs and motives. According to Cramer (2011), "Adaptive narcissism is characterized by healthy ambitions, energy, creativity, and empathy supported by an underlying sense of self that is firm and cohesive." Note the description of an efficient right hemisphere.

In contrast, Cramer cites both Kohut's and Kernberg's studies which show that "maladaptive narcissism is characterized by self-aggrandizement, power seeking and condescension in which an inflated sense of self masks underlying feelings of vulnerability and insecurity" (2011, pp. 19–20). Note the allusion to a right brain insecure attachment. Kohut (1971) theorized that pathological narcissism is associated with an early history of the infant receiving nonempathic responses from the maternal self object. The observation that the mother's inconsistent attunement is an important element in the etiology of narcissistic disorders was also made by Kohut (1977). In a clinical reconstruction of a narcissistic patient's early history with his mother, he noted:

> On innumerable occasions she appeared to have been totally absorbed in the child—overcaressing him, completely in tune with every nuance of his needs and wishes—only to withdraw from him suddenly, either by turning her attention totally to other interests or by grossly or grotesquely misunderstanding his needs and wishes. (p. 52)

On the other hand, Kernberg (1975) posited that pathological narcissism emerges from unreliable, cold, and insufficiently empathic parents who express indifference or even aggression toward the child. Egan and Kernberg (1984) described a boy who saw himself as "the center of the universe" with his parents "circling around him." The mother focused her own narcissism on her son, whom she viewed as "her appendage," and neither parent confronted nor disciplined the child. The mother was intrusive, controlling, and injurious to her son's self-esteem, and "could not tolerate it when he was sad" (p. 59).

Similarly, Rinsley (1989) pointed out that the mother of the narcissist rewards the child's growth toward separation-individuation "but only and ultimately in relation to herself." When the child is in a grandiose state, mirroring her narcissism, the mother is emotionally accessible but may do little to modulate the positive, hyperaroused state. On the other hand, when the infant is in a negative, hyperaroused state such as aggressive separation protest, she either fails to modulate it (in herself or in her child) or even hyperstimulates the infant into a state of discontrol. With regard to the origins of pathological narcissism, Broucek (1991) observed,

> Such individuals often are reared by "adoring," doting, narcissistically disturbed parents who have objectified the child and through their adoring gaze have projected onto the child aspects of their own idealized self; these parents have not only failed to find adequate support for the child's true sense of self but have also failed to provide realistic and positive and negative evaluation to support some degree of tension between the actual self and the idealized self. (p. 60)

Bromberg (1986) described the later impact of these early growth-inhibiting events in the psychogenesis of pathological narcissism as a "sense of self lacking sufficient inner resources to give meaning to life simply by living it fully" (p. 441).

This duality between healthy and unhealthy narcissism is reflected in the bright and dark side of narcissism (Back et al., 2013), where these personalities can on the one hand be consciously extraverted, socially bold, and even charming (Back et al., 2010; Dufner et al., 2013), yet on another level vulnerable and insecure. A study by Reinhard et al. (2012) cites research showing that on conscious, left hemispheric self-report measures, "narcissists report high self-esteem, and low levels of depression, anxiety and loneliness," and more "happiness and subjective well-being," which on the surface sounds like but is not a secure attachment.

And yet Reinhard's neurophysiogical investigation documented that "unhealthy" narcissistic males have higher physiological levels of the stress hormone cortisol, clearly indicating an insecure attachment. The authors point out that "despite grandiose self-perceptions, many researchers find that narcissists possess fragile self-views grounded in a sense of inferiority and worthlessness. . . . To cope with these feelings of inferiority, narcissists use defensive strategies following threats to the self." Furthermore, this "defensive or repressive coping style" is associated with increased cardiovascular reactivity to stress (see earlier in Chapter 4), although narcissists are not aware of the physiological stress their bodies are experiencing. This in turn can lead to chronic hyperactivation of the HPA axis and the immune system and weaken the body's natural defenses against stress and disease.

Writing on the relationship between fragile versus secure self-esteem and defensiveness, Kernis et al. (2008) offer data showing,

> Individuals whose self esteem was stable, not contingent, or congruent with high implicit self-esteem exhibited especially low amounts of verbal defensiveness. In contrast, verbal defensiveness was consistently higher when individuals' high self-esteem was unstable, contingent, or paired with discrepant low self-esteem . . . the possession of well-anchored and secure high self-esteem obviates defensiveness directed toward enhancing, maintaining, or bolstering feelings of self-worth. (p. 477)

When others threaten their egos, individuals with fragile self-esteem are more defensive and self-aggrandizing, criticizing or attacking the source of the threat and exhibiting frequent outbursts of anger and hostility and a desire to "get even," specifically via retribution and revenge.

Neurobiological research by Jauk and his colleagues (2017) on the neural correlates of the "dark side" of fragile narcissism and shallow self-worth documents that highly narcissistic men viewing their own face experience greater anterior cingulate negative affect and emotional conflict during self-relevant processing and an oversensitivity to "ego threat." They conclude,

> Contrary to what would be expected on the basis of self-reports, we found that highly narcissistic men display brain activation patterns that point to prevailing negative affect or emotional conflict during visual self-recognition. These results are more in line with psychodynamic than social-cognitive theories on narcissism. While previous social-cognitive research used to focus on voluntary and conscious aspects

of narcissism by means of self-report, our neurophysiological results point to latent affective dysregulation in the processing of self-relevant material. (Jauk et al., 2017)

Other authors commenting on the limitations of self-reports describe a susceptibility to response bias and a difficulty in recognizing one's own limitations, specific deficits of narcissism (Bangen et al., 2013).

In a recent article, "Building Hope for Treatment of Narcissistic Personality Disorder," Igor Weinberg (2024) overviews ongoing advances in the field and discusses new directions for treatment, current updated models of the possibility of psychotherapeutic change, and novel theoretical formulations in treating this challenging clinical population. Indeed, he suggests that we are now in a new era in the treatment of pathological narcissism. Toward that end, in this chapter I describe a clinical approach grounded in affect regulation theory, right brain psychotherapy, and hemispheric asymmetry to offer a neurobiologically informed psychodynamic model of the treatment of two types of narcissistic personality disorders.

Attachment Neurobiology of Grandiose Versus Vulnerable Narcissism

It is now well established that two forms of narcissism exist (Gabbard, 1989; Wink, 1991; Jauk & Kanske, 2021): grandiose, overt, thick-skinned narcissism, and the less-studied vulnerable, covert, thin-skinned narcissism. The former thick-skinned type, associated with grandiose self-assurance, dominance, and a lack of affiliation, reflects an underlying insecure avoidant dismissive style that is defined by an *attachment deactivating strategy*. In classic developmental attachment research, Ainsworth et al. (1978) observed that after a separation, the avoidant child, who has had his or her bids for security rejected, shows little distress at reunion, turns away and refuses contact, ignores the mother's return, and fails to seek her comfort when distressed.

As adults these avoidant personalities do not acknowledge being upset, divert attention from the source of distress, and initiate self-reliant tactics to control negative affect (Kobak & Sceery, 1988). Using a parasympathetically biased right brain attachment-deactivating strategy, they inhibit their emotions, ignore, dismiss, or withdraw under stress, and suppress threat-related thoughts. They express discomfort with dependency and intimacy, inhibit support seeking, and utilize an affect regulation strategy of handling distress alone (autoregulation over interactive regulation), what Bowlby (1973) called "compulsive self-reliance." Research documents grandiose narcissism is associated with dismissive avoidant attachment (Diamond et al., 2014). According to Weinberg (2024), treatment for grandiose narcissism targets dismissive attachment, the tendency to dismiss reliance on others during distress, including the therapist. Under interpersonal stress, these dismissive avoidant personalities are defensive, cold, contemptuous, and emotionally detached. Overt, grandiose narcissists "regulate their self esteem through overt strategies" (Ziegler-Hill et al., 2008, p. 756), through left hemispheric behavior, including verbal aggression, such as devaluing the therapist.

My colleague Clara Mucci (2022) observes that these overtly self-absorbed narcissistic personalities attempt to protect their inner fragility and low self-esteem through the defense of grandiosity and omnipotent control. She states, "Narcissistic patients (inheritors of humiliation and depression) will show a dismissive attitude or even a derogatory tone toward their attachment, often idealizing their attachment figures in order to avoid the rage, wounds and humiliations experienced during childhood" (p. 176). This derogatory tone is communicated right brain to right brain to the therapist, especially in ruptures of the therapeutic alliance, when the clinician is subjected to the patient's defensive "omnipotent control." In these negatively charged heightened affective moments of the session, there is a special use of speech, where the patient's words are used as "a weapon." In response,

> The analyst often feels like an idiot who understands nothing. On such occasions, it is possible for the analyst to react with boredom, to give aggressive interpretations, to keep a persistent silence or to allow his mind to wander to irrelevant thoughts. (Rigas, 2008, p. 38)

Grandiose narcissistic aggression is projected out onto another when the false self is shamed and humiliated ("shame rage," "humiliated fury," "self-righteous rage"). Indeed, neuroendocrinological studies show that grandiose narcissism is related to increases in testosterone and externalized aggression (Lobbestael et al., 2014). Testosterone, especially in men, is known to dampen right-lateralized HPA axis reactivity to stress and cortisol production (see Schore, 2017a), inducing an emotionally detached state. These dynamics contribute to interpersonal deficits. Grandiose narcissism is also associated with long-term interpersonal problems in romantic relationships (Wurst et al., 2017), by maintaining emotional distance from romantic partners and overemphasizing autonomy and independence (Miller et al., 2011).

In fact, research shows gender differences favoring men on grandiose narcissism (Tschanz et al., 1998; Grijalva et al., 2014). These latter authors cite the classic work of Spence and Helmreich (1978), *Masculinity and Femininity*, on gender differences in narcissism: "Most gender differences can be categorized into the following two dimensions: *agentic* characteristics, which include competitiveness, dominance, assertiveness, and need for achievement of high achievement goals, and *communal* [emphasis added] characteristics, which include friendliness, nurturance, tenderness, and selflessness" (2014, p. 263). Grijalva and colleagues conclude that narcissism is high on agency (left hemispheric) and low on communion (right hemispheric). More recently, Zeigler-Hill (2021) concludes,

> Although narcissistic individuals consistently engage in agentic self-enhancement, they do not typically self-enhance with regard to communal qualities, such as being warm, friendly, kind, and honest. That is, narcissistic individuals often recognize their own lack of communal qualities despite their tendency to exaggerate their agentic qualities. This relative lack of concern regarding communal qualities for narcissistic individuals has also been observed in their social motives, goals, and fantasies as well as their general lack of concern for others. (p. 263)

Other authors assert, "The symptomatology of narcissistic personality resembles very highly the masculine sex role stereotypic of men in our culture, including physical expressions of anger, a strong need for power, and an authoritative leadership style" (Corry et al., 2008, p. 593). In dealing with the world, this highly left hemispheric dominant personality is unable to access right brain global attention and thus consciously overutilizes what my colleague Dan Hill (2024) describes as left brain deliberate, voluntary focal attention:

It has an effortful, assertiveness-aggressiveness to it. . . . The "male gaze" uses focal attention highlighting parts and their use. It is adaptive for grasping, analyzing, and mastering things in order to make things happen. And finally, the singling out of parts also sets us apart and disposes us toward exclusion and competition.

In contrast to overt grandiose narcissism, the covert vulnerable, hypersensitive, thin-skinned form is associated with vulnerability, reactivity, and insecurity. In lieu of unconscious nonverbal insecure avoidant attachment in the first two years acting as the foundation of grandiose narcissism, I now offer evidence to show that early nonverbal insecure anxious, ambivalent, resistant attachment, also characterized as insecure preoccupied attachment, lies beneath the left brain repressive false self of the vulnerable narcissist. Indeed, studies show that both narcissistic personality disorders are associated with contradictory insecure organized attachment representations, dismissing and preoccupied, that have been respectively linked to grandiosity and vulnerability (Cain et al., 2008; Meyers & Pilkonis, 2011). Again, I return to observations of insecure attachments in the right brain nonverbal period of development, this time focusing on the infant-mother insecure anxious attachment relationship.

As opposed to insecure avoidant infants (see earlier descriptions), insecure anxious, also known as insecure resistant infants, intermix proximity/contact-seeking behaviors with angry, rejecting behaviors toward the mother at reunion. When reunited with the mother, they are resistant or clinging and thus ambivalent. Due to the unreliable and unpredictable nature of the mother's emotional availability, even when she is present the infant is uncertain what to expect with regard to her being responsive to his or her signals and right-brain-to-right-brain communication. However, "In its heightened display of emotionality and dependence upon the attachment figure, this infant successfully draws the attention of the parent" (Main & Solomon, 1986). Additionally, during preseparation episodes they are often so preoccupied with the mother and with vigilantly monitoring the mother's face that they cannot play independently. More than any other group, they show high separation distress and are difficult to comfort at reunion, indicators of high negative emotion. This insecure anxious infant thus operates with a *hyperactivated attachment system* and a difficult temperament, the central attributes of which are tendencies to intense expressiveness and negative mood responses, slow adaptability to change, and irregularity of biological functions.

Unlike the mother of the insecure avoidant infant, this caregiver does successfully serve as a source of high-intensity affective stimulation enabling high-arousal positive affects. However, during these high arousal states the caregiver does not sensitively and appropriately reduce her stimulation and thereby interferes with the infant's attempt to disengage and gaze avert. Researchers observe that if the mother does not respond to the infant's dyadic affective cues of hyperarousal by diminishing her stimulation, especially during periods of infant gaze aversion, the child's aversion threshold may be exceeded. She does not alter the tempo or content of her stimulation in response to a monitoring of the infant's affective state; instead, she overloads him and interferes with his ability to assimilate new experiences. The heightened display of a painful emotionality and inefficient capacity to regulate the high levels of anger and distress which characterizes these insecure anxious and resistant infants reflects a hyperaroused sympathetically biased affective core which poorly maintains positive mood in the face of stress. Thus, insecure anxious attachments are implicitly biased to interactively regulate and not auto-regulate the right brain attachment system. They are therefore susceptible to undercontrolled developmental psychopathology and underregulation disturbances (see Figure 5.1).

Supporting the idea of a direct link between an early insecure anxious attachment and vulnerable covert narcissism, Mikulincer and Shaver (2003) described adults with a hyperactivating insecure anxious attachment style as manifesting fears of attachment separation, abandonment, vulnerability, and rejection expressed in a ready access to painful memories and an automatic spread of negative emotion. Neuroimaging studies show that rejection sensitivity is a right brain function (Premkumar, 2012). Highly anxious individuals using a hyperactivating strategy typically ruminate about worst-case scenarios, exaggerate potential threat cues, and remain vigilant to signs that their partners might leave them. Indeed, covert narcissistic women experience high levels of anxiety and rejection sensitivity in intimate, romantic relationships. Other studies showed that women high in rejection sensitivity behave negatively toward a male romantic partner during a close interaction in order to elicit rejection, and are therefore prone to self-fulfilling prophesies of expected rejection (Downey et al., 1998).

FIGURE 5.1
Bihemispheric model of insecure anxious attachment

As opposed to Figure 2.1, note the top-down activation of the right brain attachment system and states of emotional hyperarousal, overactivation of the right hemisphere and underactivation of the left, and imbalance between the hemispheres. Under stress, insecure anxious personalities show a bias for right hemispheric interactive regulation over left hemispheric autoregulation and a susceptibility to underregulation disturbances.

Illustration by Beth Schore

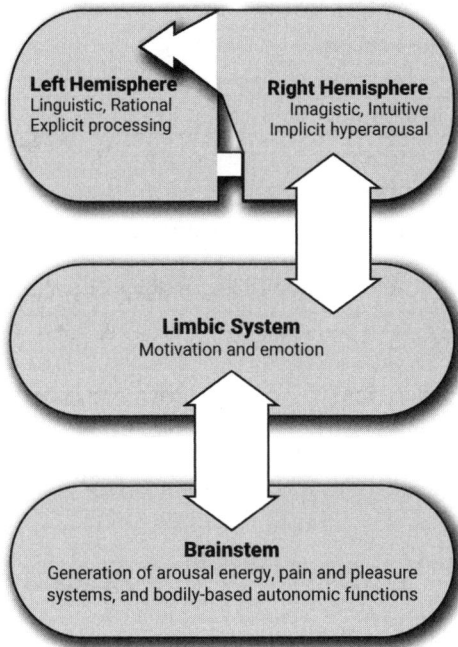

Note that vulnerable narcissists, like grandiose narcissists, also experience difficulties in relationships.

Research on the precursors of narcissism, attachment in the first two years and early parenting at three, reports that vulnerable narcissism is associated with insecure preoccupied attachment (Cramer, 2019). According to Anderson and Guerrero (1998), vulnerable narcissists with anxious-preoccupied attachments dwell on painful negative affect, worry about their well-being in their relationships, seek comfort and support in a hypervigilant state, and rely on their partners for interactive self-regulation. Preoccupied attachment is expressed in clinging, neediness, and an intense focus on the partner (Pistole, 1995). Insecure anxious preoccupied personalities are thus biased to seek interactive regulation and not access autoregulation during emotional stress. In neurobiological terms, this affect-regulatory strategy is associated with a hyperactive emotional right brain, a sympathetically biased, hyperaroused, dysregulated right orbital prefrontal cortex, and a strong attachment protest response. Hyperactivating relational strategies involve very energetic and insistent efforts to elicit a partner's support through demanding and clinging behavior. Under relational stress these covertly self-absorbed individuals detect threats in nearly every interaction, intensify emotional responses to attachment threat and loss, and keep them active in conscious explicit working memory.

Studies show that self-reports of insecure anxious (preoccupied) attachment are associated with intense emotional reactions, chronic distress, rumination, and negative views of self (Berant et al., 2005). Similarly, vulnerable narcissism is also associated with experiencing more negative and less positive emotion, and internalizing symptoms such as anxiety and depression (Miller et al., 2018). Rotenberg (2004) concludes, "In depression the physiological overactivation of the right hemisphere reflects the unsuccessful effort to overcome its functional insufficiency." This deficient regulatory capacity of an insecure vulnerable weak right hemisphere compensated by a strong positively valenced left hemisphere is capable of defensively callosally blocking and thereby repressing right-brain negative affects from dysregulating the conscious mind. Pathological grandiose narcissists are associated with a strong repression system, and pathological vulnerable narcissists with a weaker repression system. When the defense of repression fails, one of these two insecure attachment styles is exposed, and the narcissistic patient may become symptomatic.

Furthermore, in cases of vulnerable narcissism aggression is internalized and directed inwardly toward the victimized unconscious self, attacking both the subjective mind and the psychosomatic body, while in grandiose narcissism aggression is directly outwardly toward the mind and body of a devalued other. Kernberg (2010) notes that in the latter, power dynamics are extremely competitive with the therapist and suspicious of what they see as the clinician's exploitative attitude toward them. As opposed to vulnerable narcissists who are more sensitive to social rejection, grandiose narcissists are more sensitive to achievement failures. Note that the former is an exposed right brain deficit, the latter a left brain deficit.

Confirming this model of the relationship between different attachment orientations and the two forms of narcissistic personality disorders, Meyer and Pilkonis (2011) document that avoidant attachment is associated with grandiose narcissism, while anxious attachment is associated with narcissistic vulnerability. That said, both of these two forms of narcissism involve a bihemispheric asymmetry of a left brain compensatory reaction to right brain insecurity and insufficiency, and thereby a narcissistic self-facade, an exaggerated false self. This narcissistic entitlement acts as a motive for revenge and a barrier to forgiveness, as they are "too proud to let go" (Exline et al., 2004). They can't mourn, nor grieve a loss, unmet needs, and unfulfilled dreams or fantasies (Weinberg, 2024). This deficit is due to an insufficient right brain, which is necessary to recall dreams and fantasies (Benedetti et al., 2015; see discussion in Chapter 1 of the role of the right brain in dreams). According to Kernberg (1975), pathological narcissism is conceptualized as a limited ability to mourn. Furthermore, both the grandiose and vulnerable forms of narcissism also share a conscious sense of entitlement, uniqueness, self-importance, and an inflated sense of self, and therefore an amplified left hemispheric false self that generates a fantasized, idealized positive cognitive illusion about one's intra- and interpersonal emotional abilities.

Neurochemistry can now identify the brain system involved in generating the positively valenced false self as the previously discussed late-maturing left-lateralized nigrostriatal dopamine system that generates rewards for motor and verbal behavior (as opposed to the early-maturing right brain ventral tegmental mesolimbic dopamine system associated with the emotion-processing limbic and autonomic nervous system). In classic research, Tucker and Williamson (1984) cited data showing that the left hemisphere is relatively richer in processes that depend on dopamine (while the right is more organized around the noradrenergic system). The subjective experience of pleasure increases dopamine activity (Schultz, 2002), and greater positive motivation and approach behavior are associated with higher striatal (D2) dopamine receptors in the left hemisphere relative to the right hemisphere (Tomer et al., 2008).

Furthermore, basic research suggests that "increased testosterone at adolescence may change dopamine responsivity of the nigrostriatal pathway by modulating, at a molecular level, the capacity of neurons to transport and respond to dopamine" (Purves-Tyson et al., 2014). Narcissism levels peak in adolescence and then decline (Grijalva et al., 2014). Adolescent boys and adult men produce far more testosterone than do adolescent girls and adult women, and during adolescence boys' testosterone levels increase at a more accelerated rate than girls' (Shirtcliff et al., 2002). I suggest that dopamine from the substantia nigra, adrenaline, and testosterone associated with left hemisphere power dynamics are major determinants of the male-dominated gender differences of grandiose narcissism as well as the source of the strength of the positively charged defense of the left hemispheric false self. The early-forming narcissistic temperament is also directly influenced by genetic factors (Livesley et al., 1993; Luo, Cai, & Song, 2014).

Writing on adult attachment and pathological narcissism, Fossati and her colleagues (2015) assert, "Grandiose narcissism is likely to defend against perceiving the deeply rooted fears and associated negative intense negative emotions (e.g., anxiety, depression, anger) that arise when the inflated self is threatened, potentially eliciting a deep sense of vulnerability" (p. 423). In offering a dynamic self-regulatory model of narcissism, Morf and Rhodewalt (2001) conclude,

> The most striking feature of narcissism is that in their endless efforts to construct and maintain a grandiose self they engage in behaviors that concurrently undermine and erode their advances, virtually at the same rate as they make them. Indeed the narcissist seems much like Sisyphus doomed to build on the self that keeps crumbling underneath. (p. 250)

These authors observe that at the same time that narcissists hunger for self-affirmation, "they destroy the relationships on which they are dependent" (p. 179).

Mucci and Scalabrini (2021) assert,

> Narcissists damage their own resources (e.g. time and intelligence) in order to protect, through the defense of grandiosity and omnipotent control, their own inner fragility and low self esteem. . . . *They behave disruptively against common rules shared by others and enforced by institutions*, toward which they feel a sense of entitlement that makes them act beyond the normal constrictions that affect the others in society [emphasis added]." (p. 4)

Narcissism is also associated with exploitative and unethical behaviors, including white-collar crime (Blickle et al., 2006), academic dishonesty (Brunell et al., 2011), and counterproductive work behavior, such as harassing coworkers, theft, and sharing confidential company information (Grijalva & Newman, 2014). Importantly, research documents that narcissists tend to attain roles as leaders (Grijalva et al., 2014) and show elevated levels of testosterone that are linked to dominance and aggression (Archer, 2006) and as reported by Herman et al. (2006), reduced empathy (more on narcissistic leaders in Chapter 10). Narcissism is associated with compromised moral functioning, including dishonesty, lack of responsibility or commitment, a deficit of the capacity for remorse, and exploitation (Weinberg, 2024). The most maladaptive form of narcissism, exploitativeness, expressed in toxic aggression and unethical behavior, is seen in the "Dark Triad" of narcissists, Machiavellians, and psychopaths (Rauthmann & Kolar, 2013) and in "toxic masculinity," a massive unconscious repression of the feminine side of human nature, the right brain.

A central theme of this chapter is that both forms of narcissism are the product of a late-appearing left brain compensatory reaction to an early right brain insecurity, an amplified false self, and that this hemispheric asymmetry, which onsets at the end of the second and into the third year, generates the bihemispheric defense of repression. Recall Levin's (1991) work on the development of the neuropsychology of repression and his observation that left-to-right interhemispheric commissural transmission is clearly defined at three and a half years. He proposes that in this time frame of human childhood, "a system of two properly functioning cerebral hemispheres with a high level of interhemispheric (i.e., left-right and right-left) connectedness comes into being." Three to four years is a critical period of growth for the cognitive left hemisphere, which now interacts with and can callosally inhibit the emotional right hemisphere. At this time there exists two interacting hemispheric regulation systems of narcissistic self-esteem. One acts in unconscious self-regulation via classical conditioning in the right brain, the other in the conscious mind by instrumental, operant reward-punishment learning in the left brain.

In classical work on narcissism, both Kernberg (1975) and Kohut and Wolf (1978) held that narcissism is related to cognitive-affective patterning and structuring of the intrapsychic self (note the allusion to hemisphericity). In terms of modern neurobiology, this specifically refers to the involvement and interactions between the early-developing unconscious emotional right brain and the later-developing cognitive left brain, a bihemispheric model of narcissism. Further support of this involvement of the dual cerebral hemispheres is found in research showing that narcissism, grounded in attachment dynamics of the first two years, is operational in preschool-age children at 3 to 4 years (see above) or early childhood (Cramer, 2011), that is also evident at age 23 as young adult narcissism (Carlson & Gjerde, 2009). Interestingly, maladaptive narcissism was related to maternal (and not paternal) authoritarian parenting, where the mother is overcontrolling and requires obedience, thereby interfering with the child recognizing his own feelings, thoughts, and skills. In reaction, "the child remains dependent on external approval to maintain the false self, which may be a source of pride and gratification for the parent" (Cramer, 2011, pp. 20–21). In discussing parenting styles associated with the development of narcissism, Cramer concludes that unresponsive parenting styles "might create a sense of neediness and an expectation that others will not naturally be responsive to those needs. To obtain this gratification, the child might develop compensatory defensive behaviors, including the development of the grandiose self" (p. 20).

Continuing this longitudinal model of the childhood precursors of the narcissistic personality, Cramer (2017) reports that narcissistic traits of 11-year-old children (late childhood) predict both grandiose and vulnerable narcissism in adults:

> Pathological narcissism in childhood has been described as including impulsivity, poor tolerance for frustration, mood swings, excessive effort to control and manipulate, and irritability (Bleiberg, 1988, p. 504). These children are also described as having an unstable self-esteem. On the one hand, their overvaluation of the self is seen in the need for constant admiration, attention, and/or self-aggrandizement. At the same time, undervaluation of the self may be observed in their tendency to experience feelings of inferiority and worthlessness. (Beren, 1992, p. 679)

She concludes that "the possibility of intervention at an early age is important, before maladaptive behaviors become entrenched in the child's personality" (p. 683).

Weise and Tuber (2004) offer a study of self and object relations of 11-year-old narcissistically disturbed children, who exhibit

> . . . a profound self-preoccupation and lack of concern for feelings of others. An unevenness of self-feelings, which vary from omnipotent to helpless, is also evident in the relationships of narcissistic children, as is a difficulty in the management of aggressive impulses (e.g., narcissistic rage). These children, even before school-age years, replace developmentally appropriate efforts to regulate self-esteem with a defensive fantasy. . . . Experiences of helplessness, envy, or pain are completely denied when feasible. When this is not possible, they may fly into a rage or strike out at others in a desperate attempt at self-protection. (p. 254)

Clinically working with a subset of children and adolescents (ages 12, 17, and 19) that he calls "brainy kids skating on thin ice," Graham Music (2023) describes their reliance on an "intellectual defense," a "false self, a personality built on a quick mind that has come to realize that it is not safe to trust, that there is only oneself to rely on. Underneath the dazzling exterior is a self that will do anything to avoid further pain, despair, or anxiety" (p. 16). I suggest "brainy" and "quick" refer to an elevated level of left hemispheric verbal intelligence and a high IQ that is a central source of their academic success. This clinical formulation of the role of superior intellect in certain childhood narcissists complements research on narcissism in adults who display "soaring grandiosity" on agentic domains such as "intelligence, extraversion, dominance, and attractiveness" but low on communion traits such as warmth and affiliation (Luo et al., 2014). Recall Ogden's (1994a) observation that certain adults with a compulsive reliance on a false self frequently attain academic success.

Thus throughout the lifespan narcissistic personalities defend against negative affective feelings of unworthiness and self-contempt by unconsciously assuming an attitude of left brain positive affective grandiosity and entitlement. Cain and her colleagues (2008) assert,

> These narcissistic defenses from Kohut's theory involve two forms of "splitting" that represent the themes of grandiosity and vulnerability. The first form, horizontal splitting, is similar to repression in that it involves the barring of unacceptable selfobject needs and concerns from

consciousness. The individual is thus able to maintain overt displays of grandiosity while chronically denying any feelings of low self-esteem or shame. In contrast, vertical splitting uses denial and disavowal of needs, allowing the conscious experience of vulnerability and helplessness to alternate with feelings of omnipotence. Individuals employing vertical splitting exhibit narcissistic vulnerability through their access to chronic feelings of emptiness, low self-esteem, and shame. (pp. 640–641)

Note that in grandiose narcissism, shame is overregulated and barred from consciousness but still exists as unconscious shame, while in vulnerable narcissism shame is conscious and underregulated. Also note the similarity of horizontal splitting to my neuropsychoanalytic model of rigid repression as a defense that blocks unconscious painful affects from intruding into the conscious mind (see Figure 4.1). Neurobiologically, repression represents the left frontal verbal cognitive callosal inhibition of right frontal nonverbal emotions. This hemispheric asymmetry bars entry of right brain dysregulated emotional states into left hemispheric consciousness. When repression is characterologically rigid or heavy, it reflects an imbalance of the hemispheres in favor of the left, a compensatory strong left hemisphere over a weak, insecure right hemisphere. Recall that repression is an unconscious mechanism that places unwanted feelings away from the conscious mind because of shame, guilt, or fear (Diseth, 2005).

Despite this defense, Helen Lewis, a pioneer in shame studies, points out that "narcissistic personalities are clearly suffering from shame and its brittle defense of grandiosity" (1971, p. 63). It is now thought that the continuous activation of the grandiose self in overt narcissistic personalities minimizes the conscious experience of shame and depression. Furthermore, shame, the keystone affect in narcissism dynamics (Schore, 1991; Gramzow & Tangney, 1992), is highly repressed in grandiose narcissistic personalities, and they are therefore behaviorally shameless. In contrast, vulnerable narcissism clinically presents as an "inhibited, shame-ridden, and hypersensitive shy type, whose low tolerance for attention from others and hypervigilant readiness for criticism or failure makes him/her more socially passive" (Ronningstam, 2009, p. 113).

That said, both forms of narcissism have "grandiose fantasies and expectations about the self, harbor feelings of entitlement, and display a willingness to exploit others for their own gain" (Ziegler-Hill et al., 2008, p. 756), and each exhibits a reduced capacity for empathy (Jauk & Kanske, 2021). Both are heavily reliant on defense mechanisms, specifically repression, and when continually intensifying stressful life events overwhelm and disable repression and the left hemisphere false self, the ensuing pathological dysregulated regression represents a "return of the repressed," reexposing the narcissist's underlying dysregulated organized-insecure attachment and painful shame dynamics, "the dark side of narcissism" (Back et al., 2013).

In this highly dysregulating life context, the failure of the repression defense may be a primary driver of suicide in narcissistic personality disorder, characterized by suddenness, determination, and high risk for lethal outcome, often associated with deficits in emotion processing, self-esteem dysregulation, and loss of internal control (Ronningstam et al., 2018). Jauk et al. (2017) discuss the relationship of narcissism to suicide:

> The ancient myth of Narcissus comes in several different versions. In Ovid's classic version, the beautiful young hunter Narcissus, who rejects the love of the nymph Echo, is deemed by the gods to fall in love with his mirror image. Fully entranced by his own reflection in a pool of water, Narcissus eventually realizes that his love cannot be reciprocated, which leads him to commit suicide. In another prominent version by Pausanias, the myth has a different ending: Narcissus is gazing at himself when suddenly a leaf falls into the water and distorts the image. Narcissus is shocked by the ugliness of his mirror image, which leads him to commit suicide.

More generally, failures of the repression defense are responsible for the release of unbridled hidden internal suffering that is accompanied by self-hatred (Kernberg, 1992), intense narcissistic rage (Kohut, 1972), and primitive shame (Broucek, 1982) that are outwardly blocked and turned against the self, and are thereby self-destructive. Indeed, shame-prone narcissistic personalities are known to frequently suffer from narcissistic injury–triggered overwhelming internal self-shaming tendencies (Morrison, 1984) and repetitive oscillations of self-esteem, which necessitate obsessional "endless attempts at repair" (Reich, 1960). Bursten (1973) notes the task of the narcissistic repair mechanism is to rid the self of shame, an affect state that tends to linger for quite a long time until the subject recovers (Nathanson, 1987), and which spreads out from one specific content to all of "inner reality" and thereby to the entire function of expressing oneself (Wurmser, 1981). This regression can potentially drive the narcissistic personality into psychotherapy. Although affect dysregulation intensifies the patient's symptomatology, it may also allow for more accessibility to working directly with the exposed underlying right brain insecure attachment dynamics. Recall that a weakened right brain attachment bond precedes and underlies the early development of the left brain false self (Meares, 1993).

In treatment, covert vulnerable narcissists hide their aggression and behavioral tendencies, while overt grandiose narcissists do not conceal but express these directly. Bringing the right-lateralized insecure anxious (preoccupied) attachment of vulnerable narcissism that overuses interactive regulation and the insecure avoidant (dismissive) attachment of grandiose narcissism that overuses autoregulation beneath the common left-lateralized compensatory false self into awareness is a central mechanism of psychodynamic right brain psychotherapy. Clinical research shows that vulnerable narcissists are more likely to seek treatment than grandiose narcissists (Pincus & Lukowitsky, 2010). That said, both types are difficult to treat. Narcissistic patients have a very high risk for dropout in therapy (Ellison et al., 2013), with rates of up to 64% (Hilsenroth et al., 1998). Increased rates of narcissistic personality disorders have been reported in outpatient private practices (Dodge et al., 2002; Westen & Arkowitz-Westen, 1998).

The therapeutic goal of short-term treatment is to change a stressful symptomatic dysregulating insecure attachment to a previously familiar defensively regulated insecure attachment. The goal of symptom-reducing psychotherapy with grandiose and vulnerable narcissistic disorders is to respectively improve the regulation of insecure avoidant and insecure anxious preoccupied attachments. This therapeutic change is due to right brain interactive affect regulation within a strengthened therapeutic alliance. When the symptoms are reduced, the patient may end therapy, or continue into the deeper realm of long-term treatment. The goal of this work is to change the patient's insecure into an "earned secure" attachment. It entails working directly with the defensive or repressive coping style of both forms of narcissistic personality disorders, reducing rigid repression and downsizing the grandiose false self, which in turn may generate a more balanced symmetry between the hemispheres.

Right Brain Psychotherapy of Repressed Unconscious Affects

Psychotherapy with all patients, including both types of hemispherically asymmetrical narcissistic personalities, focuses on the cocreation of a therapeutic context that can facilitate a more adaptive and flexible repressive defense. Repression describes content capable of symbolic mental representation that is sequestered from conscious awareness because of its distressing and conflictual nature (Robbins, 2018). This conflict between the two cerebral hemispheres first appears with the onset of their left-right interactions around the beginning of the third year. Patients with these more developmentally advanced organized attachment histories, including secure attachments, can access not only symbolic and self-reflective functions but also volition and voluntary behavior, verbal secondary-process cognition, metacognition, mentalization, abstraction, and, most importantly, the later-forming defense of repression against negative affect. These complex cognitive functions are available to the patient, especially during voluntary regressions of psychotherapy.

In classic writings, Wolitzky and Eagle (1999) asserted,

> Both Winnicott (1958a) and Guntrip (1969) refer to the importance of the patient returning to an earlier point at which psychological development went askew and to that point at which development turned in the direction of a "false self." The basic idea behind these various formulations seems to be that under the impact of trauma, certain defensive and defective structures (e.g., *false self, a pseudo-adult self masking an underlying ego weakness* [emphasis added]) developed that are at the heart of the patient's pathology. According to this view, what needs to be accomplished in treatment is a regression to the point at which these structures developed and a resumption of developmental growth along new and better pathways. (pp. 60–61)

As previously mentioned, the time period of this resumption of developmental growth occurs at the end of the second year, when the right hemisphere subjective self ends a growth spurt and the left hemisphere begins its growth spurt and the creation of the left-lateralized false self. The necessary regression into the early-developing right hemisphere, the locus of

Winnicott's true self, occurs in synchronized shifts from the patient's and therapist's conscious left minds into their unconscious right minds, allowing for new and more complex right-brain-to-right-brain communications within the expanding therapeutic alliance.

In working with highly repressed personalities, as the therapeutic relationship strengthens and safety and trust increase, these patients who overvalue left hemisphere control can begin to participate in regulated, synchronized mutual regressions with the empathic therapist into the right hemisphere. According to Gill and Brenman (1959), this adaptive form of regression is voluntarily sought by the individual and entered only when the person judges the situation to be safe. The patient's regression has a beginning and end and is terminable and reversible, with a sudden and total reinstatement of the previous ego organization. Bach (1985) emphasizes the active role of the patient: "He submits himself voluntarily to regression because he has some confidence that it is, in fact, reversible. With these patients it is of the utmost clinical importance that the regression be engaged voluntarily and that they feel free to discuss their anxieties and to control the situation" (p. 185).

In these voluntary mutual regressions, the reduction of the repression defense occurs on both sides of the therapeutic alliance. The repression defense is universal, and therefore also exists in the clinician. Russell (1998) points out the importance of not just the patient's but the therapist's defenses, clearly alluding to a two-person psychology of mutual defense. He notes, "The most important source of resistance in the treatment process is the therapist's resistance to what the patient feels" (p. 19). In this paradigm shift, what is needed is a relational, intersubjective model of affect defenses that addresses how the patient's and therapist's defenses interact with each other, communicate with each other, and synchronize or desynchronize with each other. Like mutual dissociation defenses, left hemispheric repressive defenses of both the patient and therapist need to be lifted in order to activate regulated, synchronized mutual regressions of right brain attachment dynamics.

An essential task of the burgeoning therapeutic relationship with these more developmentally advanced patients is to cocreate a right-brain-to-right-brain communication system beneath the left hemisphere false self and to follow not only the conscious but the unconscious affect generated by the repression defense. Neuroscience is now describing "unconscious negative emotion." As I discussed in previous chapters, in order to empathically attune to the patient's conscious and especially repressed unconscious negative affective states, the creative clinician surrenders to a Freudian intrapsychic topographical regression, a horizontal switch from a left prefrontal cortical to a right prefrontal cortical system, a left hemispheric to right hemispheric shift in dominance from the rational conscious left mind into the intuitive unconscious right mind (see Figure 2.1, horizontal arrows).

In *The Science of the Art of Psychotherapy* (Schore, 2012), I discussed the classical psychoanalytic work of Theodor Reik (1948) and Ernst Kris (1952) on a creative "regression in the service of the ego," defined as the production of an idea that is both novel and useful in a particular social setting. Kris (1953) elaborated two phases of this regression: an inceptive *inspirational phase* in which unconscious and preconscious primary-process ideation surge into attention and goal-directed thinking is at a minimum (right brain divergent thinking that generates many new ideas and more than one correct solution), and a subsequent *elaborational* phase in which the inspirational processes are subjected to critical scrutiny and revised into secondary-process ideation (left brain convergent thinking that generates one possible solution). Kris stated that in the moment of a regression, a well-integrated individual who regresses has the capacity to regulate and utilize some of the primary process creatively. He further suggested that in the psychotherapeutic context of this regression, the barriers separating unconscious from preconscious or conscious processes have been loosened.

In *Right Brain Psychotherapy* (Schore, 2019b), I described the fundamental role of the clinician's right brain creativity in psychotherapy, and now I apply it to working with the repression defense. Creativity is defined as the production of an idea that is both novel and useful in a particular social setting. According to Mihov et al. (2010), creativity is the ability to "think outside the box." These researchers report a meta-analytic review of lateralization studies that support right hemispheric superiority in creative thinking. This reversible transient topographic regression from the experienced clinician's left hemispheric rational thinking to right hemispheric intuitive emotion is expressed in her ability to feel and not think her way through stressful, negatively valenced heightened affective moments of the session when the repression defense loosens.

In turn, this allows the intuitive therapist access to creative new ways of strengthening safety and trust with overregulated insecure avoidant dismissive and underregulated insecure anxious preoccupied personalities. According to Weinberg (2024), dismissive attachment is defined by a tendency to dismiss reliance on others (interactive regulation), including an avoidance of reliance on the therapist. The avoidant patient's strong bias is to rigidly stay in left hemispheric control and autoregulate relational stress, to talk about emotion rather than experience emotion, and so the empathic clinician's ability to shift right allows her to synchronize with the right brain avoidant attachment pattern beneath the left hemispheric words and provide a new experience—to seek and share attachment interactive regulation. In order to subliminally regulate the patient's relational stress, the creative therapist must access her right brain to be able to learn new ways of forming a working relationship and repairing ruptures of the therapeutic alliance with left-dominant highly repressed personalities.

The neuroscience literature holds that "the left hemisphere is more involved in the (conscious) processing of information, whereas the right hemisphere is more involved in the background-holistic (subconscious) processing of information" (Prodan et al., 2001, p. 211). Therapeutic mutual topographic regressions, transient callosal shifts in hemispheric dominance, underlie the previously mentioned clinical descriptions of the therapist's entrance into a regression by a "creative surrender" (Ehrenzweig, 1957), passively letting go, out of the left hemisphere, dominant for control, into the right hemisphere, dominant for both creativity and vulnerability (Hecht, 2014). McGilchrist (2009) describes this hemispheric shift: "We must inhibit one in order to inhabit the other," clearly implying that the left prefrontal must be inhibited (taken "offline") to bring the disinhibited right prefrontal from the background to the foreground of consciousness.

Even more specifically, these reversible shifts in dominance occur between dual prefrontal systems. A neuroimaging study by Huang et al. (2013) reports that the left frontal lobe is negatively related to creativity, that the right hemisphere's predominance in creative thinking may be inhibited by the left hemisphere, and that removal of this inhibition can facilitate the emergence of creativity. McGilchrist (2021a) asserts, "depressing the left hemisphere enhances creativity, probably because the mind is released from tendencies toward the linear explicit and linguistic modes of apprehension typical of the left—both rationalizing and verbalizing have a damaging effect on creativity, at least during the generative process itself" (p. 278). He states, "creativity can't be summoned at will, and the very act of attending to it inhibits it" (p. 240), which in turn involves "*letting go* . . . freedom of the unconscious from constant over-riding by conscious thought processes, and a conscious mind more open to its promptings" (p. 256). In this manner, the process of creativity "depends on unconscious processes, flexibility, openness to the unknown and undetermined, relinquishing control, making imaginative leaps, seeing analogies, metaphors and images—all elements that are more characteristic of the right hemisphere than the left" (p. 242). In order for these right brain processes to occur, "both the unconscious mind and the body play an important role in creativity" (p. 278).

Furthermore, the prefrontal executive functions of the right and left hemispheres are respectively mediated by the early-maturing orbital prefrontal and later-maturing dorsolateral prefrontal cortices (Schore, 1994/2016). Research shows that in contrast to the emotional orbitofrontal (ventromedial) cortex that forges two-way connections with the amygdala, the cognitive dorsolateral prefrontal system has no direct neural connections with the amygdala (Ongur & Price, 2000; Ghashghaei & Barbas, 2002). The left dorsolateral prefrontal system, which is overactivated in repression, is fundamentally involved in executive functions such as abstract thinking and self-reflective consciousness (Courtney et al., 1998; Dehaene & Naccache, 2001; Posner, 1994). I suggest this hyperactivated left-lateralized prefrontal cortex is also the neuroanatomical location of the false self.

The dorsolateral and orbitofrontal systems reciprocally inhibit each other's functions; their callosal connections are centrally implicated in interhemispheric relationships. Thus in working with the patient's repression defense that characterologically blocks entry of right brain emotional states into left brain consciousness, the empathic intuitive clinician transiently takes her left hemispheric rational dorsolateral cortex offline. This in turn disinhibits the orbitofrontal emotional system and its direct connections to the right brain, the psychobiological domain of the unconscious, and activates its capacity to perceptually sense the patient's nonverbal right-brain-to-right-brain nonverbal communications. In this manner, regression in the service of the self fundamentally involves a regression from the later-forming executive functions of the left hemisphere to the earlier-forming executive functions of the right hemisphere.

The experienced therapist's regression thus describes a partial, temporary, controlled lowering of the level of psychic functioning of the cognitive left dorsolateral cortex executive system that releases the dominance of the right orbitofrontal executive system, the major emotion-regulatory system of the therapist's right brain. This topographical left-right shift allows the empathic clinician to follow changes in the patient's affect, to track, synchronize with, and regulate the patient's unconscious affect beneath the patient's defense, especially in heavily repressed personalities. Carl Rogers (1975) asserted that empathy "involves being sensitive, moment-to-moment, to the changing felt meanings which flow in this other person" (p. 4).

The right orbitofrontal system is centrally involved in the processing of affect-related meanings (Teasdale et al., 1999; Roy et al., 2012). Because its activity is associated with a lower threshold for awareness of sensations of both external and internal origin, it functions as an "internal reflecting and organizing agency" (Kaplan-Solms & Solms, 1996). The right orbitofrontal system, the "thinking part of the emotional brain" (Goleman, 1995), functions to integrate and assign emotional-motivational significance to cognitive impressions and the association of emotion with ideas and thoughts (Joseph, 1996), clearly alluding to its connections into the left hemisphere.

Further elaborating this idea, I suggest that Freud's preconscious, the link between the conscious and unconscious mind (see Figure 2.3), represents the locus of Bowlby's unconscious internal models of secure and insecure attachment that encodes strategies of affect regulation encoded in implicit, procedural memory. Bowlby proposed that psychotherapy is directed toward altering these unconscious internalized representations of early relationships. The preconscious has been classically defined as that part of the mind below the level of conscious awareness, from which memories and emotions that have not been repressed can be recalled. In classic psychoanalytic conceptualizations, Freud's notion of repression is understood to filter affects at an unconscious level. Indeed, the right orbitofrontal cortex, the executive system of the right brain, plays a fundamental role in preconscious functions, specifically acting as a dynamic filter that implicitly tracks the arousal rhythms and flows of emotional stimuli (Schore, 2019b). I further suggest that this right prefrontal system is the anatomical locus of "the hidden observer," described as a preconscious system "that the person had registered and stored in memory without being aware that the information had been processed" (Hilgard, 1984, p. 248). The preconscious also stores and generates what Dan Stern and his colleagues (1998) call "implicit relational knowledge" (see Figure 2.3).

Note the preconscious right orbitofrontal system plays a fundamental role in the hierarchical regulation of body and motivational states via its monitoring and regulation of the duration, frequency, and intensity of affective states of emotional arousal. In this manner, it implicitly regulates the lower levels of the right brain unconscious system that generates strong negative and positive affect. But in addition, it is also centrally involved in the preconscious horizontal transmission of regulated and dysregulated affective states to the conscious left hemisphere, as well as in the processing of emotion-evoking stimuli without conscious awareness and controlling the allocation of attention to possible contents of consciousness. Joseph (1992) postulated, "The preconscious contains information and memories that exist *just below the surface of consciousness,* and in this respect, it is part of the unconscious. Once affective information reaches the preconscious, it becomes relatively accessible to the conscious mind" (see Figure 2.3). Research demonstrates that the orbitofrontal cortex acts as "gateway to subjective conscious experience" (Kringelbach, 2005, p. 699). The right orbitofrontal preconscious self-system of the emotional brain, forged in attachment dynamics, thus acts as a major determinant of which affects that support different self-states can reach right subjective and then left hemispheric objective consciousness.

Applying these data to a clinical model, in a heightened affective moment of a synchronized mutual interaction between the therapist's and patient's right orbitofrontal preconscious systems, the patient's affectively charged right brain experiences can be communicated to the left brain for further conscious processing. The objective left hemisphere can now process subjective right brain communications, allowing for a linkage of the unconscious nonverbal and conscious verbal representational realms. This facilitates the evolution of affects from their early form, in which they are experienced as bodily sensations, into subjective states that can gradually be verbally articulated and semantically encoded by the left mind.

In their writings on the right hemispheric "integrated self," Kuhl and his colleagues (2015) contend,

Expressing emotional contents through language may be one way in which communication between psychological systems may be facilitated. . . . Such verbalizations may facilitate a transfer of the right hemisphere's implicit information into the analytical left hemisphere. This transfer may be crucial for nurturing integrative competencies, especially when verbalizations are accompanied by emotional and self-related feelings. (p. 124)

Note that in this therapeutic context, affects are intrapsychically transferred within the patient's right implicit preconscious and left explicit conscious self-systems, as well as communicated and relationally shared between the patient and the empathic therapist. Left to right regressions into the orbitofrontal preconscious system allow the intuitive clinician to synchronize her preconscious with the patient's preconscious in order to receive and regulate unconscious negative affects, such as repressed unconscious shame.

Shame Dynamics in Early Human Development and Working with Repressed Unconscious Affect in the Therapeutic Alliance

In the developmental context, the mother's right hemisphere psychobiologically imprints the toddler's emerging preconscious system in the second year, a time of the emergence of the social emotion of shame, the keystone affect in narcissistic dynamics, especially in narcissistic personality disorders (Schore, 1991). The potent negative affect of shame is "a powerful modulator of interpersonal relatedness" (Nathanson, 1987). Due to the strength of this negative affect, right brain bodily-based nonverbal shame that evolves in infancy can be dissociated, while left brain verbal humiliation that begins at the end of the second year can be repressed. Dysregulated shame is thus associated with emotional abuse. Although much has been recently written on conscious shame, little attention has been placed on working with unconscious shame in the psychotherapeutic relationship.

Sylvan Tomkins (1963), the great 20th-century pioneer of the study of emotion, describes the unique properties of this painful bodily-based affect:

Though terror speaks of life and death and distress makes of the world a veil of tears, yet shame strikes deepest into the heart of man. While terror and distress hurt, they are wounds inflicted from outside which penetrate the smooth surface of the ego; but *shame is felt as an inner torment, a sickness of the soul* [emphasis added]. It does not matter whether the humiliated one has been shamed by derisive laughter or whether he mocks himself. In either event, he feels himself naked, defeated, alienated, lacking in dignity or worth. (p. 118)

The "ubiquitous and unrelieved" experience of shame, "one of the least tolerable affects for humans" (Malatesta-Magai, 1991), becomes associated with an expectation of a painful self-disorganizing state and is therefore consciously avoided or "bypassed" (Lewis, 1971), that is, defensively dissociated or repressed. Acting at unconscious levels, dysregulated humiliation inhibits the positively valenced left-lateralized grandiose false self, while shame inhibits the positive right brain affects of interest and joy, an area of difficulty for avoidant personalities. The shame dynamic is reenacted in rupture and repair transactions of the therapeutic alliance, where it sunders the emotional connection between the patient and therapist.

For example, the cocreation of an adaptive topographical mutual regression between the dismissive-repressed patient and the empathic intuitive therapist can potentially transform unconscious negative affect such as repressed shame into a domain of the preconscious where it can enter consciousness as a discrete, negatively valenced painful feeling, one that can be experienced, interactively regulated, shared, and consciously communicated between the patient and the empathic therapist. In this work, repressed unconscious shame becomes a central focus of the treatment, especially in grandiose narcissistic personality disorders where the individual is "shameless," and, like other defended negative affects, it needs to come into the patient's conscious awareness to be adaptive.

In my very first work, "Early Superego Development: The Emergence of Shame and Narcissistic Affect Regulation in the Practicing Period" (Schore, 1991), I proposed that the parasympathetic state of shame, a highly visual affect subjectively experienced as a "spiraling downward," represents a sudden decelerative shift from autonomic sympathetic energy-expending hyperarousal into energy-conserving parasympathetic dorsal vagal hypoarousal. I then expanded this model (Schore, 1994/2016), when I offered a developmental model of the interpersonal attachment origins of the primary social emotion of shame in socialization dynamics that begin in the second year. According to Erikson (1950), the central psychological dynamic of the second year is "autonomy vs. shame and doubt."

I have suggested that the origins of shame are centered in the primary attachment relationship. As such, shame is evoked not in separations that evoke fear and protest but in attachment reunion transactions, when the newly mobile toddler's excitement is met with indifference or disapproval. At about 14 months,

> the toddler, in an activated, hyperstimulated, high arousal state of stage-typical ascendant excitement and elation, exhibits itself during a reunion with the caregiver. Despite an excited expectation of a psychobiologically attuned shared positive affect state with the mother and a dyadic amplification of the positive affects of excitement and joy, the infant unexpectedly encounters a facially expressed affective misattunement, thereby triggering a sudden shock-induced deflation of narcissistic affect. The infant is thus propelled into an intensified low arousal state which he cannot yet autoregulate. Shame represents this dysregulating rapid transition from a preexisting high arousal positive hedonic state to a low arousal negative hedonic state. (Schore, 1994/2016, p. 203)

In this rapid transition of state, the nonverbal toddler experiences a sudden shift in dominance from right corticolimbic sympathetic energy-expending autonomic hyperarousal to parasympathetic energy-conserving hypoarousal. Phenomenologically experienced as a subjective implosion of the self, this instantaneous depletion of psychic energy reflects a rapid deceleration of ventral tegmental dopaminergic reward functions and a state of hypoarousal and thereby depression. In this rupture of the attachment bond, the stressed toddler needs the caregiver's repair and provision of upregulating interactive regulation, which, depending on the attachment history, may or may not be available. In the latter context, these painful dysregulating attachment dynamics of shame are frequent and unrepaired during the critical period of development of the right orbitofrontal cortex in the second year. This same time period, the "terrible twos," is a time of verbalized negativism, excessive use of the word *no*, and separation behaviors. In secure dyads, these behaviors are accompanied by repair, reunion, and rapprochement, but in insecure dyads they may encounter harsh or indifferent parenting and increased stress. On the other hand, this period of socialization may involve sensitive limit setting.

In classical studies, Mahler et al. (1975) observed that at the end of the practicing period and the onset of the rapprochement period at 17 to 21 months, "the toddler's elated preoccupation with locomotion and exploration *per se* [is] beginning to wane" (p. 90). Pine (1980) referred to the "rapprochement crisis" involving the collapse of the illusion of omnipotence: "Now he is small and alone in a big world, rather than sharing in the (imagined) omnipotence of the mother–child unit." Parkin (1985) described the transition from the exhilarated practicing state, which represents the highest point in the development of primary narcissism and the overestimation of the child's powers, into rapprochement. He defines the "narcissistic crisis" (Mahler's rapprochement crisis) as "the necessity of yielding up to reality the child's illusory claims to omnipotence" (Parkin, 1985, p. 146). Freud (1914/1957) speaks of the reluctant "departure from primary narcissism."

This critical developmental transition emotionally tests the mother–child dyad (as well as the emerging father–child relationship) and the ability to remain connected during the stage-specific narcissistic distress that unfolds. More specifically, although during the crisis the ambitendent toddler moves away from the mother, he returns during periods of dysregulating distress. The mother's "quiet availability" in these reunions for regulation of distressing affects (arousal modulation) is an essential caregiver function. During this period of developmental crisis, narcissistic rages and tantrums are used by the child to regain control. The response of attachment figures to the downregulation of this behavior is critical, in terms of both empathy and limit setting.

The markers of a successful developmental passage through this stage transition are well known. Kohut (1971) underscored the principle that a true sense of self is a product of the accommodation or neutralization of the individual's grandiosity and idealization. Parkin (1985) emphasized that "with this resolution there is a subsidence of the child's rages and of his external struggles with his mother for power." Settlage (1977) asserted that one of the major developmental tasks of the rapprochement phase is the modulation of infantile rage (noradrenergic sympathetic hyperarousal). By the end of the second year, the essential transformation in right brain affect regulation that marks the rapprochement crisis is the deflation of practicing elation and exhilaration that supports the illusion of omnipotence. Mahler (1980) emphasizes that during the rapprochement crisis, which is essentially an emotional crisis, the toddler shows "an increasing differentiation of his emotional life."

The interactive regulation of the emotion of shame, the regulator of hyperstimulated (excited, elated, grandiose, manic) states, is critical to the modulation of high-arousal narcissistic affects characteristic of the practicing period, and is thereby required for the deflation of omnipotence and resolution of the narcissistic rapprochement crisis. On the other hand, in less than optimal insecure attachment histories, the resulting deficit in narcissistic affect regulation lays the groundwork for an amplified grandiose false self and later-forming narcissistic personality disorders that involve an interaction between the right and left hemispheres in the third year. With the onset of a critical period of growth in the third year, the young child may be a parental target of stressful and painful verbal humiliation. Indeed, in my 1991 article on shame I discussed at length "implications for the early etiology of narcissistic disorders."

Authors have described psychobiological descriptions of "the more primitive, biologically based nature of shame" (Broucek, 1982). Note the evolutionary arousal-regulating mechanism of the social emotion of shame appears in the early origin of human nature. Perhaps more than any other emotion, shame is intimately tied to the physiological expression of an organismic stress response. The activity of the autonomic nervous system, which is an effector channel of the emotion-mediating limbic system, is the basis of the acute phenomenology of shame. Over the lifespan, shame acutely reduces hyperaroused and hyperstimulated states; diminishes positive narcissistic affective coloring of self-representations; contracts the self; lowers expectations; decreases self-esteem, active coping, interest, and curiosity; increases passive coping, blushing, gaze aversion, and depressive affect-toned mood; and interferes with not only right brain emotional and social functions but also left brain cognition. For much more detail I refer the reader to Chapter 5 of *Affect Regulation and the Repair of the Self* (Schore, 2003).

Darwin (1872/1965) characterized shame as a hyperactive physiological state. Freud's (1905/1953) original conceptualization of shame was that it acted as a superego counterforce or reaction formation against exhibitionistic excitement and overstimulation, which have potential ego-disruptive effects. This underscores the requisite preexisting state of hyperarousal for shame induction, and the function of shame as an arousal blocker, a regulator of hyperstimulated (elated, excited, grandiose, manic, euphoric) states. Tomkins (1963), who identified the function of shame as an "affect auxiliary," a specific inhibitor of the activated, ongoing affects of interest-excitement and enjoyment-joy, pointed out that shame reduces self-exposure or exploration powered by these positive affects. Shame signals the self-system to terminate interest in whatever has come to its attention (Nathanson, 1987). Thus the "superego-mediated flight from positively experienced exhibitionism to negatively experienced shame" (Miller, 1985) changes the affective valence and diminishes the arousal level of the organism, thereby blocking the further escalation and intensification of stimulation. The end result is a painfully stimulated state of shame. Kohut (1971) presents a similar model: At a moment of exhibitionism of the self, the sudden unexpected impact of shame is to ground the person who is overstimulated by omnipotent, grandiose affective states.

In the therapeutic alliance, the stressful, painful social emotion of shame, a powerful modulator of interpersonal relatedness, is triggered in the nonverbal right-brain-to-right-brain communication of a psychobiologically dysregulating misattunement. The eye is the prevailing organ in shame exposure, and shame triggers the involuntary defense of gaze aversion (Tomkins, 1963), which instantly breaks face-to-face eye contact. This induces a response of hiding the face "to escape from this being seen or from the one who sees" (Wright, 1991) and a state of withdrawal (Lichtenberg, 1989). Under the lens of a "shame microscope" that amplifies and expands this negative affect (Malatesta-Magai, 1991), visible defects, narcissistically charged undesirable vulnerable aspects of the self, are exposed (Jacobson, 1964). It is as though something we were hiding from everyone is suddenly under a burning light in public view (Izard, 1991). Shame throws a "flooding light" upon the individual (Lynd, 1958), who then experiences "a sense of displeasure plus the compelling desire to disappear from view" (Frijda, 1988) and "an impulse to bury one's face, or to sink right then and there, into the ground" (Erikson, 1950), which impels him to "crawl through a hole" and culminates in feeling as if he "could die" (Lewis, 1971).

The sudden shock-induced deflation of positive affect that supports grandiose omnipotence has been phenomenologically characterized as a whirlpool—a visual representation of a spiral (Potter-Effron, 1989) and as a "flowing off" or "leakage" through a drain hole in the middle of one's being (Sartre, 1957). The individual's subjective conscious experience of this affect is thus a sudden, unexpected, and rapid transition from what Freud (1914/1957) called "primary narcissism"—a sense of being "the center of and core of the universe" to what Sartre (1957) described as a shame-triggered "crack in my universe."

Thus, shame is associated with a sudden, rapid, painful implosion of the subjective self that is beyond conscious control (Schore, 1991, 1994/2016, 2003b, 2012). This intensely dysregulating negative affect inhibits the expression of any specific emotion (Tomkins, 1987), and indeed the expression of emotion per se (Kaufman, 1992), including aggression, in the form of "shame rage." Shame has long been known to be associated with anger (Tangney et al., 1992). Kohut (1971) wrote about shame-induced "narcissistic rage," which results from an angry reaction to an injury to self-esteem and the subjective experience of psychological vulnerability. In addition to anger, other emotions such as malicious envy (Lange et al., 2016) and hubristic pride (Tracy et al., 2009) are associated with narcissism. These dysregulating affects are communicated in right-brain-to-right-brain transference-countertransference communications.

Discussing the pivotal role of shame in the treatment of narcissistic adults (Black et al., 2013) and adolescents (Guile et al., 2004), Weinberg (2024) describes the clinician's countertransferential stressors in working with grandiose narcissistic personality disorders:

> Narcissistic patients tend to provoke negative feelings in their therapists (Tanzilli et al., 2017). Typically, therapists of narcissistic personality disorder patients struggle with such powerful reactions as feeling annoyed, used, close to losing one's temper, mistreated, resentful, and walking on eggshells. They experience sexual tension or feel dread or dislike the patient, feel criticized, dismissed, competitive and envious, bored, hopeless, and cruel or mean toward the patient. (p. 2)

Citing Bromberg (1992), Weinberg (2024) offers the important observation that therapeutic stalemates are jointly created in collusion by the patient and the therapist. This unconscious dynamic, a "mutual enactment of devaluation, competitiveness, or envy due to underlying narcissistic vulnerability in both therapist and patient can escalate to treatment interfering proportions."

Weinberg (2024) concludes that some of the difficulties in the narcissis-tic therapeutic alliance are cocreated, in specific relational configurations. I suggest these enactments are expressed in dysregulated transference-countertransference communications, frequently delivered in the clinician's critical tone of voice. These obstacles to the process of change develop with mutual contributions of both parties occurring outside the awareness of both.

As an example, Epstein (1994) described the iatrogenic effects of the therapist's inability to "take the transference," specifically projections of the patient's "shame rage":

> The projected affects often involve the therapist's hidden feeling of shame, envy, vulnerability, and impotence. The hidden shame is sig-naled by the therapist's use of "attack other" defenses such as sarcasm, teasing, ridicule, and efforts to control the patient in some way. Later on, the tragic projection comes full circle when the patient feels humil-iated, exploited, betrayed, abandoned, and isolated. (p. 100)

Thus, Gabbard (2022) points out that in long-term treatment of narcissis-tic patients, "therapists need to allow the patient to draw them into their internal world." This clearly suggests that in order to take the transference, the clinician must be in his or her right and not left brain.

Furthermore, according to Ornstein (1999), treatment of narcissistic rage, which is repressed and unconscious, addresses the patient's vulnera-bility, the soil in which this anger arises, through an empathic entry into the subjective inner world of the individual rather than through direct con-frontations. At continuous chronic high levels, shame is maladaptive and produces a constriction of an individual's affective states. That said, not conscious shame but chronic dysregulated repressed unconscious shame is maladaptive, while well-regulated shame is adaptive. It is important to note that shame is a moral emotion and that shamelessness is associated with immoral and destructive human behavior. Davis (1987) concluded that repression is motivated, in particular, by affective experiences of heightened self-consciousness in which the self is exposed to a negative evaluation, specifically citing shame. Dysregulated shame has been proposed to be a potent motive force for not only repression but also dissociation.

Alluding to the difference between repressed and dissociated shame, DeYoung differentiated *"bad-me* shame that can be brought out of dark psychic hiding places into the light, and *not-me* shame that must remain dissociated and unknowable" (2015, p. 154; see DeYoung's superb volume for working with dissociated chronic shame). She also pointed out that although "not-me" states have never been symbolized, "bad-me" states have been symbolized (and are thus accessible to affectively, relationally focused repression psychodynamics). The implicit avoidance of the recognition of shame "directly opposes derepression and the integration of unconscious material within the conscious ego" (Ward, 1972). Note that not conscious but unconscious repressed and dissociated shame blocks this integration. This principle applies not only to the patient but to the therapist. On numerous occasions in this volume I have focused on the clinician's defenses, shame, self-awareness, and blind spots. The deeper exploration of one's own right brain unconscious self is essential to the psychotherapist's clinical efficacy and expertise, especially in working with intense emotions like shame and its unconscious defenses.

In classic clinical studies, Broucek (1991, p. 85) observed, "The affect of shame is characterized by painful self-consciousness in which there is a strong wish to *hide* the face from the gaze of the other." And yet when shame is not acknowledged but remains hidden and repressed, it is almost impossible to alter the isolation of the subjective self. Thus the key to altering the gaze aversion of shame dynamics is direct intimate eye contact and authentic self-revelation with a trusted other. Recall Jung's "shadow self"—the part of our psyche that we seek to hide and repress. In his poem "Revelation," Robert Frost alludes to shame:

We make ourselves a place apart
Behind light words that tease and flout,
But oh, the agitated heart
Till someone find us really out
'Tis pity if the case require
(Or so we say) that in the end
We speak the literal to inspire
The understanding of a friend
But so with all, from babes that play
At hide-and-seek to God afar
So all who hide too well away
Must speak and tell us where they are.

The research of Kuchinke and his colleagues (2006) documents that the processing of spoken positive and negative emotional words activates the right and not left prefrontal cortex. Attachment words, especially those associated with positive interpersonal relationships, are more efficiently processed by the right hemisphere (Mohr et al., 2007).

Affectively focused, intuitive psychotherapy that initiates left-right frontal shifts in order to induce synchronized mutual regressions to access unconscious affects can thus potentially bring repressed affects, including unconscious shame, into conscious awareness. Referring to *preconscious* functions, Welling (2005) describes intuition as "a factory of pieces of thoughts, images, and vague feelings, where the raw materials seem to float around half formless, a world so often present, though we hardly ever visit it. However, some of these floating elements come to stand out, gain strength, or show up repeatedly. When exemplified, they may be easier to recognize and *cross the border of consciousness* [emphasis added]" (p. 33). Damasio (1999) asserts that a conscious sense of self is capable of "stepping into the light," which he describes as "a powerful metaphor for consciousness" (p. 3). This occurs in a heightened affective moment in the burgeoning therapeutic alliance that generates increased levels of safety, trust, and hope when the patient's right frontal preconscious system synchronously resonates with the therapist's right frontal preconscious system. Recall that the therapeutic alliance is the most powerful predictor of change in all types of psychotherapy (Baier et al., 2020; Muran & Barber, 2010; Ovenstad et al., 2020). Weinberg (2024) asserts, "The alliance provides leverage for change but also provides patients with a lived experience of a collaborative, respectful, and emotionally attuned relationship that on its own is conducive to emotional growth and self-exploration, and the discovery of new forms of relating."

There is now agreement that "the alliance is not stationary, but rather oscillates over the course of a session, between sessions, and over the course of therapy" (Wampold & Fluckiger, 2023). Over time the creative clinician, sensitive to even low levels of the patient's shifts into and out of affective states, learns how to fluidly synchronize his or her shifts in hemispheric dominance with the patient's shifts. As the therapy progresses and the therapeutic alliance strengthens, the empathic therapist is now able to acquire a felt sense of the patient's unconscious affects, not just beneath the surface of the preconscious, but repressed affects deeper within the patient's unconscious mind (see Figure 2.3). These heavily repressed affects may be activated when the patient is reexperiencing and recounting an emotionally difficult, stressful, shameful, painful, and highly conflictual past experience in right-lateralized autobiographical memory. The ability to tolerate what was once intolerable, the release of repressed material, is critical to growth-promoting psychodynamic treatment. The clinical dictum "safe but not too safe" means not staying too entrenched in the left mind, which processes the familiar, versus the right mind, which processes the novel, the unexpected. In this heightened affective moment, the patient and therapist need to synchronously lower defenses and take more risk.

Psychodynamic right brain psychotherapy focuses upon bringing repressed unconscious affects into awareness, especially as it is affectively played out in mutual regressions of right-brain-to-right-brain transference-countertransferential ruptures and repair of the continually developing therapeutic alliance. In this work, the empathic therapist may have a sense of the patient's affective state, but the central question is how can an unconscious affect emerge into conscious awareness in the patient's right-lateralized preconscious mind? The creative clinician facilitates this alteration in the patient's subjective consciousness not so much by offering explicit left brain mutative interpretations to make the unconscious conscious as by coconstructing a right brain context in which the patient begins to subliminally feel enough implicit safety and trust in the developing therapeutic relationship to risk transiently taking the left hemisphere repression defense offline, thereby potentially allowing for shared right hemispheric affects, including repressed unconscious affective states, to come into being. The *Oxford English Dictionary* defines *creativity* as "bringing into being."

The master psychoanalyst Susan Sands (1997) offered a creative clinical example of a "return of the repressed" and a "coming into being" of repressed aggression in a voluntary mutual regression of a vulnerable narcissist with an insecure anxious preoccupied attachment, where aggression is directed inwardly toward the victimized unconscious self (repressed and therefore bypassed). Although I presented this case vignette of an attachment reenactment in a heightened affective moment in a previous volume (Schore, 2019b), in the following I offer a more extensive analysis based on the new ideas in these chapters.

Almost from the beginning of the three-year-long therapy, I had had the persistent feeling that I was never "doing enough" for this particular patient. It was not clear to me why this should be so, for the patient was very bright, verbal, responsive to and interested in me, and able to use the therapy well.

But as I focused in more and more on my experience of him, I became aware of a "pull," like something tugging on the center of my chest. As this bodily experience became more conscious, I realized that I had in fact felt this pull from the first moment I met him. I also became more aware of a subtle countermovement in myself to resist this pull, to dig in my heels. One day the patient started (as he often did) with, "I'm not sure what I want to do today," and we both sat there for a while in *silence, staring at each other,* my *feeling the pull more and more.* I felt myself becoming irritated and resistant. I told him, "I am feeling a strong pull to do something, and yet I'm not sure what there is to do." He responded *immediately* that he felt resentful about having to have all the responsibility for this relationship.

He felt *I* was withholding, and he wanted to "demand—no, *command*" me to do what he wanted. Then he said, his *eyes filling with tears,* "*When's it going to be my turn?*" At this point *we both felt a major shift in the therapy,* that we had uncovered something that had been going on forever but had never before been made conscious.

Suddenly it was easy for *both of us* to make the connections to his childhood, where his depressed and self-doubting mother had relied on him not only to guide himself but also to guide her and reassure her that she was being a good mother. He had felt this impossible pull all his life—as well as his resistance to it.

The most striking evidence to me that we had reached a new, more fundamental level of understanding was that, after this series of interchanges, for the first time since the beginning of therapy, my own sense of "pull" completely disappeared. (Sands, 1997, pp. 652–653)

Note in Sands's opening comment she describes an evolving intimate therapeutic alliance, now over three years, in which the patient is using the therapy well. This clearly indicates numerous regulated, synchronized mutual regressions that have reduced shame, the keystone affect of narcissism, diminished the false self, and strengthened the therapeutic alliance and evolving right-brain-to-right-brain communication system between herself and the patient. As the session begins, she reads her own right brain nonverbal psychophysiological responses to being in his presence. In this reunion transaction at the beginning of the session, note the intuitive therapist's self-revelation when she authentically expresses her uncertainty about how to be with the patient, as well as her ability to take the negative transference, feel irritated and resistant, and then feed back to the patient and share her interoceptive awareness of her physiological countertransference. These bodily-based communications instantly trigger an increased assertiveness in the patient and a spontaneous demand or command expressed back to the therapist. This is followed by what had always been repressed—the externalized expression of an attachment protest, of anger outward to the mother, and the request to be the recipient and not the source of interactive regulation for the mother. Note the redirection of aggression outward and not inward toward the self in this adaptive reenactment of an interactively regulated insecure preoccupied attachment.

I suggest that in this synchronized left-right callosal shift both the patient's and the clinician's repression defenses are lifted, and the psycho-biologically attuned therapist's and patient's autonomic nervous systems are synchronized and communicating with each other in an energy-expending sympathetic-dominant state of aggression. The empathic therapist "surrenders" and takes the aggressive transference projected out (communicated) by the patient and shares it with him. In this moment, the therapist for the first time becomes interoceptively aware of not only the patient's but her own aggression in her defensive resistance to the pull, as part of her countertransference. Note her ability to implicitly physiologically synchronize and resonantly amplify the patient's unconscious aggressive state and the ensuing emotionally marked moment when what's defensively unconscious becomes conscious in both.

In the heightened affective moment of the session, the synchronized mutual regression facilitates a right brain Eureka moment in the patient, an "Aha!" self-recognition and insight, which is then immediately followed by his spontaneous strong assertion, "When's it going to be my turn?" This sudden intuitive insight and spontaneous release of repressed anger occurred in a two-person reenactment of his insecure attachment dynamics, a protest response to being controlled by the mother's role reversal, where instead of the mother being his affect regulator, he was the affect regulator of her depression and had the responsibility to reassure her that she was a good mother. He also experiences ("eyes filling with tears") the repressed sadness for the child who was deprived of his mother's interactive regulation. Notice the common progression of "coming into awareness" of sympathetic anger before parasympathetic grief and sadness. Music (2023) observes, "Often anger and murderous rage need to appear before grief and mourning and, eventually, ease and relaxation can find a place" (p. 15). At this point of change in his repression dynamics, he experiences a major shift in the therapy—the patient now openly expresses and is more able to deeply explore his newly found assertiveness, an increase in autoregulation.

Each of these elements of the heightened affective moment are accompanied by an intimate, reciprocal, bidirectional right-brain-to-right-brain communications system of safety and trust. These unconscious right brain communications are initiated in the moment of silence, when they are staring at each other. Music (2023) emphasizes the importance of state shifts toward quieter and less verbal states in which deep relaxation and "just being" can occur. Note that in this shared nonverbal right brain moment when the therapist's left brain is offline and thereby not inhibiting the right, the pull and intensity of her right-lateralized autonomic sympathetic arousal increased. Thus the repression defense of aggression is synchronously lifted in both members of the therapeutic dyad. Unconscious emotion from a primitive presymbolic sensorimotor level of an autonomic physiological pull is elevated to a mature symbolic representational level and a conscious recognition of a repressed agentic self-state that occurs in the joint reenactment of insecure attachment dynamics. When this occurs, the countertransferential bodily-based pull and the resistance to the pull disappears.

Synchronized mutual regressions that transiently release left hemispheric inhibition of strong right hemispheric affect thus promote a coming into consciousness of repressed emotion, in this case anger. These enactments act as a regulatory mechanism in expanding the patient's affect tolerance for adaptive assertive anger. The creative mutual regression thus generates a progression of the treatment, a new beginning. This includes not only a new, more fundamental level of understanding but also a coming into being in the therapeutic relationship. Carl Rogers (1954) defined creativity as "the emergence of a relational product" that allows for discovering new forms of human relationship. The therapist's interpersonal creativity relationally catalyzed unconscious, undeveloped repressed aspects of the patient's self to come into being. According to T. W. Downey (2001), "Therapeutic change is analogous to developmental change in that both involve the *crucial presence of another to release energies* [emphasis added]. In therapeutic change these are energies that have been repressed beyond the reach of developmental dynamics" (p. 56).

In this case vignette, the more fluid "reversible dominance" of the hemispheres allowed both Sands's and her patient's energy-expending left hemisphere to reduce its active inhibition of the energy-conserving right hemisphere, thereby increasing right brain emotional energy to be used for creativity. Neuroscience mirrors the common intuitive notion that repression inhibits creativity. Indeed, in repression the path from right to left hemisphere is blocked (Basch, 1983), while the illumination stage of creativity represents "a sudden, temporary increase above normal in the flow of information from right to left" (Kane, 2004). These data support the clinical propositions that creativity is shaped by activities of the preconscious and that regulated mutual regressions impact repression dynamics. I suggest that the "major shift in the therapy" in Sands's case of vulnerable narcissism represents the moment of a transformation of an insecure anxious preoccupied attachment into not only an emergent earned secure attachment (Phelkos et al., 1998) but a new expansion of the right brain. This therapeutic change alters the balance of the two prefrontal systems and reduces the characterological overactivation of the left mind in maladaptive repression, allowing more access to the adaptive functions of the patient's right mind.

Weinberg (2024) discusses recent advances in our understanding of the possibility of change in both types of hemispherically asymmetrical narcissistic personality disorders. Citing longitudinal studies, he concludes,

> The facet of hypersensitivity, that includes such characteristics as resentment, depletion, sense of entitlement, and roughly corresponds to vulnerable narcissism, continues to improve throughout the person's life, while the facet of willfulness that includes external grandiosity and exhibitionism and roughly corresponds to grandiose narcissism, improves until middle age and tends to plateau thereafter (Cramer, 2017; Edelstein et al., 2012). Taken together these studies show that pathological narcissism is associated with a slow pace of change and

that compared to vulnerable narcissism traits, traits associated with grandiose narcissism are more persistent.

Weinberg concludes that we are now in a new era in the treatment of narcissistic disorders, mentioning new directions, including a common-factor approach to therapy (Wampold & Imel, 2015) and a transactional perspective that is grounded in a good patient-therapist match (Kantrowitz et al., 1989). This synchrony allows for the coconstruction of a therapeutic alliance that enhances the patient's and therapist's ability to work together, especially in enactments jointly cocreated by both members of the therapeutic dyad (Bromberg, 1992). To these new directions in understanding and treating narcissistic personalities I would add recent information about hemispheric asymmetry, the defense of repression, interpersonal synchrony, and the change mechanisms in the right brain, as well as a return to the psychoanalytic unconscious of Freud, Winnicott, Kohut, and Kernberg.

Chapter 6

Therapeutic Synchronized Mutual Regressions and the Rebalancing of the Hemispheres

As I have discussed in previous chapters, psychodynamic psychotherapy focuses upon bringing repressed unconscious affects such as shame and aggression into awareness. In emotionally focused psychotherapy, the interpersonal neurobiological mechanism of a mutually synchronized and interactively regulated right-brain-to-right-brain communication system underlies a relational amplification of a state of consciousness, especially at moments when an unconscious affect comes into awareness. This "dyadic expansion of consciousness" (Tronick et al., 1998) increases and sustains the affect in time. The unconscious affect is synchronously held within the dynamic energized intersubjective field long enough to reach conscious awareness in both members of a resonating psychobiologically attuned dyad, and thereby shared between their right brains. The importance of this coupling of two emotional right brains is stressed by Whitehead:

> Every time we make therapeutic contact with our patients we are engaging profound processes that tap into essential life forces in our selves and in those we work with. . . . *Emotions are deepened in the intensity and sustained in time when they are intersubjectively shared. This occurs at moments of deep contact* [emphasis added]. (2006, p. 624)

Carl Rogers (1957) proposed that therapeutic change occurs in moments of "psychological contact," when the therapist is in a "highly altered state of consciousness" (note the left-right hemispheric shift). In these moments, both he and the patient are in a special condition of receptivity to each other, outside of conscious awareness. Alluding to a context of nonverbal communication and interpersonal synchrony, he observes, "The feelings the therapist is experiencing are available to him, available to his awareness, and he is able to live these feelings, be them, and able to *communicate* them," so that there is a *"close matching* between what is experienced at a gut level, what is present in awareness, and what is expressed to the client" (Rogers, 1958). He states that as a result of this psychological contact, "Simply my presence is releasing and available. . . . At those moments . . . our relationship transcends itself and becomes something larger" (Rogers, 1989). This expansion is echoed by Leslie Greenberg (2014): "The experience of therapeutic presence involves (a) being in contact with one's integrated and healthy self, while (b) being open and receptive, to what is poignant in the moment and immersed in it, (c) with a larger sense of spaciousness and expansion of awareness and perception."

I suggest that, in line with the principle that emotion acts as an "analog amplifier" that extends the duration of whatever activates it, the clinician's resonance with the patient's preconscious affect state allows for an energetic increase in the intensity of an unconscious positive or negative affect coming into consciousness, expanded into awareness in both patient and therapist. In heightened affective moments when such synchronized preconscious affects just beneath the surface of consciousness are interactively regulated, dyadically resonated, amplified, and held in short-term implicit procedural working memory long enough to be felt and recognized, they can come into awareness and shape the subsequent conscious processing of an emotional stimulus.

The key to transforming a repressed dysregulated unconscious affect into a conscious affect is implicit right-brain-to-right-brain affect communication, the intersubjective sharing of experienced affect, and interactive regulation. Research now shows that "subliminal" (Jostmann et al., 2005) or "intuitive" (Koole & Jostmann, 2004) implicit regulation of negative affects is highly sensitive to context, is nonrepressive—because unlike defensive repression it does not interfere with automatic vigilance for negative affect—and is incorporated into an accessible subjective self.

Other authors report, "Mere verbalization of unpleasant circumstances without experiencing concomitant emotions constitutes defensive rather than integrative coping," and "emotion regulation supported by the right prefrontal cortex is integrative rather than defensive and unconscious rather than conscious" (Kuhl et al., 2015).

Psychodynamic therapy attempts not control but the acceptance or facilitation of particular emotions, including defensively avoided repressed emotions in order to allow the patient to tolerate and transform them into adaptive emotions. Due to increasing feelings of safety and trust, the right brain is strengthened and the left brain false self is weakened. In repeated left-to-right synchronized and regulated regressions, the patient enters more fluidly into a right brain state of receptivity and is thereby open to right brain emotional contact with the therapist. According to Rotenberg (1993), the creative right hemisphere is open to real-life occurrences, as opposed to the left hemisphere that constructs logical structures that are shut off from the outside world. Over the course of the therapy the patient is implicitly learning how to tolerate reducing defenses to negative and positive affect, and how to be more open to his own and others' affective experience.

Furthermore, repeated left-to-right therapeutic mutual regressions that access right brain states of openness to experience allow for a more permeable boundary between the patient's preconscious and deeper repressed unconscious system (see Figure 2.3). This change mechanism, an emergent function of the expanding therapeutic alliance, allows for more direct work with the unblocking of repression, that is, a more fluid and sudden access into consciousness of right frontal "Aha!" moments of emotional as opposed to cognitive insight, as we saw in the Sands (1997) case. In that clinical vignette, note the emotionally marked moment when what was defensively unconscious became conscious in a moment of right brain "Aha!" self-recognition.

McGilchrist (2021a) observes, "Insight, the ability to see suddenly to the core of a problem when it is not obvious, and resolve it, is a process often accompanied by an 'Aha' moment." Domash (2010) describes "sudden bursts" of insight in "Aha!" or "eureka" therapeutic moments:

> From a neuroscience point of view, the emotional 'Aha' is in part a right brain phenomenon, the intuitive spontaneous, emotional, and

imagistic aspect of mind that allows us to access our unconscious, that is, to bypass rational thought and in an instant surprise ourselves with a new or different idea. (p. 316)

I suggest that these subjective positively valenced "Aha!" moments are accompanied by the affect of surprise and are fueled by sudden high levels of dopamine.

In this creative work, the therapist's synchronized and therefore well-timed left-right callosal regression is critical. With respect to regressions, Kane (2004) states that the shift in hemispheric dominance in a creative moment of a regression in the service of the ego involves a callosal disinhibition, "a sudden and transient loss or decrease of normal inter-hemispheric communication, removing inhibitions placed upon the right hemisphere." This horizontal shift allows access to right-lateralized vertical cortical-subcortical circuits. McGilchrist (2021a) cites evidence showing that "moments of insight are robustly associated with activity in the right amygdala, an ancient structure involved in emotional reactions" (p. 176). Giovacchini (1991) describes the creative process as "a broad range of functioning [that] traverses various levels of the psyche, frequently reaching down to the very earliest, primary process-oriented parts of the self. Ego boundaries, in turn, can become quite fluid and permeable, even though they are ordinarily firmly established and well structured" (p. 187).

Schiepek and his colleagues (2014) conclude that stable boundaries

. . . result from consistent experiences, in particular stable relationships and attachment to important others. . . . A stable relationship between client and therapist yields the solid boundary conditions, which in turn allow for a destabilization . . . as well as restabilization process. . . . Those patients who experience at least one instability and a constantly positive atmosphere reached the best psychotherapy outcome. (p. 7)

Domash (2010) observes,

We . . . need to be both "neat" with well-differentiated boundaries and a strong sense of self and also "sloppy" in order to tolerate relaxation of boundaries, sudden surprises, playfulness, ambiguity, uncertainty, and paradox—all at the same time. These are the ingredients of unconscious freedom. (p. 320)

In terms of hemispheric asymmetry, these clinical data are describing a more balanced interaction between the conscious left and unconscious right hemispheres. Neuroscientists assert,
.

> A balance model has been proposed between the left and right cerebral hemispheres. . . . The two hemispheres exist in a reciprocally balanced relationship, with each hemisphere opposing and complimenting the other. Thus, increased activation in a hemispheric region will result in decreased activation in the homologous other. (Foster et al., 2008, p. 2846)

That said, a central theme of McGilchrist's (2009) *The Master and His Emissary* is that at this point in time the hemispheres are out of balance: The left hemisphere is increasingly dominating Western civilization, right hemisphere empathy is reducing, and the integration of the hemispheres is being devalued. These disturbing data reinforce the importance of the psychotherapeutic alteration of maladaptive left hemispheric defensive repression of right brain states as a source of the rebalancing of the two hemispheres.

Creative Mutual Regressions and the Adaptive Rebalancing of the Right and Left Hemispheres

Over the course of the treatment, synchronized clinical regressions allow for an integration not only within the patient's right hemisphere but also between his or her right hemispheric unconscious and left hemispheric conscious minds. These adaptive creative mutual regressions facilitate structural alterations of the relationships of the hemispheres to each other, including a transformation from excessive left hemispheric rigid repression and inhibition of right hemispheric functions to a more balanced flexible interhemispheric interaction. The focus of therapy with highly asymmetrical repressed personalities is thus on improving right hemispheric attachment deficits and reducing left hemispheric defensive compensation of a false self. Over time, therapeutically lowering repression is associated with a more efficient and creative right brain and a diminution of the left brain grandiose false self.

Thus, the reduction of the patient's defensive rigid repression and the emergence of an adaptive, more flexible repression allow the patient more direct access to the adaptive functions of his or her right brain. This enables the patient to not only initiate but share creative regressions in the service of the ego, which Kris (1952) described as a generator of fantasy, imagination, and the appreciation of wit and humor, and Schafer (1958) associated with advances in interpersonal relations, such as empathy, intimacy, and communication. Rogers (1954) characterized the patient's emergent capacity for "constructive creativity" and an increased ability to play that results from a therapeutic alteration of a rigid repression defense. He suggested this leads to "the creative seeing of life in a new and significant way" (p. 255). Rotenberg (2004) describes the role of the right hemisphere in creativity, "the ability to bring something new into existence": "Ingredients of the creative way of thinking include the following: seeing things in a new way, making connections, taking risks, being alert to chance and to the opportunity presented by contradictions and complexities, and recognizing familiar patterns in the unfamiliar" (p. 3). McGilchrist (2015) contrasts the adaptive functions of the right brain intuitive "creative unconscious" with the left brain analytic conscious mind. He describes this essential role of the right hemisphere in the creative processing of novelty, something new:

For creativity to succeed . . . there needs to be breadth of vision; the capacity to forge distant links; flexibility rather than rigidity; a willingness to respond to a changed or changing context; as well as tolerance of ambiguity and of knowledge that is, at least at the outset, inherently imprecise. This all makes possible *a quest for something that is truly new* [emphasis added] . . . breaking out of the mold of the inauthentic, the stale and the familiar. And all this is terrain better traversed by the right hemisphere than the left. (McGilchrist, 2021a, p. 245)

Note this description also characterizes new expanded relational and emotional contexts of implicit change mechanisms, including those emerging in the self-discovery of deep psychotherapy. According to Marcel Proust, "The real voyage of discovery consists not in seeking new lands but in *seeing with new eyes.*" In each of our lifetime journeys, we are all explorers of the origins of our own human nature, our own unconscious minds, making new discoveries with and about our subjective right brains.

On a clinical level, in long-term psychotherapy, the therapeutic transformation of rigid repression into resilient repression can allow for a creative rebalancing of the right and left hemispheres. Mayseless and Shamay-Tsoory (2015) demonstrate that altering the balance between the right and left frontal lobes can modulate creative production. Therapeutically reducing left frontal and enhancing right frontal activity lessens left brain cognitive control, thereby increasing access to right brain creativity. This therapeutic callosal growth enables the patient to have more direct access to the adaptive functions of both cerebral hemispheres.

According to McGilchrist (2009), the right and left hemispheres create coherent, utterly different, and often incompatible versions of the world with competing priorities and values. He refers to

> . . . two ways of being in the world, both of which are essential. One was to allow things to be present to us in all their embodied particularity, with all their changeability and impermanence, and their *interconnectedness*, as part of a whole which is forever in flux. . . . We feel *connected* [emphasis added] to what we experience, part of the whole, not confined in subjective isolation from a world that is viewed as objective. The other was to step outside the flow of experience and "experience" our experience in a special way; to represent the world in a form that is less truthful, but apparently clearer, and therefore cast in a form which is more useful for manipulation of the world and another. (p. 93)

Earlier I cited Spence and Helmreich's (1978) seminal studies on two basic human motivational systems, communal and agentic. Mirroring and expanding that work, Kuhl and Kazen (2008) characterized these two different basic systems in humans, which they termed affiliation and power, describing a basic link between affiliation and right hemispheric processing and power and left hemispheric processing. Their laterality research documents that affiliation-related stimuli are associated with the left visual field and right hemispheric processing, while power-related stimuli are associated with the right visual field and left hemispheric processing. The right hemispheric affiliation system is associated with a holistic and intuitive cognitive style and is involved in intimacy and affective sharing in close relationships. On the other hand, left hemispheric power motivation accesses linear thinking and generates instrumental planning and a social hierarchy. With respect to other examples of the right lateralized affiliation system, these authors cite my right hemisphere work on empathy, affective communication, and attachment (Schore, 2001a).

In a follow-up fMRI study of power versus affiliation social motivation, this group reported that viewing a movie clip of a power scene, a conversation between a dominant Mafia boss and his subordinate in *The Godfather*, was linked with neural activity in the left hemisphere, while watching an affiliation scene, a nostalgic, intimate moment of romance and love in *Sleepless in Seattle*, was associated with increased activity in the right hemisphere (Quirin, Meyer, et al., 2013). In subsequent EEG research, they described affiliation as a basic human need that is evolutionarily rooted in parental care and social development and is located in the right prefrontal cortex, namely the right orbitofrontal (ventromedial) cortex (Quirin, Gruber, et al., 2013). Recall in the introduction I cited the *OED*'s definition of affiliation as "connection." The right-brain-to-right-brain process of interpersonal synchrony that is associated with intimacy and emotional connection has been shown to increase affiliation (Hove & Risen, 2009), as well as compassion (Valdesolo & Desteno, 2011), rapport (Miles et al., 2009), and altruism (Morishima et al., 2012). Like affiliation, interbrain synchrony is associated with social closeness (Dikker et al., 2021).

Consonant with this characterization of the dual hemispheres, Hecht (2014) cited a large body of brain laterality studies indicating that the right hemisphere mediates affiliation motivation, being closely connected with and accepted by other people, as opposed to left hemisphere power motivation, the need to maintain individuality, independence, and autonomy. He asserts, "Ideally, these two coexisting needs—for affiliation and power— would complement and balance each other. Nevertheless, oftentimes they are in conflict and lead to opposite directions." Hecht concludes that the challenge for humans is the conflict between "the longing for intimacy and closeness with significant others and the desire for some privacy and occasional solitude."

In the elegant words of the poet Rainer Maria Rilke,

For one human being to love another, that is perhaps the most difficult of all our tasks, the ultimate, the last test and proof, the work for
which all other is but preparation. I hold this to be the highest task
for a bond between two people: that each protects the solitude of the
other. (p. 3)

In these precious moments we can enjoy the unique experiences of being
alone, where we can let loose our imagination. From my point of view,
the current U.S. culture overlooks and devalues the precious, adaptive
functions of the self generated by privacy. As I have previously written,
individual cultures, at an unconscious level, shape not only the degree of
repression but the balance of right brain affiliation and left brain power
motivations in both genders (Schore, 2019b). I further suggest that at this
point in time in the United States, left hemisphere power motivation has
increased in both male and female genders.

Long-term psychotherapeutic work with the emergence of dissociated
self-states into consciousness can thus restructure the right hemisphere,
while lifting rigid, maladaptive repression of the dynamic unconscious
can creatively rebalance the right and left hemispheres. The therapeutic
rebalancing of the explicit, conscious objective self with the implicit, unconscious subjective self allows for a more harmonious relationship, yet one
that can also process the intrinsic tensions and conflicts between left hemispheric autonomy functions and right hemispheric interpersonal functions.
McGilchrist (2021a, p. 278) observes, "there is more 'decoupling' and
independence of the hemispheres in creative individuals. . . . Decreased
interconnectivity enhances hemispheric specialization, which in turn benefits the incubation of ideas that are critical for flexibility, divergent thinking and originality." This balanced hemisphericity structurally underlies
a unified sense of self that can fluidly access both the left brain conscious
self and the right brain unconscious self.

And yet within this dual system the left hemisphere acts as the "conceptual self" while the right hemisphere represents the "integrated self"
(Kuhl et al., 2015). According to Kuhl and his colleagues (2015), the conceptual self, which generates a conscious self-concept, "is mediated by
analytic thought and reasoning processes that are explicitly encoded in
language. . . . *The conceptual self has no direct access to the person's emotional functioning and somatic states* [emphasis added]" (p. 118). That said,

they observe, "In today's ego driven media society, the conceptual self is often celebrated more than the integrative self" (p. 126).

In contrast, the right-lateralized integrative self, grounded in perception and automatic behavior, has extensive connections with implicit emotion. Functionally, it "integrates a large number of the person's self aspects simultaneously" and accesses holistic feelings and intuition that implicitly guide the individual's preferences and behavior. These authors assert, "Whereas the narrow focus of analytic thinking may be confined to one emotion, the holistic feelings of the integrated self are full of emotional and somatic overtones ('emotional landscapes')" (Kuhl et al., 2015). They conclude that although parts of the integrated self can be made conscious, they are never fully conscious and can never be fully articulated.

Citing a large amount of laterality data, they show that "the integrated self is supported by parallel-distributed processing in the right anterior cortex," and its adaptive preconscious functions are specifically expressed in "emotional connectedness, broad vigilance, utilization of felt feedback, unconscious processing, integration of negative experiences, extended resilience, and extended trust" (Kuhl et al., 2015, p. 115). They conclude, in healthy personalities the unconscious, intuitive right integrative self and the conscious, analytic left conceptual self are continually interacting. I suggest that this interaction involves a bidirectional communication between the left prefrontal and the right prefrontal cortex.

Bromberg (1979) postulated that therapeutic regressions represent "a fundamental component of psychoanalysis" that act as "the royal road to new growth." He posited that "the ego (or self), in order to grow, must voluntarily allow itself to become less than intact—to regress. Empirically this is one way of defining regression in the service of the ego" (p. 653). He concluded,

> The deeper the regression that can be safely allowed by the patient, the richer the experience and the greater its reverberation on the total organization of the self. . . . For the deepest analytic growth to occur, the new experience must require that the existing pattern of self representation reorganizes in order to make room for it. (p. 654)

Bromberg asserted that regression in therapy is a naturally occurring process, if not impeded by too much interaction on the therapist's part. In the working-through stage of the treatment, this growth occurs in therapeutic regressions into the patient's deep unconscious, what Jung called the shadow self, that part of our psyche which contains our darkest fantasies, negative emotions, and desires. This entrance into the deep recesses of the human psyche occurs in an intrahemispheric structural regression, a vertical hierarchical state switch from the higher to lower levels of the right brain unconscious (see Figure 2.3).

With respect to the central theme of this book, regressions shed direct light upon the essential dynamic functions of the hidden levels of the unconscious mind. Freud (1900/1953) demonstrated that these essential unconscious functions are fundamentally involved in the deeper aspects of the human experience, and Darwin (1859/1958, 1872/1965) showed the central role of human emotion in the evolutionary origins of human nature. According to Heinz Kohut (1971), the creator of psychoanalytic self-psychology and promoter of psychotherapeutic empathy, "The deeper layers of the analyst's psyche are open to the stimuli which emanate from the patient's communications while the intellectual activities of the higher levels of cognition are temporarily largely but selectively suspended" (p. 274).

Recall my assertion in the introduction that relational psychoanalysis is a major contributor to our understanding of the depths of human nature and the deeper strata of the unconscious right mind. Citing my right brain work, Rayna Markin discusses the importance of "session depth":

> Relational therapists and their clients dive into deep waters and as a result the therapeutic process is not a shallow one. The establishment of a personal relationship in which nonverbal messages are heard and voiced in an immediate, experience-near manner is likely to engender a powerful session. Interventions that are evocative, emotionally intense, that establish an internal focus for change . . . facilitate session depth. (2014, p. 331)

In plumbing the depths of the patient's psyche, the therapist is not staying up in the left hemisphere interpreting (left brain to right brain), but rather participating in a synchronized perceptual-imagistic mutual structural regression into the deeper strata of the right, where the patient and therapist are traveling on Freud's unconscious "royal road" together (right brain to right brain). Over time, the loosening of the rigid defensive repressive top-down left hemispheric control of the conscious self over the right hemisphere unconscious self and the subsequent rebalancing of the hemispheres allows for a flexible interaction between the hemispheres but also the further development of a more complex right brain. McGilchrist (2015) observes that "the right hemisphere exhibits a more tentative and self-depreciating style, whereas the left hemisphere is confident about matters of which it is ignorant, and overestimates its capacities," clearly alluding to the left hemispheric grandiose false self. Thus, therapeutically lowering repression is associated with a more efficient right brain and a reduction of the left brain grandiose false self.

The Loosening of Rigid Repression and Growth of the Right Brain in Therapy and Later Human Development

Recall McGilchrist's (2009) description in Chapter 2 of an adaptive right-left-right sequence in Figure 2.1, in which the right hemisphere underwrites our experience of the world that the left unpacks and processes before returning it to the right, which reintegrates it into the wider picture. With a less rigid repression defense, this more flexible hemispheric interaction now allows for a holistic experience of the right brain, followed by a logical examination and categorization by the left, and then a return to the right for a final, more complex synthesis and abstract analysis and an integrated and transformed whole, a bihemispheric whole person. This now allows for an emergent function, where the rationality of the left hemisphere is subject to the broader contextualizing influence of the more emotionally complex right hemisphere.

As I have written in *Right Brain Psychotherapy*, over the course of long-term treatment, the more the patient in day-to-day life uses topographical regressions that horizontally shift left into right brain–dominant relational and emotional functions, the more he or she accesses synchronized mutual regressions to activate moments of shared, intimate deep contact with emotionally salient close others, the more the characterological highly repressed affect-blocking defense is reduced (Schore, 2019b). In the evolving psychotherapeutic relationship, this move to more flexible hemispheric defenses is expressed in increased subjective safety and trust in both members of the therapeutic dyad. As the collaborative therapeutic alliance strengthens over time, both members nonconsciously increase the use of the word *we* in spontaneous emotionally laden therapeutic conversations. Thus, inter-actively regulated mutual regressions allow for the lessening of both left hemispheric repressive and right hemispheric dissociative defenses.

The essential importance of adaptive bottom-up access of the early-maturing deeper levels of the unconscious core self over the lifespan has been described by Hans Loewald (1949/1980):

> Perhaps the so-called fully developed, mature self is not one that has become fixated at the presumably highest or latest stage of development, having left the others behind it, but is a self that integrates its reality in such a way that the earlier and deeper levels of self integration become alive as dynamic sources of higher organization. (p. 20)

This adaptive capacity allows an efficient right brain to flexibly cope with the successive emotional and social challenges to the unconsciously inte-grated self over different life stages, within changing cultural and social environments. I suggest that this interpersonal neurobiological mechanism underlies Jordan's assertion that "people grow through and toward rela-tionship throughout the lifespan" (2000, p. 1007).

Recall my assertion in Chapter 1 that the enduring legacy of a secure attachment is an efficient right brain that can implicitly regulate and inte-grate positive and negative emotional experiences and thereby cope with the novelty and stress that is inherent in all human interactions. These individ-uals have the capacity to subjectively experience complex mixed emotions in their close relationships, two oppositely valenced emotions, such as an amalgam of love and hate, or bittersweet emotions in which they simul-taneously feel a negative state of loss and sadness and a positive state of pleasure (Berrios et al., 2015), or when they are listening to sad music that induces a pleasurable feeling (Mori & Iwanaga, 2014; Sachs et al., 2015).

Earlier I cited Maunder and Hunter's (2009) description of a resil-ient, collaborative secure attachment in human adulthood: "A person with secure attachment has developed sufficient self-confidence and confidence in the value of close relationships to allow flexibility in moving comfort-ably between autonomy and dependence in a way that is realistically and effectively responsive to circumstances." In other words, secure attachment involves a flexible capacity, what Hecht (2014) terms a balance between left hemisphere power, independence, and autonomy and right hemisphere affiliation, dependence, and connection to people in intimate interpersonal relationships.

In discussing therapeutic relationships that promote change in the patient, Podolan and Gelo (2024) offer attachment research on effective clinicians:

> Unlike insecurely attached therapists, secure therapists seem to form stronger alliances, have better outcomes, respond and repair ruptures more empathically, use countertransference more effectively, and are able to intervene with more compassion. As opposed to insecurely attached therapists, secure therapists seem to be more effective in treating clients with personality disorders. . . . Securely attached therapists are also better at exploring the depths of the client's world more thoroughly and making narrative more coherent. (pp. 407–408)

Talia and colleagues show that therapists with a secure attachment use less detaching or coercive and more intersubjective and engaging interventions, such as empathically attuned self-state conjectures and disclosure of their own inner states (Talia et al., 2020).

From an interpersonal neurobiological perspective, regulated intersubjective contexts of long-term psychotherapeutic treatment allow for the evolution of an earned secure attachment in the patient and more complex psychic structure, which in turn can process more complex right brain functions (e.g., intersubjectivity, nonverbal communications, empathy, affect tolerance, stress regulation, and adaptive defenses). The growth-facilitating relational environment of a deeper therapeutic exploration can induce plasticity in both the cortical and subcortical systems of the right brain. This increased connectivity in turn generates more complex development of the right-lateralized biological substrate of the human unconscious, including alterations of the patient's nonconscious insecure internal working model that now encodes more effective coping strategies of implicit affect regulation and thereby expanded resilience and flexibility of the right-lateralized subjective self. Thus internal working models cannot be altered without clinical work on unconscious defenses, including repression.

The therapeutic change of an insecure anxious or insecure avoidant attachment into an earned secure attachment produces a more efficient right brain, and thereby alters the imbalance of the hemispheres by reducing the compensatory overactivation of the left mind, allowing more access to the adaptive functions of the patient's right mind. Clearly alluding to a securely attached right brain, Guntrip (1969) described "a profound sense of belonging, a being at one with his world which is not intellectually thought out but is the persisting atmosphere of security in which he exists within himself." Attachment workers are now defining secure attachment as "flexibly integrated" (George & Aikins, 2023). Kuhl and his colleagues (2015) assert that "the unconscious nature of the *integrated self* implies that self-access may be facilitated when people relinquish conscious control and give the self's unconscious intelligence more room" (p. 123). The coupling of our right brain–integrated self with the people we feel safe with and trust allows our relational unconscious mind to continue to grow over the lifespan.

Evidence that socioemotional functions continue to mature in adulthood is provided by De Pisapia and his colleagues, who reported a neuroimaging study of "interpersonal competence" in healthy male young adults, defined as "the capacity to interact and communicate with others, to share personal views, to understand the emotions and opinions of others, and to cooperate with others or resolve conflict should it occur" (2014, p. 1257). In this clear allusion to secure attachment, these authors documented that an increased level of interpersonal competence is associated with higher white matter integrity in several major tracts of the right hemisphere. They concluded,

> According to this line of research, the development of emotional and social intelligence in the individual—from childhood to adulthood—depends on the quality of their relationship with a principal caregiver and those socioemotional competencies heavily rely on right brain function. The finding may have implications for theories claiming that the right hemisphere plays a major role in modulating emotion and nonverbal communication during the first interpersonal relationship that every human being experiences, namely the infant–mother relationship (Schore, 1997, 2000, 2009a). (De Pisapia et al., 2014, p. 1262)

Recall that in Chapter 1 I discussed the work of Kotikalapudi et al. (2022), who reported that white matter tracts exclusively in the right hemisphere correlate with personality profiles predictive of subjective well-being, a marker of secure attachment.

Supporting these ideas, Hecht (2014) marshals a great deal of neurobiological studies to show that in adults, "the right hemisphere has a relative advantage over the left hemisphere mediating social intelligence—identifying social stimuli, understanding the intentions of other people, awareness of the dynamics in social relationships, and successful handling of social interactions" (p. 1). Indeed, the right hemisphere is dominant for social interactions (Semrud-Clikeman et al., 2011). Affectively oriented psychotherapy that impacts the deep subjective core of the personality, the origin of human nature, allows for expanded social and emotional functions of the patient's right brain. As Weinberg (2000) observes,

> Only the right hemisphere enables one to sustain experiences in their complexity and in interactive and mutually enriching connections between their various components. This ability to represent experiences in a multi-dimensional way generates a *need for new experiences* [emphasis added] in order to further enrich, deepen, and organize them.

This principle also apples to the clinician's right brain. Although the right hemisphere matures earlier than the left, the myelination of the emotional, social right hemisphere remains neuroplastic over the lifespan, and its maturation is completed later than the left (Joseph, 1996). The professional growth of the clinician reflects progressions in right brain relational processes that underlie clinical skills, including affective empathy (Decety & Chaminade, 2003; Schore, 1994/2016), the ability to tolerate and interactively regulate a broader array of negative and positive affective self-states (Schore, 2003b, 2012), implicit openness to experience (DeYoung et al., 2012), clinical intuition (Marks-Tarlow, 2012; Schore, 2012), and creativity, the production of an idea that is both novel and useful in a particular social setting (Asari et al., 2008; Mihov et al., 2010; Schore, 2012). With respect to the latter, my late colleague James Masterson (1985) concluded that creativity is an essential function of "the real self," where it is used specifically "to change old familiar patterns into new, unique, and different patterns."

These right brain functions become more complex with clinical experience, and they directly impact how we get better at the art of psychotherapy. This laterality research directly addresses the large body of research on the critical role of "common factors" (Wampold, 2015; Hess, 2019) in psychotherapy, and the skills of effective therapists associated with successful treatment outcomes. These common factors underscore the universality of the emotional bond between the patient and therapist, and the generalizability of the psychodynamic concept of the working alliance across all forms of treatment. I will speak more of these common factors as right brain skills in Chapter 8, where I use interpersonal neurobiology to address the fundamental questions, how and why are some therapists better than others (Castonguay & Hill, 2017), and how does nonverbal communication improve clinical outcomes across different treatment models (Priebe et al., 2019)?

Indeed, the psychotherapist's interpersonal and emotional skills that facilitate the patient's symptomatic improvement and emotional growth are clinically expressed in the therapeutic alliance. In an array of spontaneous, improvised, emotionally laden therapeutic conversations, collaborative interactions, rupture and repair transactions, and shared heightened affective moments within the alliance, the empathic therapist accesses a storehouse of affective and social experiences gained over the course of his or her career. An emotional and relational perspective of the development of professional expertise dictates that the continually evolving psychotherapist frequently reflects upon the subjective experiences of being with different types of patients, including not only the patients' unique personalities, but also his or her own conscious and especially unconscious intersubjective coparticipation in the therapeutic process. In various right-brain-to-right-brain synchronized mutual regressions, the therapist interacts and collaborates with the patient's unconscious psyche, leaving a unique implicit personalized emotional signature, just as the patient's unconscious penetrates the clinician's psyche and leaves its unique imprint (Benedetti, 1987).

A central construct of Freud's theory is the term *neurotic*, which refers to a conflict between internal personal wishes and external social expectations, a "superego conflict." Recall that repression is the disavowal of psychic conflict. In long-term depth psychotherapy that alters the repression defense, regulated mutual regressions promote "bearable intrapsychic conflict" in the patient between the right brain affiliation and left brain power motives, between intimacy and autonomy, what Freud termed the fundamental psychological human conflict between the two fundamental human motivations, love and work. The therapeutic rebalancing of the explicit, conscious objective self with the implicit, unconscious subjective integrative self allows for a more harmonious relationship, yet one that can also process the intrinsic tensions and conflicts between left hemispheric independence functions and right hemispheric interpersonal functions. This developmental advance is expressed in a more complex capacity for tolerating conflict between the dual modes of self-regulation, autoregulation in autonomous contexts, and interactive regulation in interconnected contexts.

In *Right Brain Psychotherapy*, I proposed that mutually regulated synchronized regressions enhance the patient's creative approaches to conflicts (Schore, 2019b). Neurobiologically, these conflicts represent the different complementary but also incompatible perspectives and motivational systems of the left and right hemispheres. In contrast to the heavily repressed personality's rigid left hemispheric inhibition of right hemispheric functions, deep psychotherapy can facilitate the growth of an adaptive interhemispheric capacity that allows more fluid access to the unique specializations of both hemispheres, including increased tolerance for left hemispheric control and anxiety, and right hemispheric uncertainty, vulnerability, novelty, and creativity. This evidence-based model of psychotherapeutic changes in hemispheric balance suggests that long-term psychotherapy can facilitate the growth of synaptic connections between the right prefrontal and left prefrontal regions. I propose that this right-to-left and left-to-right callosal growth is expressed in synchronized neuroplastic synaptogenesis between the right hemispheric orbital (ventromedial) prefrontal regions of the unconscious emotional brain and the left hemispheric dorsolateral prefrontal regions of the conscious rational brain.

The body of my work suggests that a psychotherapeutic change from imbalanced to rebalanced hemispheres can allow for a more effective social and emotional right brain, and thereby an adaptive capacity to cocreate close intersubjective pair bonds in enduring long-term intimate relationships of shared safety and trust. In such relationships, right brain mutual regressions within a synchronized reciprocal loving relationship can, over time, lead to a continuing rebalancing of the hemispheres. Recall that in Chapter 1 I suggested physiological interpersonal synchrony is associated with lowering testosterone in married men, especially those in committed romantic relationships—another example of the potential rebalancing of the left hemisphere power and right hemisphere affiliation motivation as a man becomes a husband and a father.

Chapter 7

The Fundamental Role of the Right Brain in Human Intersubjectivity, Play, and Mutual Love

Throughout these chapters I have been elaborating a psychobiological model of intersubjectivity, the nonverbal communication between two human minds. At the end of the last century, my late colleague Colwyn Trevarthen (1993) presented his groundbreaking neurobiological explorations of the origins of human intersubjectivity. In the subsequent three decades, his ongoing studies continued to confirm, elaborate, and expand upon these pioneering efforts and to make an enduring contribution to our understanding of early human development. Anchored in what has now become a large body of studies in developmental neuroscience, the central organizing principle of his work dictates that from the very beginnings of life, the infant is receptive to and aware of the subjective states of others, particularly the primary attachment object, the mother. This adaptive ability of the infant to bidirectionally communicate its affective states is especially activated in moments of dyadic intimate free play.

Trevarthen's seminal work, confirmed by other major developmental researchers, demonstrated that this capacity for primary intersubjectivity specifically emerges at two to three months. At eight weeks, human babies are ready to engage in behavioral turn-taking when they expect social contingency, which consists of predictable back-and-forth interactivity. In such face-to-face, eye-to-eye intersubjective emotional communications, the infant and mother, intently looking at and listening to each other, synchronize and mutually regulate their emotional states. Indeed, during what he refers to as "protoconversations," the emotions of both members of the dyad are expressed and actively perceived and responded to in spontaneous, reciprocal, rhythmic turn-taking interactions (Trevarthen, 1993).

Within this relational context of primary intersubjectivity, the baby, attracted to the mother's voice, face, and hand gestures, replies playfully, with affection, imitating and provoking imitations. In the same moment, the mother attentively watches and listens, anticipating the baby's expressions intuitively, and sympathetically replies to the infant's communications with emotional facial expression, prosodic motherese, and emotional touch. Thus, in this protoconversation of synchronized and coordinated visual-facial, auditory, and tactile emotional signals, the mother–infant dyad cocreates an intersubjective reciprocal system of *nonverbal communication* (see Figure 7.1). Trevarthen concluded, "The

FIGURE 7.1
Lateral view of channels of face-to-face
communication in primary intersubjectivity

Protoconversation is mediated by synchronized, intersubjective eye-to-eye orientations, vocalizations, hand gestures, and movements of the arms and head, all acting in coordination to express emotions and interpersonal awareness.

Kenneth J. Aitken and Colwyn Trevarthen, "Self/other organization in human psychological development," Development and Psychopathology, volume 9, issue 4, pages 653–677, 1997 © Cambridge University Press, reproduced with permission.

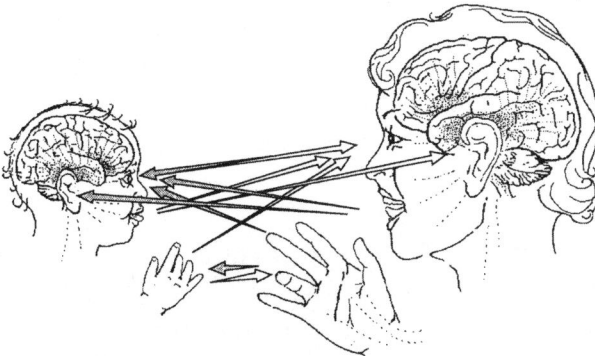

emotions constitute a time-space field of intrinsic brain states of mental and behavioral vitality that are signaled for *communication* [emphasis added] to other subjects and that are open to immediate influence from the signals of these others" (1993, p. 155).

Trevarthen observed that this synchronized two-way traffic of reciprocal nonverbal signals elicits instant emotional effects, namely the positive affects of joyful pleasure and excitement that build within the emotion-transacting protoconversation. But his synchronization model also focused on internal structure-function events. As he stated, "The intrinsic regulators of human brain growth in a child are specifically adapted to be coupled, by emotional communication, to the regulators of adult brains" (Trevarthen, 1990, p. 357). These regulated intersubjective interactions permit the intercoordination of positive affective brain states within the emotionally communicating dyad. His work underscored the fundamental principle that not only is the baby's brain affected by these relational emotional transactions, but its growth also literally requires brain-brain interaction in the context of a burgeoning positive affective relationship between the mother and her infant. This fundamental interactive mechanism requires older brains to engage with mental states of awareness, emotion, and interest in younger brains, and involves a coordination between the subjective feelings of an adult and the intersubjective motivations of the infant to forge an emotional bond with the mother.

Trevarthen emphasized the critical role of interpersonal resonance in these intersubjective communications:

> Corresponding generative parameters in . . . two subjects enable them to *resonate* with or reflect on one another as minds in expressive bodies. This action pattern can become "*entrained*," and their experiences can be brought into register and imitated. These are the features that make possible the kind of *affectionate* [emphasis added] empathic communication that occurs, for instance, between young infants and their mothers. (1993, p. 126)

Furthermore, he stated, "Adaptation of a given brain to a particular social world depends . . . on a motivated search by the young for certain target experiences (as in) expressing mental or motivational states to others, and getting into contact with their mental states" (Trevarthen, 1990, p. 335). In this dyadic state of interpersonal resonance, the infant is "able to exhibit to others at least the *rudiments of individual consciousness and intentionality* [emphasis added]" (Trevarthen & Aitken, 2001, p. 5). Thus this two-person interpersonal context of primary intersubjectivity also serves as a developmental origin of not only subjectivity but self-consciousness, the primordial consciousness of the subjective self.

In parts of this chapter, which I first published in 2021 in the journal *Frontiers in Psychology*, the largest and most-cited psychology journal in the world, I offer an interpersonal neurobiological model of Trevarthen's intersubjective protoconversations between the mother and her two- to three-month-old preverbal infant. Other parts of this chapter were published in 2017 in an interview I did with the *American Journal of Play*, where I'm on the editorial board (Schore, 2017b). In the upcoming sections I describe an operational definition of intersubjectivity as rapid, reciprocal, bidirectional right-brain-to-right-brain visual-facial, auditory-prosodic, and tactile-gestural positively valenced nonverbal communications between the mother and her developing infant. Expanding this model, I then discuss the fundamental role of interpersonal synchrony in intersubjective proto-conversations, as well as how these right-lateralized emotional transmissions generate bioenergetic positively charged interbrain synchrony within the dyad. Toward that end, I present recent brain laterality research on the essential functions of the right temporoparietal junction, a central node of the social brain, in face-to-face intersubjective nonverbal communications between two minds.

In a later section of this chapter, I offer an interpersonal neurobiological model of the continued development of right brain intersubjectivity in the second year and beyond, and the relational origins of the highly adaptive functions of mutual play and mutual love. Next, I offer thoughts on the clinical applications of Trevarthen's intersubjective positively valenced protoconversations in a reciprocal, bidirectional right-brain-to-right-brain nonverbal emotional communication system embedded in the coconstructed therapeutic relationship. I end by presenting ideas on the relationship between the affect-communicating functions of the intersubjective motivational system and the affect-regulating functions of the attachment motivational system.

Regulation Theory Models Intersubjectivity as Right-Lateralized Nonverbal Emotional Communications

There is now broad consensus that intersubjectivity exists only in the human species, and that it defines our human nature (Bjorklund, 2020; Moll et al., 2021). In my own studies on the early development of intersubjective nonverbal emotional communication, I have utilized the interdisciplinary perspectives of interpersonal neurobiology and regulation theory, a theory of the development, psychopathogenesis, and treatment of the subjective self (Schore, 1994/2016, 2003a, 2003b, 2012, 2019a, 2019b). The central focus of this psychoneurobiological model of human development is to more deeply understand the underlying mechanisms by which the structure and function of the mind and brain are shaped by experiences, especially those embedded in emotional relationships, as well as the relational mechanisms by which communicating brains synchronize and align their neural activities with other brains. With respect to this nonverbal communication between brains, I have drawn upon the overlap of Trevarthen's work on intersubjectivity and Bowlby's on attachment theory. Although the former focused on emotion-transacting events early in the first year and the latter on emotional events late in the first and second years, both offered a similar model of nonverbal visual-facial, auditory-prosodic, and tactile-gestural communications between mother and infant.

In a mirror image of Trevarthen's two-way traffic of emotional facial expressions, gestures, and vocal expressions, Bowlby proposed that mother–infant attachment communications are "accompanied by the strongest of feelings and emotions, and occur within a context of facial expression, posture, and tone of voice" (1969, p. 120). Interestingly, unlike Bowlby's, Trevarthen's neuroscience research was directly informed by extensive studies of developmental brain laterality (see Trevarthen, 1996, "Lateral Asymmetries in Infancy: Implications for the Development of the Hemispheres"). Indeed, in that publication he noted that the prosody of the voice of the mother is responded to by the infant's right hemisphere. He also concluded that "the right hemisphere is more advanced than the left in surface features from about the 25th (gestational) week and this advance persists until the left hemisphere shows a post-natal growth spurt starting in the second year" (Trevarthen, 1996, p. 582). His work on brain laterality was heavily influenced by his split-brain research in the lab of Roger Sperry.

Following these valuable leads, in my first book, *Affect Regulation and the Origin of the Self* (Schore, 1994/2016), I drew upon a large body of research on brain laterality and hemispheric asymmetries of structure and function to describe the intersubjective protoconversation as a right-lateralized, reciprocal, nonverbal emotion communication system. Toward that end, I cited a large number of extant researchers who offered evidence on the early development of the right hemisphere and concluded that the essential adaptive capacity of intersubjectivity is specifically impacted by the infant's early social experiences. Since these social interactions occur in a critical period of right brain growth, the child is using the output of the mother's right cortex as a template for the imprinting, the hard wiring of circuits in his own developing right cortex that will come to mediate his expanding socioemotional capacities to appraise variations in both external and internal information.

I further proposed that over the course of human infancy these right-brain-to-right-brain nonverbal affective communications represent a relational context in which the primary caregiver implicitly monitors the infant's affect and psychobiologically attunes to and regulates the child's internal states of central nervous system and autonomic nervous system arousal. Although Trevarthen stressed the role of intersubjectivity in positively charged play states, my work also addresses the nonverbal intersubjective communications of negatively valenced emotional states between the infant's mind/body and the mother's mind/body.

I have suggested that intersubjective mother–infant nonverbal communications directly influence the "early life programming of hemispheric lateralization" (Stevenson et al., 2008) and are a major contributor to the dominance of the right brain in human infancy (Schore, 1994/2016; Chiron et al., 1997). Neuroscientists are now asserting that one measure of healthy development in infants is lateralized behavior (Hall et al., 2008). A large body of laterality research in developmental neuroscience demonstrates the adaptive role of the infant's early-maturing right brain in processing visual-facial, auditory-prosodic, and tactile-gestural nonverbal communications (Schore 1994/2016, 2003a, 2012, 2019a). Recall, over all stages of human development, the perception of faces, voices, and gestures is lateralized in the right hemisphere.

With respect to *visual-facial nonverbal communications*, it is now established that mutual gaze is essential for early social development (Trevarthen

& Aitken, 2001). The development of the capacity to efficiently process information from faces requires visual input to the right (and not left) hemisphere during infancy (Le Grand et al., 2003). At two to three months of age, infants show right hemispheric activation when exposed to a woman's face (Tzourio-Mazoyer et al., 2002). By six months, infants express a right-lateralized left gaze bias when viewing faces (Guo et al., 2009) and significantly greater right frontotemporal activation when viewing their own mother's (as opposed to a stranger's) face (Carlsson et al., 2008). On the other side of the mother–infant dyad, a large body of research indicates that the adult right occipital-temporal cortex generates a rapid holistic face representation at 170 milliseconds after stimulus onset, beneath conscious awareness (e.g., Jacques & Rossion, 2009).

Ongoing developmental neurobiological studies of *auditory-prosodic nonverbal communications* reveal that maternal infant-directed speech ("motherese") activates the right temporal area of four- to six-month-old infants, and that this activation is even greater in seven- to nine-month-old infants (Naoi et al., 2011). Seven-month-old infants respond to emotional voices in a voice-sensitive region of the right superior temporal sulcus, and happy prosody specifically activates the right inferior frontal cortex (Grossmann et al., 2010). These authors conclude, "The pattern of findings suggests that temporal regions specialize in processing voices very early in development and that, already in infancy, emotions differentially modulate voice processing in the right hemisphere" (Grossmann et al., 2010, p. 852). As to the mother's emotional prosodic participation, recent adult research demonstrates a "right-lateralized unconscious, but not conscious processing of affective environmental sounds" (Schepman et al., 2016, p. 606).

With respect to *tactile-gestural nonverbal communications*, Sieratzki and Woll (1996) describe the effects of touch on the developing right hemisphere and assert that the emotional impact of touch is more direct and immediate if an infant is held to the left side of the body (see studies of "left-sided cradling" and activation of the right hemisphere in mother and infant in Schore, 2012, 2019a). Nagy documents a "lateralized system for neonatal imitation" and concludes, "The early advantage of the right hemisphere in the first few months of life may affect the lateralized appearance of the first imitative gestures" (2006, p. 227). Developmental research demonstrates the essential role of maternal "affective touch" on human infant development in the first year of life (Ferber et al., 2008). This allows the infant and mother to create a system of "touch synchrony" in order to alter vagal tone and cortisol reactivity (Feldman et al., 2010). The dyad thus uses interpersonal touch as a communication system, especially for the communication and regulation of emotional information.

In order to process these intersubjective nonverbal communications, the infant seeks proximity to the mother, not just physical but intersubjective emotional proximity in face-to-face, mind-to-mind, body-to-body communications. During these communications, the sensitive primary caregiver's right brain implicitly (unconsciously) attends to, perceives, recognizes, appraises, and regulates nonverbal expressions of the infant's more-and-more intense states of positive and negative affective arousal. Recall that Lyons-Ruth (1999) characterizes a "two-person unconscious" in the intersubjective dialogue. From an interpersonal neurobiological perspective, intersubjectivity represents a cocreated system of unconscious communications of positive and negative affect between two subjective minds, throughout the lifespan. My ongoing studies in the field of neuropsychoanalysis, the neuroscience of unconscious processes, continues to offer interdisciplinary evidence showing that the right brain, the psychobiological substrate of the human unconscious mind, acts as a relational unconscious that communicates with another relational unconscious (e.g., Schore, 1994/2016, 2003b, 2012, 2019b).

Furthering these ideas, I return to Trevarthen's groundbreaking descriptions of the critical role of infant-mother synchrony in face-to-face proto-conversations. Aitken and Trevarthen (1997) asserted,

> In interaction between a normal infant and a happy and receptive caregiving companion the dual intrinsic motive formation systems of the two subjects are mutually supportive in rhythmic, sympathetic engagements which demonstrate *synchrony and turn-taking* [emphasis added] in utterances and clear flexible emotionally toned phrasing with affect attunement. (p. 667)

These authors documented facial movements, voice, and gesture used by infants in their synchronized engagement with mothers. The timing and organization of playful events between them allows the child to adaptively synchronize their subjective states of mind so that purposes, interests, and feelings are shared intersubjectively. Indeed, interpersonal synchrony is a central construct that lies at the core of Trevarthen's right-brain-to-right-brain intersubjective protoconversation.

In this same time period, parallel studies using simultaneous two-camera videotape recordings of the mother–infant interaction confirmed the centrality of interpersonal synchrony, by Ed Tronick and Berry Brazelton (Tronick et al., 1977), Beatrice Beebe and Dan Stern (Jaffe et al., 2001), and Ruth Feldman (Feldman et al., 1999). These authors documented that nonverbal affective communication via facial expressions and vocalizations underlie maternal–infant interpersonal synchronization. Mother-infant face-to-face communication is studied by "microanalysis," which operates like "a social microscope," identifying "subterranean" rapid communications that are not perceptible in real time (Beebe & Steele, 2013).

As an example, Feldman's laboratory explored moments of "affect synchrony" that occur in dyadic positive affectively charged social play, clearly reflecting Trevarthen's primary intersubjectivity:

> Face-to-face interactions, emerging at approximately 2 months of age, are highly arousing, affect-laden, short interpersonal events that expose infants to high levels of cognitive and social information. To regulate the high positive arousal, mothers and infants . . . synchronize the intensity of their affective behavior within lags of split seconds. (Feldman et al., 1999, p. 223)

Feldman and her colleagues observed that in this infant-leads-mother-infant-leads, mother-follows sequence, affect synchrony affords infants "their first opportunity to practice interpersonal coordination of biological rhythms, to experience the mutual regulation of positive arousal, and to build the lead-lag structure of adult communication" (p. 223). Recall their assertion, "Synchrony in dynamic systems . . . reflects the degree to which interactants integrate into the flow of behavior the ongoing responses of their partner and the changing inputs of the environment" (p. 224).

In 1994, in my first book, *Affect Regulation and the Origin of the Self*, I cited the classic research of Lester, Hoffman, and Brazelton (1985), who asserted that "synchrony develops as a consequence of each partner's learning the rhythmic structure of the other and modifying his or her own behavior to fit that structure" (p. 24). The word *synchrony* derives from the Greek words *syn*, which means the same or common, and *chronos*, which means time, and so synchrony literally means occurring at the same time, in the same moment, simultaneous. Across literatures, the construct of synchrony is tightly associated with psychobiological attunement, affective reciprocal interchange, emotion transmission, physiological linkage, and coregulation, all aspects of an intersubjective protoconversation. In a two-way turn-taking communication system, both individuals align and synchronize a shared direction of affective change and then simultaneously adjust their social attention, stimulation, and accelerating arousal to each other.

This synchronization occurs at different levels, from neural activity, to physiological states such as heartbeat rhythm, to pupil size, to facial expressions and body postures (see Schore, 2019a, for references). Strogatz (2008) emphasizes the essential construct of synchrony across all levels of science: "At the heart of the universe is a steady, insistent beat: the sound of cycles in sync. It pervades nature at every scale from the nucleus to the cosmos." I suggest this also includes its central role in the development of human nature.

A large body of developmental research now documents mother–infant physiological synchrony at three months (Moore & Calkins, 2004), six months (Moore et al., 2009), and 12 months (Ham & Tronick, 2006) of age, a period when the mother–infant nonverbal affective protoconversations become more complex. Feldman's laboratory shows that mother and infant coordinate autonomic heart rhythms in moments of interaction synchrony (Feldman et al., 2011). These studies describe the longitudinal development of the capacity for synchronized intersubjective communications between the mother's mind/body and the infant's developing mind/body, as well as the enduring impact of early emotional communications on the adaptive capacity for intersubjectivity over later stages of human development.

Indeed, mother–child behavioral synchrony is individually stable from infancy through adolescence (Feldman, 2010). Interestingly, in a study of what Feldman now terms "social synchrony" in mother–child dyads, she is calling for a "move from focus on one-brain functioning to understanding how two brains dynamically coordinate during real-life social interactions" (Levy et al., 2017, p. 1036), or in other words, research on interbrain synchronization. Note that interpersonal synchrony refers to a synchronization of subjective states, involuntary behaviors, and physiological rhythms between the minds and bodies of two individuals, while interbrain synchrony refers to an alignment and coupling of brains between two individuals. Over three decades, my work on intersubjective right-brain-to-right-brain nonverbal communication describes the right-lateralized interbrain synchronization embedded in the mother–infant (and therapist–patient) relationship.

Prenatal Precursors of Intersubjectivity and Transition Into Early Postnatal Periods

In my ongoing writings, I continue to offer an interpersonal neurobiological model of the ontogeny of intersubjectivity over the first years of human life (e.g., Schore, 1994/2016, 2012, 2019a, 2019b, 2021a). It is important to note that the early substratum of this adaptive human capacity is laid down before birth, in the preceding prenatal period, and in the mutual regulating relationship between the fetus's and mother's physiological systems across the placenta. In the last trimester of pregnancy, a time of rapid maturation of brain architecture and functional networks (Tau & Peterson, 2010), this dyadic system is centrally involved in the fetal programming of the ANS stress-regulating sympathomedullary and hypothalamic-pituitary-adrenal axes, which are lateralized to the right hemisphere (Wittling, 1997).

Research indicates that in the third trimester, almost 40,000 new synapses are formed every second, and this process continues into early postnatal life (Tau & Peterson, 2010). At this point in development, the paraventricular and ventromedial areas of the hypothalamus are activated in stress regulation and the right insula, a structure within the temporal lobes that is essentially involved in the subjective awareness of inner body feelings and emotionality, as well as the regulatory functions of the central and medial amygdala and their dense connections to the autonomic nervous system, come online (Schore, 2017a).

During this same time frame, developing structures in the fetal brain support a critical period of growth of the rapidly maturing autonomic nervous system, what Jackson (1931) described as "the physiological bottom of the mind." Porges's (2011) work on the polyvagal system offers research evidence documenting that the early-forming, oldest, parasympathetic unmyelinated dorsal nucleus of the vagus, the later-developing catecholaminergic sympathetic nervous system, and the last-developing and newest parasympathetic myelinated ventral vagal system in the nucleus ambiguus are all functioning at the start of the last trimester. Underscoring the laterality of these ANS subsystems, he proposes a right-lateralized circuit of intrapsychic emotion regulation that underlies the functional dominance of the right side of the brain in regulating autonomic function.

Porges further states that the maturation of this "mammalian" ventral vagal system, which acts as an interpersonal social engagement system, continues well into the first year. In discussing "the development of the autonomic nervous system in the human fetus," he concludes, "The unique features of the autonomic nervous system that support mammalian *social behavior* [emphasis added] start to develop during the last trimester of fetal life" (Porges, 2011, p. 126). Well-defined sleep states, which are impacted by the ANS, appear at 32 gestational weeks in the human fetus (Prechtl, 1985; Nijhuis, 2003). The first sensory system to come online in the fetus is the vestibular system which influences fetal movement and receives input from the inner ear (Bradley & Mistretta, 1975; Johnson Chacko et al., 2016). Research indicates that the fetal auditory cortex responds to sound at 28 weeks gestation (Wilkinson & Jiang, 2006), that the fetus perceptually receives social auditory information (e.g., the mother's voice) in the final weeks of gestation, and that this input can be recognized after birth, as newborns prefer their mothers' voices (DeCasper & Fifer, 1980; Lecanue & Schaalt, 1996). Research documents that "exposure of the mother's speech *in utero* during the last week of fetal life, under sleeping 'unconscious conditions' may explain why neonates react to the impact of the maternal voice," and that "new born infants remember sounds, melodies, and rhythmic poems they have been exposed to during fetal life" (Lagercrantz & Changeux, 2009, p. 257).

I suggest that during the last trimester, the fetus's right-lateralized autonomic nervous system is synchronously communicating with the mother's right-lateralized developing autonomic nervous system, and that these dyadic experiences are stored in the fetus's right brain implicit-procedural autobiographical memory. This bidirectional maternal-fetal right-brain-to-right-brain subcortical communication occurs in psychobiological transactions of stress-related hormones such as cortisol and corticotropin-releasing hormone (CRH) across the placenta, and in communications between autonomic areas of the mother's emotional right brain and the fetus's right brain, especially the right medial amygdala, which is in a critical period of growth and has extensive connections with the autonomic nervous system. In my neuropsychoanalytic writings, I have identified the subcortical right amygdala as the deep unconscious mind.

In an essential review article published in *Pediatric Research*, "The Emergence of Human Consciousness: From Fetal to Neonatal Life," Lagercrantz and Changeux (2009) boldly assert,

> A simple definition of consciousness is sensory awareness of the body, the self, and the world. The fetus may be aware of the body, for example by perceiving pain. It reacts to touch, smell, and sound, and shows facial expressions responding to external stimuli. . . . These reactions are probably preprogrammed and have a subcortical nonconscious origin. (p. 255)

Indeed, psychoanalytic authors have proposed that the first experience of physically "being-with" another human occurs in utero, and that this precedes the capacity for being-with another *ex utero*. Over 100 years ago, Otto Rank (1924) asserted that "the real Unconscious consists only in the libidinal relation of the embryo to the womb" (p. 195). In recent writings, Amid (2024) describes this embryonic form of unconscious communication as a primal right-brain-to-right-brain nonverbal mode of emotional communication used in utero. In support of this model, the prenatal psychologist Mott concludes, "If the mother felt emotionally unsupported then this feeling of deficiency, lack of recognition and the failure of looked-for support would be just as specifically felt by the fetus" (quoted in Maret, 2009, p. 17).

Recent research documents that at 24 weeks gestation the fetus is able to perceive painful stimuli, and that facial expressions of pain similar to adults' are seen in preterm infants after 28 weeks gestation (Lagercrantz & Changeux, 2009). Note that human sentience first emerges in the last trimester of the fetal period, and for the rest of the lifespan remains operating at the deepest stratum of the human unconscious mind. In other words, consciousness, a basic human attribute, first begins not at birth but in utero. These early experiences of the developing emotional right brain are imprinted into foundational subcortical fetal circuits of the rapidly developing autonomic nervous system. For more on how these fetal autonomic affective experiences impact later development, see "Early Development of the HPA Axis, Attachment Trauma, and the Emergence of Psychiatric Externalizing Psychopathologies in Adolescence" in Chapter 4 of *The Development of the Unconscious Mind* (Schore, 2019a).

Writing on the first hour outside the womb, the neonatologist Raylene Philips (2013) describes the long-term importance of skin-to-skin contact immediately after birth. Citing my work (Schore, 1994/2016), she suggests that "babies and even fetuses are indeed capable of forming memories that remain in their subconscious for life," suggesting that "the events surrounding birth have the potential to set the stage for patterns of subconscious thought processes and behaviors that persist for a lifetime" (p. 67). In these implicit-procedural body-to-body communications, the infant processes tactile and olfactory stimuli that emanate from the mother's body.

It is now well established that at birth human infants, who have only 1/40 the visual activity of an adult, detect eye contact with the mother and that "*making eye contact is the most powerful mode of establishing a communication link between humans* [emphasis added]" (Farroni et al., 2002, p. 9602). Researchers document that at birth, infants prefer images of a human face, are sensitive to the eyes of a face, and show interest in faces that provide enjoyable eye contact (Lagercrantz & Changeux, 2009). According to these authors,

> Birth may also release an inborn "positive emotion," a "motivation" oriented toward the outside world and in particular toward the mother. . . . This first arousal drives the newborn to spontaneously explore the world. . . . The infant affective display then becomes part of an intercommunication system with the caretaker. . . . As a consequence of affect sharing, emotional contagion is already developed in the newborn. (p. 258)

This eye-to-eye communication represents an expansion of prenatal autonomic communication before birth to postnatal autonomic communication after birth. Research shows that the newborn autonomic nervous system is in a state of transition that continues its further development after birth (Takatani et al., 2018). Basch stated that "the language of mother and infant consists of signals produced by the autonomic, involuntary nervous system in both parties" (1976, p. 766), clearly describing a communication system between two social right brains.

In the ensuing perinatal postpartum stage, after birth the psychobiologically attuned mother and the neonate begin to cocreate face-to-face right-brain-to-right-brain communications that are driven by subcortical face-processing areas in the right-lateralized colliculo-pulvinar-amygdala pathway, which is responsible for the nonconscious perception of emotional signals (Tamietto & de Gelder, 2010). A structural MRI investigation of the brain of the one-month human infant documents that subcortical gray matter regions are rightward asymmetrical. According to Dean et al. (2018), "The amygdala, caudate, hippocampus, putamen, pallidum, insula, thalamus, anterior and cingulate gyrus, and parahippocampal gyrus volumes were larger in the right hemisphere" (p. 10).

In previous writings, I have offered evidence that in this earliest stage of postnatal development, an essential role is played by the central amygdala, with its deep connections to bioaminergic centers that control arousal centers deep in the midbrain and brainstem, including noradrenaline generated in the locus coeruleus, dopamine in the ventral tegmental area, and serotonin in the raphe nucleus. But in addition, the central amygdala also has direct synaptic connections with the sympathetic and parasympathetic components of the autonomic nervous system, and the maturing cortical areas of the right hemisphere (Schore, 2014a, 2017a, 2019a).

This early perinatal stage of human infancy represents the onset of a critical period for a transition from subcortical to cortical face-processing systems and from the dorsal vagal to the experience-dependent maturation of Porges's (2011) right-lateralized ventral vagal social engagement system. In these primordial implicit nonverbal communications, the mother regulates the infant's internal states of sympathetic and parasympathetic autonomic arousal, thereby facilitating a burgeoning state of autonomic sympathovagal balance and an implicit subjective sense of safety, expressed in the infant's state of "quiet alertness" or "alert inactivity" (Schore, 1994/2016).

Porges (2011) asserts, "The right vagus and, thus, cardiac vagal tone are associated with processes involving the expression and regulation of motion, emotion, and communication" (p. 140) and that "the vagal control of the right side of the larynx produces changes in vocal intonation [prosody] associated with expression of emotions" (p. 141). In this manner, the intonation of the voice reflects the physiological state that is transmitted to the other. According to Manini and her colleagues, "The autonomic nervous system seems to represent an elementary mechanism supporting

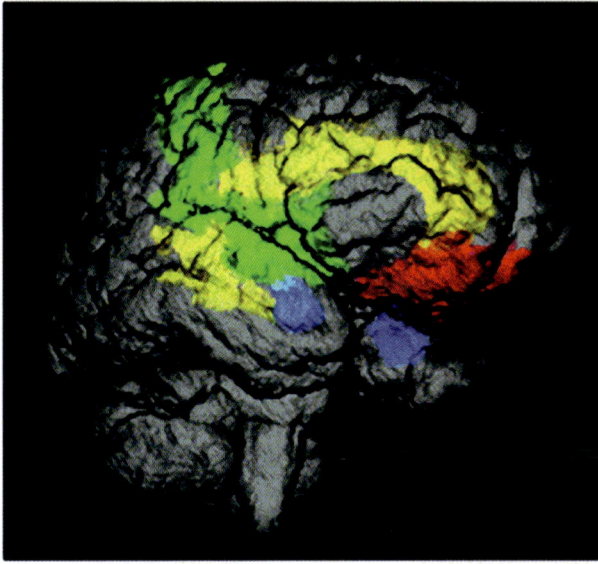

Figure 2.2: Neuroanatomy of the right-lateralized socioemotional brain and the hierarchical limbic system. Note the amygdala (blue), the anterior cingulate (yellow), and the orbitofrontal (ventromedial) prefrontal cortex (red), as well as the posterior somatosensory cortex (green) in the right hemisphere. The right insula is located deep within the lateral sulcus, which is the large fissure that separates the frontal and parietal lobes from the right temporal lobe.

Reprinted from Current Opinion in Neurobiology, Vol 11, Issue 2, Ralph Adolphs, "The neurobiology of social cognition," pages 231–239, © 2001, with permission from Elsevier.

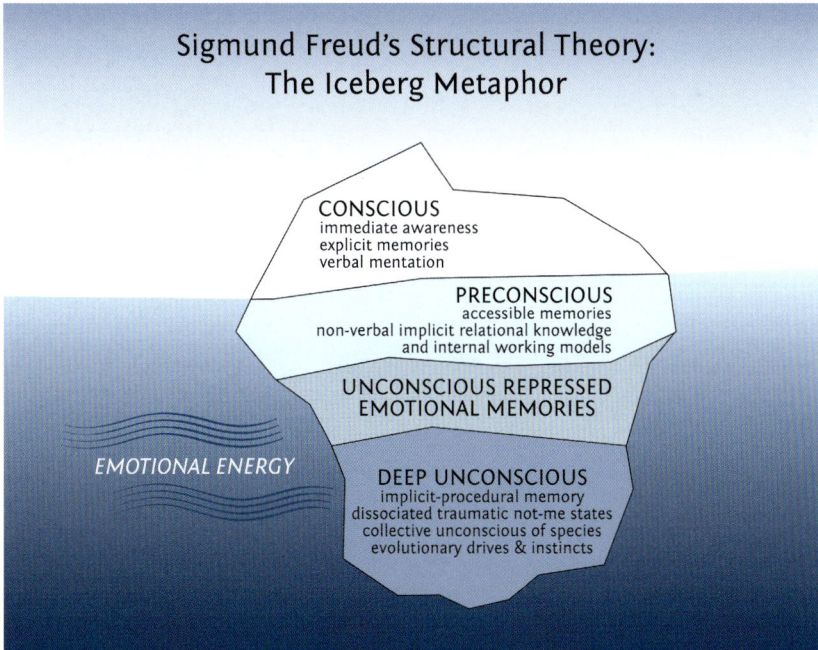

Figure 2.3: Revised update of Freud's iceberg metaphor.

Illustration by Beth Schore

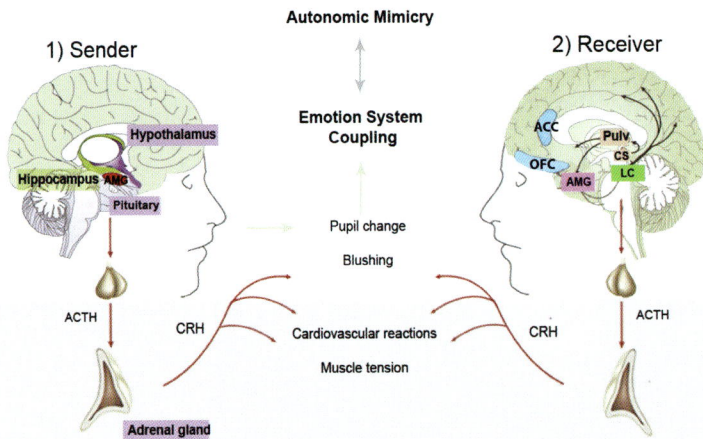

Figure 8.1: Lateral view of the neurological mechanisms of unconscious autonomic mimicry. Sender on the left: (1) Sender's stress response is initiated by hypothalamus-pituitary-adrenal axis activation. (2) Adrenal gland secretes adrenocorticotropic hormone (ACTH), increasing the level of corticotropin-releasing hormone (CRH) in the bloodstream. (3) These neuroendocrinological reactions are accompanied by cardiovascular changes, muscle tension, pupil dilation, and sweating. Receiver on the right: (4) The affective information is implicitly registered by the receiver's senses and passes through (5) the superior colliculus (CS) pulvinar (Pulv) pathway to the amygdala (AMG). (6) The amygdala and locus coeruleus (LC) activate the hypothalamic-pituitary-adrenal axis. (7) The amygdala and LC project to higher cortical networks such as the orbitofrontal cortex (OFC) and anterior cingulate (ACC), influencing social decisions. (8) Sender and receiver emotionally converge on physiological (lower gray) levels. For clinical purposes, think of the sender as patient, receiver as therapist.

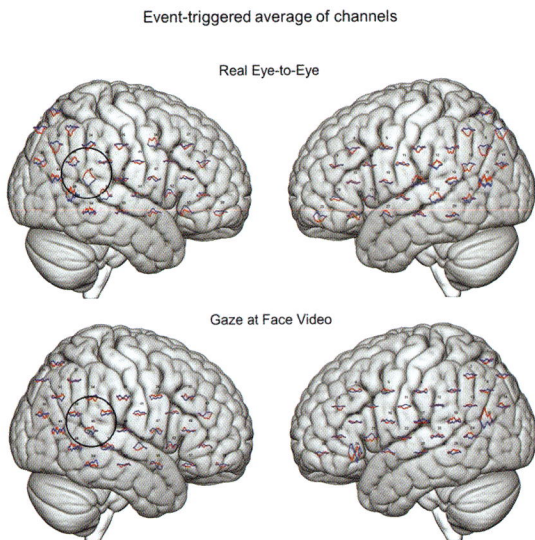

Event-triggered average of channels

Real Eye-to-Eye

Gaze at Face Video

Figure 8.2: Live real-time eye-to-eye contact compared to gaze-at-face video responses. The black circle on the right hemisphere diagrammatically represents the tight TPJ. The top row shows responses of the right TPJ for the real face-to-face task, and the bottom row responses for th video gaze task. Increased right TPJ activity is seen in the live bu not the video condition.

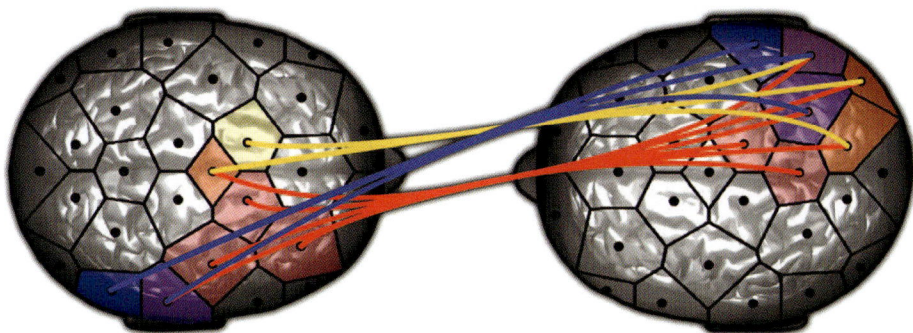

Figure 9.1: Top-down view of a hyperscanned, right-lateralized interbrain synchronization of a spontaneous bidirectional nonverbal communication of face, voice, and gesture. Adapted from "Towards a Two-Body Neuroscience," with permission from the author.

© 2011 Guillaume Dumas, taken from "Towards a two-body neuroscience," *Communicative & Integrative Biology*, reprinted by permission of Informa UK Limited, trading as Taylor & Francis Group https://www.tandfonline.com

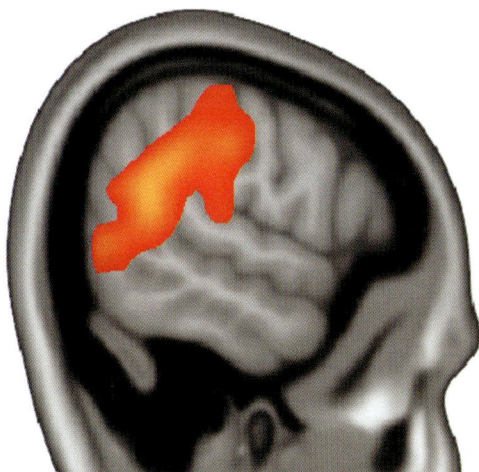

Figure 9.2: Lateral view of neural coupling sites within the right temporoparietal junction in nonverbally interacting subjects. Note location in the posterior cortical areas of the right hemisphere.

Bilek, E., Ruf, M., Schäfer, A., Akdeniz, C., Calhoun, V. D., Schmahl, C., Demanuele, C., Tost, H., Kirsch, P., & Meyer-Lindenberg, A. (2015). Information flow between interacting human brains: Identification, validation, and relationship to social expertise. *Proceedings of the National Academy of Sciences, 112(16)*, 5207–5212. https://doi.org/10.1073/pnas.1421831112 Cropped from original.

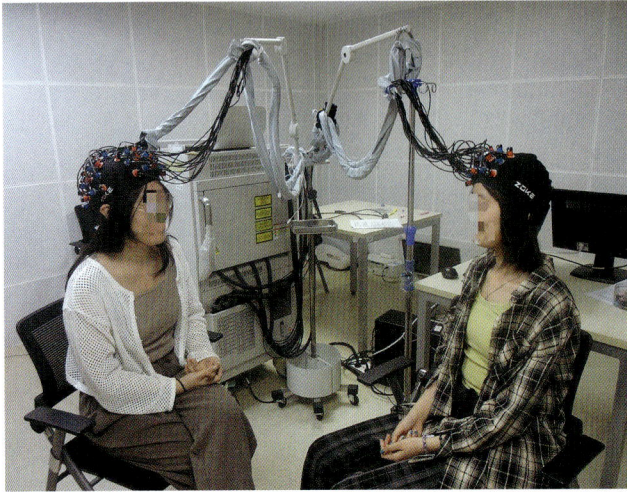

Figure 9.3: Experimental design of hyperscanning fNIRS study of right-lateralized interbrain synchronization between client and therapist during a counseling session. Notice that the optic probes were placed only over the patient's and therapist's right hemispheres. Supplied by Zhang et al. (2020) for "Interpersonal Brain Synchronization Associated With Working Alliance During Psychological Counseling" (2020).

Figure 9.4: fNIRS probe of the emitter and the sender in the posterior right TPJ.

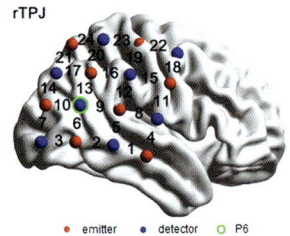

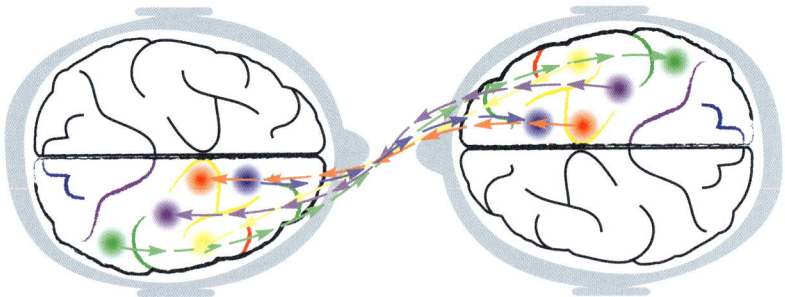

Figure 9.5: Top-down view of a right-lateralized interbrain synchronization and right-brain-to-right-brain nonverbal communication of emotion in psychotherapy, based on Dumas et al. (2011) and Zhang et al. (2018, 2020).

Illustration by Beth Schore

emotional synchrony between mother and infant" (2013, p. 2). This clearly implies that Porges's social engagement system is a two-person autonomic communication system, ANS to ANS. Safety is generated and shared by the cocreation of a synchronized resonance between two interacting right-lateralized social engagement systems.

This maturational advance heralds the onset of mother–infant right hemispheric eye-to-eye, body-to-body left-cradling bias, a tendency to cradle an infant on the left side, regardless of the mother's handedness or culture of ethnicity, that is mostly unconscious (Vervloed et al., 2011) and therefore an early expression of the depths of human nature. This evolutionary epigenetic facilitator of social cognition and the development of the right-lateralized social brain is found in 70–80% of mothers (Bourne & Todd, 2004; Forrester et al., 2018; Giljov et al., 2018; Hendriks et al., 2011; Malatesta et al., 2019; Schore, 2012, 2019a, 2019b; Vauclair & Donnot, 2005). Infants spend large amounts of their waking (and sleeping) activity in the arms of their mothers, and this makes cradling one of the main social contexts where intimate mother–infant intersubjective body-to-body interaction takes place (Suter et al., 2007). According to these researchers,

> The right hemisphere is superior in decoding facial expressions and emotional stimuli. Cradling the baby on the left side in the left visual field therefore enhances the processing of its facial expressions and affective signals, resulting in an enhanced mother–child communication and monitoring of the infant's well-being. Yet, not only is the decoding of signals of the infant by its mother facilitated, but the child also has the advantage in being able to monitor the left side of its mother's face, which is more expressive than the right side. (p. 16)

Manning et al. (1997) concluded that the tendency of mothers to cradle the infant on their left side "facilitates the flow of affective information from the infant via the left ear and eye to the center of emotional decoding, that is, the right hemisphere of the mother" (p. 327). I would add that this emotional decoding occurs in the context of an emerging synchronized intersubjective bidirectional right-brain-to-right-brain communication system cocreated in the developing mother–infant relationship. In a recent overview, authors are defining left-cradling as "the exchange of emotional information (through the respective right cerebral hemispheres) between the cradler and cradled individuals" that "during infanthood might be part of a complex biobehavioral system fostering the development of a typically lateralized brain in the child" (Marzoli et al., 2022, p. 10).

Indeed, at around eight weeks, the onset of primary intersubjectivity, there is a dramatic progression of the infant's social and emotional capacities. This postnatal period is initiated in a critical period of development of the infant's posterior right cortical areas involved in visual, auditory, and tactile sensory processing, as well as the right insula, which is one of the most rapidly growing areas in the first year, involved in awareness of interoception of visceral sensations, body movement, emotions, vocalizations, pain, and consciousness (Gilmore et al., 2012; Schultz, 2016). This structure deep within the temporal lobes (see Figure 2.2) is also essentially involved in facial processing (Berthier et al., 1987), in the subjective emotional awareness of inner body feelings, and in visceral and autonomic functions that ultimately mediate the generation of an image of one's physical state, a "sentient self" (Craig et al., 2010, 2011).

In this same time frame, expanded growth is also seen in the right basolateral amygdala and its dense connections with cortical areas (see Figure 2.2). The neuropsychologist Rhawn Joseph (1992) asserted, "The right amygdala appears to be more greatly affected by early rearing experiences." Studies reveal that a phenotype of early infancy identified at four months predicts individual differences in reactivity of the right amygdala to faces almost two decades later in adults (Schwartz et al., 2012). Neuroscientists now conclude, "The amygdaloid complex can not be thought of as a 'primitive' or vestigial brain system since it is privy to the highest levels of sensory processing that has been afforded by the expansion of association cortex in the human brain" (Schumann et al., 2011, p. 746). Other researchers observe, "The amygdala is commonly associated with the processing of fearful and unpleasant emotional stimuli, but has also been shown to play a part in processing of happy expressions of facial emotion" (Ranotte et al., 2004).

Todd and Anderson (2009) boldly assert,

> Traditionally, the amygdala has gotten a lot of "bad" press. Popular wisdom has portrayed the human amygdala as the center of an ancient animal id that drives us to rapid impulsive action before our more reasoned judgments can kick in. For a long time, it was considered to be a

fear center or threat detector that is instrumental in allocating processing resources to potentially harmful events. This was in part because, thanks to research in nonhuman animals, the amygdala's role in fear learning was extremely well mapped. More recent studies in humans suggest that it is responsive to positive and arousing rather than to strictly negative events, as well as to ambiguous events. (p. 1217)

In the second quarter of the first year, another homeostatic control system comes online that is associated with responsivity to social cues: the right anterior cingulate (medial frontal) cortex, which hierarchically controls the earlier amygdala-dominated limbic configuration. In important work, Allman et al. (2011) document that the number of evolutionarily recent von Economo neurons (VENs) or "spindle cells" in the anterior cingulate and frontoinsular cortical areas are low at birth, and but increase significantly in the first eight months of human infancy. The numbers of VEN neurons is significantly greater in the postnatal than the neonatal brain, and the authors suggest that "VEN abundance may be related to environmental influences" (Allman et al., 2011, p. 62). Intriguingly, these neurons, which are unique to humans and great apes, are much more abundant in the right hemisphere, reflecting the fact that "rightward asymmetry emerges during the first few months of postnatal life" (p. 64).

Functionally, these large bipolar neurons in the right anterior cingulate and frontoinsular areas perform essential regulatory functions, especially in processing information related to right-lateralized sympathetic arousal, and in the communication of social information. It is now thought that "VENs may relay a fast intuitive assessment of complex social situations" (Allman et al., 2005, p. 1112). I suggest that intersubjective attachment transactions directly influence the numbers and connectivity of these right-lateralized limbic-autonomic VENs, and that relational trauma in the right brain critical period interferes with their developmental experience-dependent maturation, and thereby plays an important role in socioemotional psychopathogenesis. Basic research shows that "VENs may be particularly vulnerable to dysfunction" (Watson et al., 2006), for example, in the etiology of autism (Allman et al., 2005).

Most intriguingly, research documents neuroplastic structural changes in the mother's brain during this same developmental period (Kim et al., 2010). This longitudinal study included two time points: 2–4 weeks postpartum and 3–4 months postpartum, and therefore over the onset of intersubjectivity at 2–3 months. During this period, gray matter in the mother's brain increases specifically in her right insula, hypothalamus, amygdala, and anterior cingulate, as well as in positively valenced meso-limbic dopamine nuclei. The authors conclude that interactions with the infant induce these structural changes, which are expressed in functional increases of maternal motivation and sensitivity to infant cues. Indeed, they report that these structural changes at 3–4 months "were predicted by a mother's positive perception of her baby at the first month postpartum. Thus, the mother's positive feelings for her baby may facilitate the increased levels of gray matter" (Kim et al., 2010, p. 698). This clearly implies that the mother's positive feelings for her developing baby are associated with subsequent changes and growth in not only her infant's but also her own brain.

These infant and maternal neurobiological data can be interpreted within the framework of interpersonal neurobiology's central principles that the structure and function of the mind and brain are shaped by synchronized emotional relationships, and that brains align their neural activities in social interactions. This simultaneous brain growth on both sides of the mother–infant dyad suggests a synchronized alignment between the mother's and infant's right brain cortical-subcortical limbic autonomic circuits during positively valenced intersubjective emotional protoconversations. At 2–3 months, a critical period for the onset of intersubjectivity, the mother's right basolateral amygdala and anterior cingulate are undergoing neuroplastic reorganization, at the very same time when her infant's right basolateral amygdala and anterior cingulate are in a critical period of growth. This coordinated accelerated synaptic growth in both brains occurring at the same time is another example of mother–infant synchrony, defined as coordinated timing in development (Jaffe et al., 2001).

For a much more detailed description of human right-lateralized fetal and postnatal development, I refer the reader to my recent volume *The Development of the Unconscious Mind* (Schore, 2019b).

Intersubjective Bioenergetic Transmissions Generate Positively Charged Interbrain Synchronization

As mentioned, these episodes of affect synchrony occur in the first expression of social play. I suggest that these positively charged mother–infant emotional interactions generate increasing levels of dopaminergic arousal and thereby joy (elation), a state of intense pleasure plus the urge for contact seeking. The synchronized positive arousal of mutual play is regulated by the reciprocal activation of endorphins that increase opiates and pleasure in both brains (Kalin et al., 1995). Endorphins enhance play behavior (Schore, 1994/2016), induce mirthful joyous laughter (Miller & Fry, 2009), and increase the firing rate of mesolimbic dopamine neurons (Yoshida et al., 1993). Dopamine is the most important catecholamine involved in reward effects, and in this cocreation of a reciprocal reward system, high levels of ventral tegmental mesolimbic dopamine are generated in both brains. Activation of the mesolimbic dopamine system that exerts a growth-promoting neurotrophic effect on the postnatal cortex is associated with initiation of movements toward emotional or motivational stimuli and the incentive of anticipation of reward. Trevarthen also reported an increased positive state of excited expectation in protoconversations, which I suggest is associated with states of regulated sympathetic hyperarousal.

Stern (1990) described how infants seek stimulation that arouses, excites, and activates them and find this state of heightened activation intensely pleasurable. He described the energetic capacities of dynamic "vitality affects," the positive affects that are required to build self-structure, and characterized maternal social behavior that can "blast the infant into the next orbit of positive excitation" (Stern, 1985). In such interactions of interpersonal resonance, both partners synchronize states and simultaneously adjust their social attention, stimulation, and accelerating energy-mobilizing catecholaminergic sympathetic autonomic arousal to each other's responses. On a moment-to-moment basis, the empathic caregiver's sensory stimulation synchronizes with the crescendos and decrescendos of the infant's endogenous arousal rhythms, allowing the mother to appraise the nonverbal expressions of her infant's internal emotional arousal and positive psychobiological states, to mutually upregulate them, and to communicate and intersubjectively share them with the infant.

In these essential face-to-face emotional transactions of mutual gaze, the mother initially attunes to and resonates with the infant's resting state, but as this state is dynamically activated (or deactivated or hyperactivated), she contingently fine-tunes and corrects the intensity and duration of her affective stimulation in order to maintain the child's positive affect state (see Figure 7.1). As a result of this moment-by-moment synchronization of affective direction, both partners increase together their degree of engagement and facially expressed positive affect. This interactive micro-regulation continues, as soon after the heightened affective moment of accelerating arousal and an intensely joyful full-gape smile, the baby gaze averts in order to downregulate the potentially disorganizing effect of the accelerating arousal of the intensifying emotional state. Research indicates that the unconscious communication of synchronized mimicry decreases when the gaze of the other is averted (Wang et al., 2011). In order to maintain the positive emotion, the psychobiologically attuned mother takes her cue and backs off to reduce her stimulation. She then waits for the baby's signals for reengagement in the reappearance of the infant's quiet alert state and a bid for reengagement (Schore, 2003a).

In this manner, not only the tempo of their engagement but also their disengagement and reengagement are coordinated and synchronized. In this process of contingent responsivity, "the more the mother tunes her activity level to the infant during periods of social engagement, the more she allows him to recover quietly in periods of disengagement, and the more she attends to the child's reinitiating cues for reengagement, the more synchronized their interaction" (Schore, 1996, p. 61). The sensitive care-giver who is physiologically synchronized with the child thus facilitates the infant's emotional information processing by adjusting the mode, amount, variability, and timing of the onset and offset of stimulation to the infant's actual integrative capacities (Schore, 2003a).

In such synchronized, reciprocal, turn-taking interactions, the mother must be attuned not so much to the child's overt behavior as to the reflections of the covert, involuntary physiological rhythms of his internal state, enabling the resonant dyad to coconstruct a "mutual regulatory system of arousal" that contains a "positively amplifying circuit affirming both partners" (see Schore, 1994/2016, "Mirroring Gaze Transactions and the Dyadic Amplification of Positive Affects"). In physics, resonance refers to a phenomenon whereby an unusually large oscillation is produced in response to a stimulus whose frequency is the same as, or nearly the same as, the natural vibratory frequency of the system. The capacity of the infant to experience increasing levels of positive arousal is thus amplified and externally regulated by the primary caregiver and depends on her capacity to playfully engage in synchronized emotional exchanges that generate increased positive arousal in herself and her child (see Figures 2.1 and 2.2

in Schore, 2003a). I suggest that over the lifespan this shared intersubjective state of oscillating highly positive arousal is what the Beach Boys termed "pickin' up good vibrations."

I would add that this interpersonal synchrony is also expressed in right-lateralized interbrain synchrony, simultaneous changes of emotional energy within the coupled right brains of both members of the dyad. In terms of self-organization theory, the mutual entrainment of their right brains during moments of affect synchrony triggers an amplified energy flow that allows for a coherence of organization that sustains more complex states of consciousness within both the infant's and the mother's right brains. Recall Trevarthen and Aitken's (2001) assertions that in synchronized primary intersubjective transactions, interpersonally resonated positive states of arousal are amplified, that this impacts the infant's capacity to generate "rudiments of individual consciousness," and that this two-person interpersonal context serves as a developmental origin of not only subjectivity but "self-consciousness."

In parallel writings, Tronick et al. (1998) described the cocreation of an expanded "dyadic state of consciousness" within the mother–infant dyad, when the emergent state of consciousness becomes more coherently organized and more complex. Tronick hypothesized that "the capacity to create dyadic states of consciousness with another, and the quality of those states, depends in part on the history the individual had in creating these states early in development with his or her mother (and others)" (Tronick et al., 1998, pp. 298–299). He also proposed that dyadically expanded states of consciousness represent an "unconscious force driving social engagement" (p. 296). In earlier writings, I suggested that Tronick is referring to a relational expansion of a state of affective consciousness, what Edelman (1989) called "primary consciousness," that relates visceral and emotional information pertaining to the biological self to stored information processing pertaining to outside reality, and which is specifically located in the right brain (Schore, 2003a). Similarly, Trevarthen's "rudiments of individual consciousness" refers to this intersubjective right-lateralized primary consciousness within the infant's early-developing right mind.

I propose that the source of primary consciousness is in the previously mentioned bioaminergic noradrenergic, dopaminergic, and serotonergic arousal centers in the deep brainstem and midbrain. These three bioaminergic arousal-generating systems in the midbrain and brainstem continue to evolve in postnatal periods, when they send axon collaterals up the neuraxis, thereby exerting trophic, energetic, and regulatory roles on the development of large areas of the cerebral cortex and limbic system. In his recent book, the neuropsychoanalyst Mark Solms (2021) also attributes the source of consciousness to brainstem and midbrain systems. Furthermore, I propose that right brain primary consciousness is generated in right-brain-to-right-brain primary intersubjectivity. Note the intersubjective interbrain synchronization between two right-lateralized subjective minds and its impact upon a cardinal function of the human mind, the generation of states of consciousness.

In basic neurological research on the impact of deep brain stimulation on specific brain regions involved in consciousness, Lu and colleagues (2024) documented that stimulation in right brain regions triggered stronger enhancements of consciousness than left brain regions. Using functional near-infrared spectroscopy to evaluate levels of consciousness, they conclude,

> One potential explanation for our finding is that the brain regions in the right hemisphere primarily engage in interactions with components of the ascending arousal system. These interactions are responsible for regulating behavioral arousal, consciousness, and motivation, as they receive and process information from this system. . . . Therefore, the variability features in the right brain regions may achieve better reflections of the consciousness-related brain functional variations than those in the left brain regions. Another possible explanation is that the right hemisphere may have the potential to promote communication (Schore, 2020; Hartikainen, 2021). . . . Motivation to engage in communication related to the right hemisphere is paramount and may precede the execution of verbal and motor functions during communication involving the left hemisphere. (p. 9)

I suggest this intensification of right brain activity is primary consciousness, which according to Edelman (1989) precedes what he termed left-hemisphere higher-order consciousness. Thus in the right-brain-to-right-brain communication system of an interactive protoconversation, a state of consciousness is shared between the three-month-old infant and the mother. The emergent ability to share energetic states of right brain primary consciousness with another human being is a central aspect of human evolution and a defining quality of the depths of human nature.

Furthermore, Feldman et al. (2011) highlighted the relational context of "intense moments" of "interaction synchrony" cocreated by three-month-old infants and their mothers:

> Face-to-face exchanges are short events spread across the daily routine of parent and child that mark purely social moments and involve *higher levels of positive arousal and social coordination*, as compared to episodes of caregiving and feeding. The brevity and intensity of such moments appear to initiate a process of biological concordance between the partners' heart rhythms. As seen during episodes of high positive arousal—for instance, moments of vocal or affective synchrony which are accompanied by *high positive energy—the tightness of the biological synchronicity increased* [emphasis added]. . . . Gaze synchrony in [and] of itself . . . without a rise in positive arousal, did not increase biological synchrony. (p. 573)

These emotional transactions of heightened affective moments involving synchronized, ordered patterns of energy transmissions (directed flows of electromagnetic energy) represent the fundamental core of the right brain systems of communication and regulation (see Schore, 1994/2016, 1997b, 2003a, 2012). Synchrony in dynamic systems, including social systems, is viewed as a complex, emergent, and indeterminate process. A central tenet of dynamic systems theory holds that at particular critical moments, a flow of energy allows the components of a self-organizing system to become increasingly interconnected, and in this manner organismic form is constructed in developmental processes. As the patterns of relations among the cortical and subcortical components of a self-organizing system become increasingly interconnected and well ordered, it is more capable of maintaining a coherence of organization in relation to variations in the environment. This description applies to the interconnectivity of the cortical-subcortical components of the early-developing right brain subjective self-system.

More specifically, in right-brain-to-right-brain emotion-transacting intersubjective communications, organized patterns of information emanating from the caregiver's face, voice, and gestures trigger synchronous energy shifts in the infant's brain and body, central nervous system, and autonomic nervous system. The caregiver is thus modulating changes in the child's energetic state, since physiological arousal levels are known to be associated with changes in cellular metabolic energy controlled by brain mitochondria, as I described in Chapter 3. Within a cocreated intersubjective field, these regulated emotional exchanges between the mother and infant in turn elicit synchronized increased energy shifts in both of their right brain limbic systems.

Recall that intersubjective maternal-infant bioenergetic transmissions during mutual play (and mutual love) generate a positively charged dynamic electromagnetic intersubjective field created by the synchronized coupling of the infant's and mother's emotional right brains, especially during the infant's critical period of right brain neuroplasticity and growth. This right-lateralized interbrain synchronization generates dynamic bioenergetic "vitality affects." The science of bioenergetics studies the vital activities of living systems. The *OED* defines *vital* as "full of life or energy." All of this is occurring in a critical period of accelerated metabolic activity and growth of the infant's emotional right hemisphere, especially his or her limbic system. In all biological systems, the primary limiting factor for growth is energy, the metabolic energy needed for life processes.

In Chapter 3, I discussed the role of deficits of metabolic energy in less-than-optimal early highly stressful dysregulating attachment experiences that interfere with critical-period right brain development. Here I describe the role of energy in positively valenced attachment experiences that optimize right brain development. Recall that the biological source of this emotional energy is mitochondria, which control brain metabolism (Naviaux, 2020). This powerhouse of the cell is the critical site of oxidative phosphorylation, the primary biological oxidations that generate cellular and thereby organismic metabolic energy in the form of adenosine triphosphate (ATP), the energy-carrying molecule found in the cells of all living organisms (Wilson, 2017). Large amounts of ATP are generated in the brain to maintain membrane ion gradients and processes regulating synaptic transmission. Researchers are now demonstrating that "ATP synthesis is required for synaptic function" (Rangaraju et al., 2014) and describing "*synaptic energy use and supply*" (Harris et al., 2012). Mitochondria thus supply the energy for the right brain critical period of accelerated synaptogenesis.

Indeed, mitochondria are known to have important biosynthetic activities, and the developmental increase of bioenergetic capacities of synchronized populations of mitochondria in neuronal synaptogenesis supports early brain development, since this early critical period of growth is coupled to a source of energy. This expanded capacity to generate mitochondrial synaptic energy fuels the significant bioenergetic demands of myelination, axonal and dendritic growth, and synaptogenesis, especially in right brain critical periods of neuroplasticity. Although the adult brain consumes nearly 20% of the adult human body's basal metabolism, an infant's brain consumes more than 40% of the infant's basal metabolism. It is long established that almost 25% of the infant's energy intake goes to brain growth, and that 75% of brain size develops after birth.

During these periods of rapid growth, different right brain areas undergo a transition from anaerobic glycolysis to aerobic glycolysis (Goyal et al., 2014), as well as aerobic growth supported by mitochondrial oxidative phosphorylation, and thereby an increase in levels of energy metabolism in the critical period of human right brain development (Schore, 1994/2016). This metabolic energy is delivered into circuits of synaptic connectivity between the cortical and subcortical levels of the infant's developing right brain, including the midbrain and brainstem bioaminergic generating systems that generate emotional arousal, allowing the right-lateralized social-emotional brain to act as a dynamic system, a cohesively organized self-regulating integrated whole. In 1994 I suggested that right brain emotional arousal is associated with changes in mitochondrial metabolic energy (Schore, 1994/2016).

Over the lifespan, all emotion is composed of two dimensions: valence (positive-negative, pleasant-unpleasant, approach-avoidance of discrete emotions) and arousal (energy, intensity, calm-excited). Theoretical and clinical models of psychotherapeutic change need to focus more on the role of energy in both developmental and clinical contexts, and on the intensity of emotional arousals, especially in strong and weak emotional bonds and affective communications in the attachment and therapeutic relationships.

Freud postulated that the mind has a fixed amount of psychic energy, or libido, and that the id was the source of the psychic instinctual energy or force that powered the mind. Although the word *libido* has since acquired overt sexual implications, in Freud's theory it stood for all psychic energy. For Freud, in addition to sexual urges, energy fuels perception, memory, imagination, and thought processes, but I would add emotion, the intensity of emotional energy and thereby the strength of love (and hate), and the durability versus the fragility of the attachment bond embedded in the cocreated therapeutic alliance. The biological construct of energy needs to return to psychological theories, as a neuropsychoanalytic reformulation of Freud's psychic energy.

In fact, energy shifts are the most basic and fundamental features of emotion, discontinuous states are experienced as affect responses, and nonlinear psychic bifurcations are manifest as rapid affective shifts. Such state transitions result from the activation of synchronized bioenergetic processes in central nervous system cortical and limbic circuits that are associated with concomitant homeostatic adjustments within the autonomic nervous system's anabolic energy-conserving parasympathetic and catabolic energy-mobilizing sympathetic branches, in a yin-yang relationship of autonomic sympatho-vagal balance. Furthermore, interpersonal physiological synchrony is expressed in the coupling of the sympathetic and parasympathetic components of the autonomic nervous systems not only within but between individuals. Physiologically synchronized and mutually regulated emotional mind-body states thus reflect the nonlinear pulsing of positively charged energy within the components of a dynamic, self-organizing right-lateralized mind-body system of the subjective self, as well as between one right-lateralized intersubjective self and another intersubjective self. For more on the role of mitochondria and energy dynamics, see Chapter 36 in *Affect Regulation and the Origin of the Self* (Schore, 1994/2016), and Schore (1997b), reprinted in Chapter 5 of *Affect Dysregulation and Disorders of the Self* (Schore, 2003a).

Right Temporoparietal Cortex: A Central Node of the Social Brain

The 1997 article I just mentioned discussed the organization of the early-developing nonlinear right brain, in which I described the rapid, implicit, nonconscious emotional energy-dependent imprinting of regional cortical and subcortical circuits during critical periods of infancy (Schore, 1997b). Subsequent research confirmed the early development of the right brain, before the left (e.g., Gupta et al., 2005; Mento et al., 2010; Ratnarajah et al., 2013; Sun et al., 2005). Supporting the idea of an early period of accelerated growth at two to three months, research indicates that in the first three months brain growth increases by 64% (Holland et al., 2014) and that the total number of cortical neurons in the human brain increases by 23% to 30% from birth to three months (Shankle et al., 1999). In light of the well-documented observation that the onset of primary intersubjectivity occurs at two to three months, specifically what cortical right brain structures are in a critical period of growth and synaptic connectivity at this time? Since the infant's visual-facial, auditory-prosodic, and tactile-gestural sensory processing occurs in the posterior cortical areas of the early-developing right hemisphere, the social brain, this right-lateralized posterior cortical region is such a candidate.

In previous writings I reported extant developmental neurobiological studies of the infant brain showing that regional differences in the time course of cortical synaptogenesis exist, and that the metabolic activity that underlies regional cerebral function is ontogenetically highest in the posterior sensorimotor cortex and only later rises in anterior frontal cortex (Schore, 1994/2016). In the first months of life, association areas of the posterior parietal somatosensory cortex (see the left side of Figure 2.2) mature as a result of high levels of tactile bodily sensation provided by the maternal environment, with visual input secondary (Chugani et al., 1987). Yamada and colleagues' (1997) fMRI research demonstrated that a milestone for normal development of the infant brain occurs at about eight weeks. At this point in time, a rapid metabolic change occurs in the visual cortex of infants. These authors interpret this rise to reflect the onset of a critical period during which synaptic connections in the occipital cortex are modified by more complex visual experiences, including processing of the mother's face. Another study documented a large, robust cerebral asymmetry in the infant right superior temporal cortex at three months (Glasel et al., 2011). These researchers suggest that this rapid growth is specifically associated with visual processing, voice perception, and non-verbal social communication.

With respect to the processing of auditory prosody, a near-infrared spectroscopy (NIRS) study by Homae and colleagues (2006) revealed that prosodic processing of a female emotional voice occurs in three-month-old infants, specifically in the right temporoparietal region. Indeed, auditory information emanating from the mother's face, embedded in the affective tone of her emotionally expressive voice, is known to be processed in the right temporoparietal cortex (Ross, 1983). In discussing the mother–infant interaction, Dissanayake (2017) emphasizes how much all sensory modalities or "languages" of the intersubjective engagement—facial, vocal, and body—are processed as a whole, a gestalt in the infant's brain during these interactions. The right temporoparietal junction (right TPJ) is known to be activated in the experiencing of positive affect associated with synchronous multisensory stimulation (Tsakiris et al., 2008).

This right-lateralized system, a heteromodal association area located at the intersection of the posterior end of the superior temporal sulcus, the inferior parietal cortex, and the lateral occipital cortex, integrates four sensory modalities (the face, voice, touch, and smell of the mother). Indeed, the right temporoparietal system integrates input from auditory, visual, somesthetic, and emotional limbic areas and forges critical-period connections with the right ventral anterior cingulate, involved in responsivity to social cues and play behavior, and the right insula with its extensive connections to the ANS, which generates a representation of visceral responses accessible to awareness, thereby providing a somatosensory substrate for subjective bodily-based emotional states experienced by the corporeal self. The right TPJ forges direct synaptic contacts with the right basolateral amygdala and its extensive connections with cortical association areas, and with the right-lateralized sympathoadrenal system and the hypothalamico-pituitary-adrenocortical systems involved in subcortical autonomic activity.

During the early postnatal critical period of posterior cortical development, the right TPJ cortical-subcortical system also increases its reciprocal connections with the right locus coeruleus, which generates states of noradrenergic arousal and attention, via "a right hemispheric ventral attention network" that detects salient and behaviorally relevant stimuli in the external social environment as well as internally directed processes in order to deal with environmental changes, thereby playing an essential role in social cognition (Corbetta et al., 2008). In total, this increased interconnectivity of the right TPJ sensoriaffective system allows for the infant's developing right brain to form more complex implicit visual-facial, auditory-prosodic, and tactile-gestural nonverbal communications, and thereby even greater capacities for intersubjectivity.

A large body of recent studies now indicates that the functions of the right TPJ strikingly mirror the central functions of Trevarthen's primary intersubjectivity. Recall his description of the interpersonal context of protoconversation: face-to-face, interactively synchronized, reciprocal, rhythmic turn-taking social interactions embedded in an intersubjective nonverbal communication system that evolves in intimate free play that cocreates a positive affective relationship and interpersonal awareness between mother and infant (see the posterior area of the infant's brain in Figure 7.1). Researchers are emphasizing "the importance of the right temporoparietal junction in *collaborative* social interactions" (Tang et al., 2016, p. 23) and are documenting its fundamental involvement in the building of *positive relationships* (Kinreich et al., 2017). Hill (2024) posits that an intersubjective affectively attuned positive state of hyperarousal that fuels further exploration is the "magic elixir of psychotherapy." I suggest that this right-lateralized system represents the early relational source of the positive transference within the therapeutic alliance and in everyday life.

Interdisciplinary studies now indicate that this posterior right cortex, a central node of the social brain that enhances social ability (Santiestaban et al., 2012), is activated in face-to-face transactions (Redcay et al., 2010), where it functions in "attention and social interaction" (Krall et al., 2015, p. 587) in a social context of a "basic interpersonal interaction" (Goldstein et al., 2018, p. 2532). The right TPJ serves as a convergence zone of sensory and contextual information which is then integrated to create a social context with other social agents (Lee & McCarthy, 2016). This multifunctional system is centrally involved in updating one's internal model of the current environment (i.e., contextual updating) and adjusting expectations based on incoming sensory information (Geng & Vossel, 2013). It responds to visual, auditory, and tactile stimuli and is specialized for the detection of personally relevant social stimuli, particularly when they are salient or unexpected (Corbetta & Shulman, 2002). Indeed, the right-lateralized TPJ has been designated as the hub of human socialization (Carter & Heuttel, 2013).

Furthermore, authors are now asserting that this right hemispheric temporoparietal polysensory area "plays a key role in perception and awareness" (Papeo et al., 2010, p. 129) and in "the unconscious guidance of attention . . . outside of conscious awareness" (Chelazzi et al., 2018, p. 2). This right-lateralized implicit system is essential to "the control of self- and other representations" (Santiestaban et al., 2012, p. 2274) and to the ability to "switch between internal, bodily, or self-perspective and external, environmental, or other's viewpoint" (Corbetta et al., 2008, p. 317). These functions clearly imply the central role of the right TPJ in psychoanalytic internal object relations between self and other.

More recently, McGilchrist (2021a) concludes that "both the sense of an integrated self and the differentiation between the self and world depend on the integrity of the right temporoparietal region" (p. 335). This posterior area of the right hemisphere is also a pivotal neural locus for multisensory body-related information processing, for "maintaining a coherent sense of one's body," and for a "subjective feeling of body ownership" (Tsakiris et al., 2008). These latter authors observe that this structure generates "an *internal model of the body* that would function as a stored template against which to compare *novel* stimuli, playing a role in maintaining a basic sense of *embodied self* [emphasis added]" (p. 3015).

In seminal studies, Decety and Lamm (2007) wrote on the central role of the right TPJ in social interaction and self-functions, and in another Decety and Chaminade (2003) concluded that "self-awareness, empathy, identification with others, and more generally intersubjective processes are largely dependent upon . . . right hemisphere resources, which are the first to develop" (p. 591). Indeed, this right-lateralized system is known to be fundamentally involved in face and voice processing, as well as "making sense of another mind" (Saxe & Wexler, 2005, p. 1391). Over the lifespan, the right TPJ is activated in affective empathy, and via its direct connections with the ANS "in instantiating autonomic and subjective aspects of responding to others' emotional suffering" (Miller et al., 2020). As I have shown, the synchronized, dynamic, intersubjective interaction of one right temporoparietal system with another right temporoparietal system in a collaborative social interaction is expressed in an intersubjective face-to-face, affect-regulating right-brain-to-right-brain nonverbal communication with another mind. Indeed, there is now agreement that *"the right temporoparietal junction is a central hub for interpersonal synchronization* [emphasis added]" (Konrad & Puetz, 2024).

Note the remarkable complexity of the subjective and intersubjective functions of the right TPJ cortical-subcortical system in the early postnatal period. As mentioned, these adaptive, indeed essential primordial psychobiological functions include a developing ability to engage in nonverbal emotional communications with another human being and a shared positive emotional state, a responsiveness to social relational cues, a capacity to integrate sensoriaffective stimuli, and an ability to detect personally relevant stimuli, particularly when they are salient or unexpected, as well as perception, attention, awareness, consciousness, and a representation of an embodied self. These recent discoveries in neuroscience underscore the central importance of this right-lateralized system in human development. Yet I suggest that this early-appearing psychic structure, what Stern (1985) calls a core self and Damasio (2012, 2018) calls a protoself that operates beneath conscious awareness, has previously been extensively described by Sigmund Freud, and that its adaptive functions lie at the foundation of psychoanalytic theory.

Utilizing a neuropsychoanalytic perspective, I deduce that the multifunctional right temporoparietal system is isomorphic with Freud's early-developing unconscious corporeal ego. In *The Ego and the Id*, Freud (1923/1961) concluded, "The ego is first and foremost a *bodily ego*." Freud spoke of an early-developing unconscious ego and a later-developing conscious ego that "is in control of voluntary movement" and is "located in the speech area on the left-hand side" (1923/1961), clearly alluding to the posterior regions of the left hemisphere and Wernicke's receptive language area, and what neuroscientists are now describing as a "verbally driven ego-bound mode of ordinary consciousness" (Flor-Henry et al., 2017). Yet Freud also stated, "A part of the ego—and heaven knows how important a part—may be unconscious, undoubtedly is unconscious" (1923/1961). He further asserted, "The processes in the Ego (they alone) may become conscious. But they are not all conscious, nor always so, nor necessarily so; and large parts of the Ego may remain unconscious indefinitely" (Freud, 1926/1961).

These neuropsychoanalytic data suggest that the early-developing coherently organized unconscious ego is neuroanatomically located in the posterior right hemisphere (as opposed to the conscious ego located in the posterior left hemisphere). They indicate a significant modification of Freud's theory—this right posterior cortical-subcortical system is involved in not just intrapsychic but also interpersonal functions of a relational unconscious that intersubjectively communicates with another relational unconscious. In optimal interpersonal contexts, at two to three months the human bodily-based unconscious ego can nonverbally communicate with another unconscious ego via intersubjective, synchronized, reciprocal, right-temporoparietal-to-right-temporoparietal, positively and negatively charged social-emotional interactions. Furthermore, science now documents that the earliest expression of the human unconscious mind is not solely a Freudian intrapsychic cauldron of untamed passions and destructive drives but an interpersonal generator of amplified joy and shared love.

This research also confirms Freud's fundamental discoveries, demonstrating that this right-lateralized system of social connectedness, a deep core of the personality, operates implicitly, beneath awareness as an unconscious ego in everyday life, across the lifespan (as opposed to the later-maturing left TPJ and the conscious ego in mentalization). These findings underscore the fact that the human unconscious, a central construct of psychodynamic theory and clinical practice for the past hundred years, needs to be reinserted into academic developmental psychology from which it has almost been banished. Recall, Bargh and Morsella (2008) concluded, "Freud's model of the unconscious as the primary guiding influence over everyday life, even today, is more specific and detailed than any to be found in contemporary cognitive or social psychology."

Development of Intersubjectivity, Love, and Play Over the First Year and Beyond

During the two- to three-month transitional period of the human brain growth spurt, new adaptive functional advances of the rapidly maturing right brain emerge, including the capacity to intersubjectively emotionally communicate with other minds and the ability to share intense emotional states with another human being. In classic developmental research, the psychoanalyst-psychiatrist Daniel Stern (1985) described the transition from an early-forming "emergent self" at birth into a "core self" at two to three months, the exact interval of Trevarthen's primary intersubjectivity. He observed, "At the age of two to three months, infants begin to give the impression of being quite different persons. When engaged in social interaction, they appear to be more wholly *integrated* [emphasis added]. It is as if their actions, plans, affects, perceptions, and cognitions can now all be brought into play and focused, for a while, on an interpersonal situation" (Stern, 1985).

Stern noted that with the onset of this emergent developmental function, the subjective social world is altered and interpersonal experience operates in a different domain, a domain of "core-relatedness." He concluded that at this developmental stage, the infant participates in shared "observable interactive events" involved in "bridging the infant's subjective world and the mother's subjective world" (1985, p. 119), and that now "there are many ways being with an other can be experienced . . . such as *merging, fusion . . . symbiotic states* [emphasis added]" (p. 100). At the same time, the mother simultaneously responds in an attuned way "to be with" the infant, "to share," "to participate in" or "join in" with the infant's subjective experience (Stern, 1985).

In classic developmental psychoanalytic studies, Margaret Mahler (1967) posited that in an early symbiotic phase, the mother and infant share a *dual unity*. Bergman and Fahey (1999) documented that mothers at this time describe a symbiotic state in themselves similar to the symbiotic states of the baby, and this reciprocal attunement leads to a sense of openness, mutual sensitivity, and *oneness* to each other's feelings, which Pine (1992) described as "meaningful moments of *merger*." G. Benedetti (1987) proposed, "the birth of the self is composed of a mixture of interchangeable parts of oneself and others" (p. 194). More recent studies of this period of early infancy show that self-other boundaries become blurred in these attuned caregiver–infant interactions (Stumpfogger & Panagiotopoulou, 2021). I suggest that these early-evolving intersubjective functions of Stern's core self and Freud's bodily-based unconscious ego are associated with the infant's developing right temporoparietal self-system, and its central involvement in nonverbal communication and interpersonal synchrony.

In their research on the transition at two to three months, Ammaniti and Gallese (2014) reported,

From the second month after birth, parents and infant begin to show a temporal structure in their interactions. . . . In this period, the sharing of social gaze between parent and baby is the expression of coordinated [synchronized] interactions, which can occur between 30% and 50% of the time. At the same time, mutual gaze can be integrated with parents' and infants' affectionate touch. . . . At around 3 months, parents tend to touch their baby in an affectionate way and infants tend to respond with an intentional *affectionate touch* [emphasis added]. (p. 147)

Note the increases of the mother's loving touch that emerge at this time period and the appearance of what I have termed "quiet love" (Schore,

2019b). Quiet love has been characterized as "a mutual dwelling of baby and mother where one and one makes not two but one" (Ulanov, 2001, pp. 49–50). Note the merger state and a shared state of "oneness."

Confirming this same transitional critical period, Miall and Dissanayake (2003) documented changes in the mother's behaviors:

> Over time, mothers subtly adjust their sounds and movements to what the baby seems to want (or not want), and to its changing needs and abilities. They gradually move from the gentle, cooing reassurance of the first weeks to trying to engage the baby in increasingly animated *mutual play*. At 8 weeks utterances and facial expressions have become more *exaggerated* [emphasis added], both in time and space. (p. 342)

"Animated mutual play" accompanies "excited love," which occurs in moments of thrilling excitement and intense interest in interaction with the mother and contains an energetic potential (see Schore 2019b).

Dissanayake (2017) also described changes in prosodic motherese at this time as dyadic in nature, where both partners influence each other, and multimodal, where multiple senses and more than one communication modality can operate at the same time. Frame-by-frame microanalyses of videotaped mother–infant interactions showing the faces and torsos of both partners side by side reveal that the interactions of dyadic vocalization are as significant as facial expressions and head and body movements (Murray & Trevarthen, 1985). In another study of the cocreated positively valenced nonverbal communication system between mother and infant that evolves in this same time, period Dissanayake (2001) asserted,

> It should also be emphasized here that although mothers "talk" to their babies, the multimodal messages in early interactions are nonverbal. What mothers convey to infants are not their verbalized observations and opinions about the baby's looks, actions, and digestion—the ostensible content of talk to babies—but rather positive affiliative messages about their intentions and feelings: You interest me, I like you, I am like you, I like to be with you, You please me, I want to please you, You delight me, I want to communicate with you, I want you to be like me. (p. 91)

In this intimate context of intense positive affective arousal, these are the early nonverbal communications of love. The *Oxford English Dictionary* defines *love* as "deep affection, strong emotional attachment."

Raymond Bradley (2024) describes love as the arousal and regulation of affective energy that propels and guides our growth and development as social beings. This social bond of interdependence is expressed in a tacit field of affective connection that underlies the development of adaptive psychosocial organization in all stages of human life. He cites my work on how the mother–infant interaction shapes the brain and thereby has enduring psychosocial consequences: "The child's first relationship, the one with the mother, acts as a template for the imprinting of circuits in the child's emotion-processing right brain, thereby permanently shaping the individual's adaptive or maladaptive capacities to enter into all later emotional relationships" (Bradley, 2024, p. 5; Schore, 1997, p. 30). The author proposes that these intimate, loving interactions are structured along two dimensions—love/affect and regulation/modulation—and are organized as a socioaffective dialogue in which the mother stimulates her baby's positive emotional states and then regulates the infant's aroused affective energy. This occurs in a patterned, highly synchronized series of reciprocal exchanges that generate a coherent state of bodily-based socioemotional attunement between the pair. He observes,

> Signaled primarily by mutual eye contact ("mutual gaze dialogue")—bodily gestures and movements, and especially changes in facial emotional expression—enormous quantities of information are exchanged in split-second sequences of highly coordinated communication between the two. The information not only encodes data on their internal psychophysiological states as individuals, but also encodes information on the socioemotional structure of their dyadic interactions. (Bradley, 2024, p. 5)

Bradley adapts Trevarthen's (1993) maternal-infant protoconversation in the upper part of Figure 7.2, adding the physiological synchrony of sympathetic and parasympathetic autonomic states on the bottom of the figure.

Bradley suggests that love acts as a guide to parents for raising a psychosocially healthy infant well equipped for adult life. He concludes,

FIGURE 7.2
Socioaffective dialogue between infant and a loving mother within Trevarthen's intersubjective protoconversation

Face-to-face socioaffective channels of nonverbal communication in which coordinated eye-to-eye orientations, vocalizations, gestures, and movements of the hands, arms, and head all act in concert to signal emotional states and interpersonal awareness. Psychophysiological processes (e.g., heart rhythm patterns and communicating bodily-based autonomic nervous systems) are synchronized and coordinated through entrainment with the mother's systems. Note the heart-to-heart communications.

Figure 1-Socioaffective Dialogue. From R.T. Bradley, "Harnessing the Force of All Creation: Part One. The Power of Love to Shape Reality," World Futures (1-35, June 21, 2024). Adapted and redrawn from "Figure 8.1. Chapters of face-to-face communication in protoconversation, and three phases in the cycles of expressions between mother and baby," C. Trevarthen, "The self born in intersubjectivity." In Ulric Neisser (Ed.), The Perceived Self, pp. 121–173. New York: © Cambridge University Press 1993, reproduced with permission of Cambridge University Press through PLSclear.

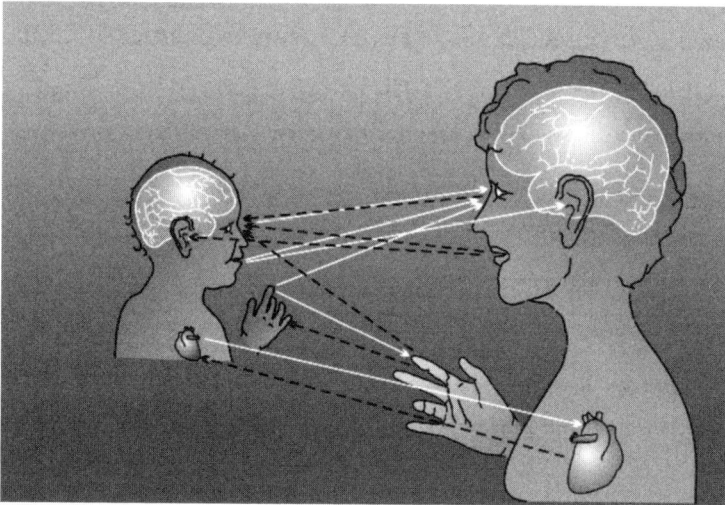

"Appropriately modulated love generates optimal neuropsychosocial development, creating the requisite foundation for psycho-social autonomy and self-conscious agency for life" (2024, p. 6).

In my own recent writings, I describe how intersubjectivity evolves in an intimate, loving context of interpersonally synchronized mutual play, a shared positive affective relationship that amplifies intense joy and excitement, and that this same intimate context of maternal affection also interactively generates the tender emotions of mutual love (Schore, 2019a,

2019b). *The Development of the Unconscious Mind* (Schore, 2019a) includes a chapter, "The Association of the Right Brain and Mutual Love Continues Across the Lifespan: What's Love Got to Do With It?" In that work, I contend that although love is mostly thought to be the province of the arts, poets and writers, actors, dancers, and musicians, from the very beginnings of modern biology and psychology, science has also explored its origins and emotional expressions.

Indeed, in his seminal work *The Expression of Emotions in Man and Animals*, Charles Darwin proposed, "The emotion of love, for instance that of a mother for her infant, is one of the strongest of which the mind is capable. . . . No doubt, as affection is a pleasurable sensation, it generally causes a gentle smile and some brightening of the eyes. A strong desire to touch the beloved is commonly felt" (1872/1965, pp. 224–225). Specifically referring to the origins of this most fundamental attribute of the human species, he speculated, "The movements of expressions in the face and body . . . serve as the first means of communication between the mother and her infant; she smiles approval and thus encourages her child on the right path or frowns disapproval" (p. 385).

At the end of the 19th century, Sigmund Freud began his pioneering studies in psychoanalysis and initiated the field's long history of interest in the essential role of love in human function and dysfunction. Referring to his evolving position on the developmental origins of love, I've suggested, "Although for much of his career [Freud] seemed ambivalent about the role of maternal influences in earliest development, in his very last work he stated, in a definitive fashion, that the mother–infant relationship 'is unique, without parallel, established unalterably for a whole lifetime as the first and strongest love-object and as the prototype of all later love relations'" (Freud, 1940/1964, cited in Schore, 2003a, p. 256).

In the middle of the past century, John Bowlby (1953), a psychoanalytic follower of Freud, began his seminal writings on what would become attachment theory in *Child Care and the Growth of Love*. In that volume, he asserted that a mother's love in infancy and childhood is as important for mental health as are vitamins and proteins for physical health. In his later writings, he concluded, "Many of the *most intense emotions* arise during the formation, the maintenance, the disruption, and the renewal of attachment relationships. The formation of a bond is described as falling in love, maintaining a bond as loving someone, and losing a partner as grieving over someone" (Bowlby, 1969, p. 130). Recall Freud asserted that the primary human motivational systems are love and work. Expanding Freud's idea, I suggest that over the lifespan, love, an essential driver of human nature, is generated in the implicit, automatic, effortless processes of the unconscious right brain while work represents the explicit, intentional, effortful operations of the conscious left brain.

Also in the mid-20th century, another of Freud's disciples, Erich Fromm, wrote the classic *The Art of Loving*, in which he described love as "the experience of union with another being" and "becoming one with another." In that volume, Fromm described what he deemed to be the central problem in individual development: "What meaning—in both women as well as men—does our longing for a mother have? What constitutes the bond to the mother?" (1956, pp. 26–27). He stated that motherly love is an unconditional affirmation of the child's life and needs, and that it is expressed in two different aspects:

> One is the care and responsibility absolutely necessary for the preservation of the child's life and his growth. The other aspect goes further than mere preservation. . . . Motherly love, in this second step, makes the child feel: it is good to have been born; it instills in the child the love for life and not merely the wish to remain alive. . . . Mother's love for life is as infectious as her anxiety. (pp. 46–47)

Supporting Darwin, Freud, Bowlby, and Fromm, in *The Development of the Unconscious Mind* I cite neuroimaging research of love in mother–infant as well as in romantic dyads. These studies show the central role of the right brain, including specifically the right orbitofrontal cortex, the control system of attachment, in the enduring impact of the emotional communications of the loving mother on her infant's developing right brain (see Schore, 2019b). For example, Bartels and Zeki (2004) authored an MRI study, "The Neural Correlates of Maternal and Romantic Love," showing activation in the mother's lateral orbitofrontal cortex as she looks at a picture of her own infant's face. They conclude,

> The tender intimacy and selflessness of a mother's love for her infant occupies a unique and exalted position in human conduct. . . . It provides one of the most powerful motivations for human action, and

it has been celebrated throughout the ages—in literature, art and music—as one of the most beautiful and inspiring manifestations of human behaviour. (p. 1155)

Neuroscientists are currently asserting that the first expression of intimacy, the love between a mother and her infant, represents "one of the most powerful and evolutionarily preserved forms of positive affect in the emotional landscape of human behavior" (Nitschke et al., 2004), that "the phylogenetically ancient role of maternal care . . . appears to be underpinned by evolutionarily ancient structures" (Abraham et al., 2014), and that maternal love for the infant is "a biologically essential mechanism for the preservation of the human species" (Noriuchi et al., 2008). The OED defines intimacy as "inner or inmost nature." In other words, early intimate intersubjective experiences shared with a loving mother positively shape the right brain evolutionary depths of human nature.

Describing these first moments of close intimate contact, the psychoanalyst Heinz Kohut (1971) observed, "The most relevant basic interactions between mother and child usually lie in the visual area: The child's bodily display is responded to by the gleam in the mother's eye." He also referred to the energizing effects of the loving mother's maternal gleam on the infant. In 1994 I suggested that the maternal gleam may literally be a sparkle, that is, a flash of light processed by and reflected off of the mother's hyperexposed foveal area of the retina and onto the infant's fovea (Schore, 1994/2016). The fovea provides the highest visual acuity and contains cone cells that detect colors. Indeed, optic system structure-function relationships may provide a neurophysiological basis for this hidden phenomenon.

It is known that "ideoretinal light" represents excitations of optic neurons arising from within the retina without benefit of light from the external world. Basic research documents that the experience of an "inner light" is associated with biophoton emission and activity in the right and not left hemisphere (Dotta & Persinger, 2011; Saroka et al., 2013). The latter authors observe that the perception of inner white light is commonly reported in practitioners of Buddhism as spiritual experiences of "inner energy," an expression of "the radiance of the fundamental nature or true self in human beings" (Saroka et al., 2013).

Other data indicate that the loving mother's and infant's synchronized face-to-face, eye-to-eye right-brain-to-right-brain intimate, playful nonverbal communications generate high levels of accelerating, amplified, positive emotional arousal, which is fundamentally associated with changes in mitochondrial metabolic energy. The emotional energy embedded in this intense positive affective state of the deep affection of mutual love is available to the infant's developing right brain while exposed to high levels of spontaneous interpersonal and intrapersonal novelty, allowing for the multimodal integration of external and internal sensations. In this manner, the energized intersubjective field of mutual love structuralizes Stern's "core self" that appears at two to three months, a critical period of right brain development, and thus the core self, operating at levels beneath conscious awareness, has an enduring influence on the capacity to cocreate an emotional loving bond with a valued other at later stages of the lifespan.

Ammaniti and Gallese (2014) offered an evocative portrayal of Stern's model of the similar interpersonally synchronized expressions of mutual love in early and later development:

> As Daniel Stern has written, expressions of love begin early in an astonishing way. Mother and child behavior overlaps with the behavior of two lovers. For example, mother and child look at each other without speaking, hold a physical closeness with faces and bodies in constant contact, display alterations in vocal expressions or *synchrony of movements*, and perform particular gestures like kissing each other, hugging, touching, and taking the face or the hands of the other. . . . When parents speak to their child, or lovers talk with one another . . . they emphasize the musicality of the words instead of the meaning, they use baby talk, and they express a wide range of nonverbal vocalizations. . . . Facial expressions assume a special register also, altering and emphasizing the facial mimic. There is also a choreography in the movements of mother and baby, like those of two lovers; *they move in synchrony, getting closer and more distant on the basis of a common rhythm* [emphasis added]. (pp. 110–111)

Authors are asserting that over the first year, "intersubjective behavior continues to grow significantly over the semesters" (Muratori et al., 2011, p. 19). The synchronized right-brain-to-right-brain mother–infant intimate, playful, intersubjective protoconversation continues throughout human infancy in mutual play, songs, lullabies, and nursery rhymes. In peek-a-boo episodes, maternal affect matches, synchronizes, and amplifies infant joy and excitement. A mother playing peek-a-boo will delay the removal of her hands from her eyes in order to provoke surprise, amusement, and laughter from her baby, or similarly when reciting "This Little Piggy" will wait to utter what the fifth piggy squeals—"wee, wee, wee, all the way home."

Recall that the right temporoparietal system responds to visual, auditory, and tactile stimuli and the detection of personally relevant stimuli, particularly when they are salient or unexpected. Indeed, the right amygdala processes emotionally salient attachment sounds such as laughter (Tschacher et al., 2010), and the right frontal lobe processes humor (Shammi & Stuss, 1999), common accompaniments of play. In this early mutual play, repetition in the mother's exaggerated facial expressions, vocal utterances, and body movements and the affect of surprise coordinates and synchronizes the minds and brains of two bodies, mutually regulating the infant emotionally and uniting mother and child temporally (see Schore & Marks-Tarlow, 2018). Thus over the course of the first year, intersubjective play occurs in a relational context of what Tronick (2007) terms "mutual regulation," what I term "interactive regulation."

The perspective of interpersonal neurobiology suggests that mother–infant play is more socioemotional than cognitive, and that, fundamentally, the underlying mechanism of this arousal-altering, pleasurable, dopaminergic, rewarding mutual activity facilitates the experience-dependent maturation of right brain cortical and subcortical systems. This primordial form of intersubjective play generates the neurobiological substrate on which all forms of play evolve—mother–infant and solitary, spontaneous and controlled, active and passive (see Schore, 2017b). During the first year, intersubjective, synchronized mutual play expands the infant's affect array and facilitates the dyadic amplification and transformation of mildly pleasurable enjoyment into joy and the intensification of mildly pleasurable interest into excitement. At 10–12 months, the onset of a critical period for the right orbitofrontal cortex and the emergence of upright locomotion, fully 90% of maternal physical and verbal behavior consists of affection, play, and caregiving, and by one year of age, curiosity and stimulation-seeking exploratory play time increases to as much as six hours of a child's day (Schore, 1994/2016).

My colleague Russell Meares asserts, "The mother–infant protoconversation represents an interplay between two right brains" (2016, p. 52).

He argues that in optimal developmental contexts, the right-brain-to-right-brain protoconversation continues in the second year, a time when a toddler develops a burgeoning playful imagination and shows an expanded need for novel experiences. With the ongoing expansion of higher right brain functions, the intersubjective protoconversation takes the emergent form of intersubjective imaginative games, then intrasubjectively internalized dialogues, and finally what Meares calls "conversational play." This creative game, which the toddler plays while alone, is grounded in the child's burgeoning capacity for make-believe and is expressed in the expressive use of emotional words and analogy.

Indeed, Meares describes it as right hemispheric analogical or protosymbolic play, which is imbued with the affective dimension of joy and pleasure. The creative game consists of a miniature story, told as if to the child himself or herself but also to someone else, who is not there except as a feeling of the background presence of the internalized, protoconversational mother. This conceptualization fits nicely with Winnicott's (1958a) observation that the first real experience of being alone in the presence of the mother occurs in this same time period of right orbitofrontal maturation in the second year. The earliest form of symbolic play allows the toddler to play with ideas and generate fantasies, including imagined interactions with other minds (Schore, 2017b). Functional magnetic resonance imaging shows that the recall of fantasies and imagination activates a right hemisphere network including the inferior frontal gyrus and superior and middle temporal gyrus (Benedetti et al., 2015).

I would add that upon entering early childhood, these emergent products of right brain symbolic imagination can also be shared with a valued other in the intersubjective play of creative storytelling. The right inferior gyrus is also involved in detecting the moral implications of stories (Nichelli et al., 1995). Moral reasoning, like symbolic processing, is also supported by activation of right-lateralized orbitofrontal, ventromedial, anterior cingulate, and amygdala circuits (Ferrario et al., 2024). Indeed, researchers document this hemispheric asymmetry: "In most people the analytical . . . verbal component being associated with left-hemispheric structures, while the nonverbal, symbolic, and unconscious components are associated with activity in structures of the right hemisphere" (Aftanas & Varlamov, 2007, p. 71). My colleague Darcia Narvaez (2014) discusses the essential role of the right brain in her superb volume on the neurobiology and development of human morality. According to McGilchrist (2009), right brain symbols convey an array of implicit connotations "which ramify through our physical and mental, personal and cultural, experience in life, literature and art" (p. 51). Note that the cortical-subcortical circuits of symbolic processes, imagination, and moral reasoning are essential markers of human nature.

The psychoneurobiological substrates of these complex symbolic abilities, heavily influenced by right brain cortical-subcortical activation, appear at the end of the human growth spurt, late in the second year (Dobbing & Sands, 1973). These two right-lateralized adaptive functions, plus another, mutual love, are higher right brain functions built upon shared common lower-level processes, primary intersubjectivity and protoconversation, which begin at the early postnatal stage of the right brain critical period. In this manner, the interpersonally synchronized right-brain-to-right-brain intersubjective communications that begin to structuralize the right temporoparietal core self at two to three months represent the primordial developmental crucible of the adaptive capacities of mutual symbolic play, imagination, and love (see Schore, 2012, 2019a, 2019b). These fundamental expressions of what it means to be human can not only be accessed within a mind but also intersubjectively shared between human minds.

Tying together the developmental and adult contexts, Daniel Stern (2004) described the special state of integrated assembly of feelings, behaviors, and thoughts that are associated with the intersubjective context of falling in love. Note the references to right brain nonverbal processes:

> Following are some of the elements of falling in love that are driven by an intersubjective motive (many of these are shared both by lovers and by parents with their young babies): Lovers can look into each other's eyes, without speaking, for minutes on end—a sort of plunging through the "window of the soul" to find the interior other. . . . There is also an exquisite attention to the other's attentions and feelings, not only to read them correctly but even to anticipate them. There is a playfulness that involves much facial, gestural, and postural imitation. And there is the creating of a private world, a sort of privileged intersubjective space to which they have the keys. The keys are special words with specific meanings, secret abbreviations, sacred rituals and spaces, and so on.

All these things create a psychological niche in which intersubjectivity can flourish. (pp. 108–109)

The association of the right brain and mutual love continues across the lifespan. Maslow (1968) proposed, "Beloved people can be incorporated into the self." Baumeister and Leary suggested that "love aspires to a mutual dissolving of personal boundaries, leading to an egalitarian merging into a new whole" (1995, p. 522). According to Paladino and her colleagues,

> Relationships with loved ones are often described as a blurring of self-other boundaries and the metaphorical expressions "you are part of me" and "we are one." Research shows that such merging can occur at the conceptual level and the bodily level. . . . Social psychology studies show that in close interpersonal relationships, the other becomes cognitively confounded and merges with the self. (2010, p. 1202)

The *OED* defines *intimate* as "thoroughly mixed, united." In Chapter 8 I equate this merger state with synchronous "at-one-ment" (Amid, 2024).

This aspect of close relationships has been most extensively investigated by the psychological research of Elaine and Arthur Aron. They assert, "The model treats love (the desire for a relationship with a particular other) as arising from a desire to expand the self by including that other in the self, as well as by associating expansion with that particular other" (Aron & Aron, 1996). This enlargement of the self is mutual, and not at another's expense. They posit that in addition to love being emotional, it is also fundamentally motivational, and that love involves a motivation of expansion toward a state of wholeness and integration.

According to Baumeister and Leary, "People seem to need frequent, affectively pleasant or positive interactions with the same individuals, and they need these interactions to occur in a framework of long-term, stable caring and concern" (1995, p. 520). All forms of mutual love, deep and lasting close friendships, long-term romantic relationships, and strong spiritual connections involve a right-brain-to-right-brain reciprocal intersubjective context that implicitly communicates and interactively regulates intense positive and negative bodily-based affective states. Synchronized, shared right brain states of reciprocated mutual love thus generate the most intense states of emotional arousal and positive affects in the human experience.

This intimate, right brain bodily-based nonverbal communication system of resonance, amplification, mutual regulation of physiological rhythms, and cocreation of the fundamental human process of interpersonal synchrony is evocatively described by Emily Dickinson in her poem, "The Lovers," published in *Poems by Emily Dickinson, Series Two*.

The rose did caper on her cheek,
Her bodice rose and fell,
Her pretty speech, like drunken men,
Did stagger pitiful.

Her fingers fumbled at her work,—
Her needle would not go;
What ailed so smart a little maid
It puzzled me to know,

Till opposite I spied a cheek
That bore another rose;
Just opposite, another speech
That like the drunkard goes;

A vest that, like the bodice, danced
To the immortal tune,—
Till those two troubled little clocks
Ticked softly into one.

Note the right-lateralized autonomic nervous system dysregulation, interpersonal physiological synchrony, mutual implicit affect regulation, and shared state of oneness. Kane (2004) shows that poetry is fundamentally right hemispheric language.

The interpersonal neurobiological mechanisms of resonance and amplification of intense emotional arousal allow both members of all close relationships to experience the strongest, most intense subjective emotional states, and thereby to intersubjectively share with a valued other the intense pleasure and pain that accompany the most emotionally significant aspects of human life. This becoming one with another, experience of union with another being, or symbiotic merger in turn cocreates a subjective state of not only safety and trust, but also of wholeness, self-expansion, and integration in both partners of a loving pair bond, including the long-term patient–therapist relationship. Bromberg (2017) describes psychotherapy as the growth of wholeness.

In recent clinical literature, the child psychotherapist Graham Music (2023) concludes, "As therapists, we are aiming to build personalities with solid foundations, people who no longer need to skate on thin ice to avoid a perilous emotional abyss, who are able to discern who it is safe to trust, to love, and to be loved by" (p. 16). In the adult literature, Langer (2024) now asserts, "At its deeper levels, the therapeutic relationship can become a kind of love. 'Love' describes the deepest sort of relationship between two beings. If we know anything about love, we know it is an implicit, right brain to right brain process." With respect to the central theme of this book, the pursuit of mutual love involves the right brain depths of human nature. It is not only a focus of psychotherapy but also a major motivational system expressed from the beginnings to the final stages of human life. From its relational onset in early infancy, mutual love increases right-lateralized emotional plasticity on both sides of any loving dyad, whether parent-child, adult romantic, or intimate friendships. According to Porges and Carter (2010), "Although the brain retains plasticity and adaptability throughout life, early experience may set the parameters for that plasticity. Attachment may be said to set up social and emotional homeostasis, deigning future patterns of intimacy" (p. 200).

This intimacy is later expressed as a host of adaptive states of being, including to be young at heart and loving within an intensely close emotional bond with a highly valued other; to have a childlike capacity to be unselfconsciously playful with an equally animated other, thereby remaining "forever young"; to be mutually creative when interacting with another open, curious mind; to share private moments of daydreaming and imagination within a stimulating relationship; to jointly develop a unique, shared, spontaneous sense of humor with another private self; to laugh out loud with an emotionally engaged other with so much gusto that one nearly comes to tears; to be able to vulnerably communicate deeply personal hopes and dreams with a safe, trusted companion; to be capable of quietly reveling with another in the precious little pleasures of life; to respect the quiet solitude of the other; to share the joy of a love of being alive with another emotionally communicating subjective self; and to intersubjectively cocreate a long-lasting, mutually loving opposite- or same-sex relationship across the lifespan, wing to wing, oar to oar.

I'd like to end this chapter with some last thoughts about the affect-communicating functions of the right brain intersubjective system and the affect-regulating functions of the right brain attachment system. I have described how the posterior right temporoparietal system is centrally involved in synchronized nonverbal communications, when partners are in the same state at the same time. This essential function of the early-forming right brain core self is expressed over the lifespan as an adaptive capacity to enter into intersubjective, reciprocal, right-brain-to-right-brain nonverbal interactions with another human, beneath the words. Recall that previously cited research demonstrated the importance of the right temporoparietal junction in *collaborative social interactions* in a social context of a *basic interpersonal interaction*.

Feldman and her colleagues now assert that "brain coordination may be supported by the *non-verbal* [emphasis added] rather than verbal aspects of social interactions" and that "brain-to-brain synchrony localizes to temporal-parietal regions and highlights the role of attachment and social connectedness in the coordination of two brains" (Levy et al., 2017, p. 6). Brain-to-brain synchrony allows for a deeper understanding of a spontaneous social interaction between two dynamically synchronized, nonverbally communicating brains, including face-to-face, moment-to-moment right-brain-to-right-brain emotional communications at levels beneath awareness. The "ultrarapid" unconscious detection of a human face takes place in just 100 milliseconds (Crouzet et al., 2010).

In earlier chapters I have contrasted healthy attachment dynamics and regulated right brain emotional functions with less than optimal attachment and right brain psychopathogenesis expressed in deficits in intersubjectivity and disturbed relationships. Indeed, like the developmental process of attachment, intersubjectivity is currently seen as a critical construct within psychopathogenesis and psychotherapy. Although Trevarthen stressed the role of intersubjectivity in positively charged play states, psychotherapists also address the nonverbal intersubjective communications of negatively valenced and even traumatic emotional states. Indeed, early stressful ruptures of the attachment bond that are routinely not followed by relational repair are commonly found in patients with an early history of right brain attachment stressors. In my work, I continue to offer clinical and interdisciplinary research evidence demonstrating that all psychiatric disorders show deficits in right brain affect regulation (Schore, 1994/2016, 2003b, 2012, 2014a, 2014b, 2019a).

There is now general acceptance that in addition to affect dysregulation, intersubjective relational deficits are a central focus of all forms of infant, child, adolescent, adult, and group psychotherapy (see Schore, 1997, 2000c, 2003b, 2019b, 2021b). In terms of the dyadic psychotherapeutic relationship, right brain deficits of intersubjectivity are expressed in an inability, especially under relational stress, to nonverbally emotionally communicate and interpersonally synchronize with another brain (e.g., see Schore, 2014a, for deficits of intersubjectivity in autism spectrum and borderline personality disorders). Along with the patient's symptomatology, these intersubjective difficulties lie at the core of the treatment of the patient's relational deficits that operate outside of conscious awareness. From the perspective of modern attachment theory, patients' organized and disorganized attachment styles refer not only to different implicit strategies of emotion regulation but also reduced abilities for entering into intersubjective synchronized right-lateralized nonverbal emotional communications with others.

In the clinical literature, Meares (2012) directly refers to Trevarthen's intersubjective protoconversation and asserts that the dynamic "interplay between two right brains provides a structure for the therapeutic relationship" (p. 312). Face-to-face interpersonal synchronization of right brain patterns enables the therapeutic dyad to intersubjectively communicate and implicitly share their conscious and unconscious emotional states in a "protoconversation," what I have termed "a conversation between limbic systems," a "spontaneous emotion-laden conversation" (Schore, 2012). This right-lateralized interpersonal neurobiological mechanism embedded in the positive transference allows the clinician to act as an interactive regulator of the patient's emotional states, which in turn facilitates a reduction in the patient's presenting symptomatology. In this work, the clinician interactively downregulates negative affect in stress-reducing therapeutic contexts, and upregulates positive affect in playful therapeutic contexts.

It should be noted that the intersubjective motivational system and the attachment motivational system are both central mechanisms involved in the therapeutic relationship and in psychotherapeutic change, and that both are expressed in adaptive right brain interpersonal neurobiological functions. Developmentally, the former system, located in the right temporoparietal regions and its subcortical connections, enters a critical period of maturation at the beginning of the first year, while the latter, located in the right orbitofrontal regions and its more extensive cortical and subcortical connections, at the end of the first year. In the second year, the posterior right temporoparietal cortical areas form reciprocal bidirectional synaptic connections with the anterior right orbitofrontal cortical areas, the hierarchical apex of the limbic system and the locus of the attachment control system, the most complex affect- and stress-regulating mechanisms, thereby allowing the right brain to act as an integrative self-regulating system.

The early-maturing right-lateralized intersubjective system of reciprocal nonverbal communication between two right minds structurally and functionally evolves at the beginning of the human brain growth spurt, in contrast to the later-maturing right-lateralized system of regulation of emotional states that structurally and functionally evolves at the terminus of the growth spurt. Throughout the lifespan, the early-developing capacity for intersubjectivity acts as a right-lateralized nonverbal positive emotion-communicating and mutually regulating system, while the later-maturing attachment system builds upon the intersubjective system and functions as an adaptive right brain regulation system that can self-regulate and interactively regulate positive and negative emotions.

Thus I have described how interactively regulated affect transactions that maximize positive and minimize negative affect cocreate a secure attachment bond between mother and infant. The construct of interpersonal synchrony is a central communicational element of both right brain protoconversation and attachment dynamics. The evolutionary mechanism of attachment fundamentally represents the regulation of biological synchrony between and within organisms. These dual right brain processes underlie the right-lateralized subjective self's capacity for communicating with other minds (intersubjectivity), as well as for attachment, interactively regulating emotion between and within brains, minds, and bodies. Each of these are activated by the skilled clinician in the psychotherapy relationship.

The research I've cited throughout this chapter challenges and disconfirms a long-held incorrect assumption that only the left and not the right hemisphere is dominant for positive emotions. A large body of research indicates that strong positive emotions such as joy, excitement, and love are generated in the right brain. The deeply human construct of love, almost banished by science in the last century, needs to reemerge at the core of the human experience and become a central focus of scientific and clinical studies.

Chapter 8

Right-Brain-to-Right-Brain Communications: Recent Developmental and Clinical Advances

The background of sections of this chapter, first published as an invited article in the *Annals of General Psychiatry* in 2022, was my acceptance address for a Lifetime Achievement Award from Sapienza University of Rome for Recognition of Outstanding Contributions to Psychotherapy and Neuroscience, and my response to this honor, an overview of over three decades of my work on the right brain and its central role in development, psychopathogenesis, and psychotherapy to a large psychiatry audience (Schore, 2022). In the following I significantly expand that work and briefly summarize the body of my studies over time, offer some comments on what I view as the major current trends in developmental research and clinical practice, and share what I see as changes and future directions that result from the integration of neuroscience into modern attachment theory and right brain psychotherapy. As in all my work, I frequently use the literal voices of scientists and clinicians to show convergence and common language now being used to describe the underlying psychobiological mechanisms central to the change processes in mother–infant attachment and therapist–patient psychotherapy relationships.

In my first book, *Affect Regulation and the Origin of the Self*, published in 1994 (rereleased as a Classic Edition in 2016), I explored the neurobiology of human emotional development, concluding that affective processes, especially unconscious right-brain-to-right-brain nonverbal communications acting beneath levels of awareness, lie at the core of the subjective self (Schore, 1994/2016). The focus was on the early-developing right brain in bodily-based attachment dynamics and in psychotherapy. In a subsequent volume at the beginning of this century, *Affect Dysregulation and Disorders of the Self*, I discussed attachment trauma and the etiology of psychiatric and personality disorders (Schore, 2003a), and in another, *Affect Regulation and the Repair of the Self*, I focused on the psychotherapeutic treatment of the emotional right brain in early-forming self-pathologies (Schore, 2003b). By this time in the Decade of the Brain, an "emotional revolution" was occurring in psychotherapy, and clinical models that integrated psychology and biology were moving toward brain-mind-body conceptualizations. In the books, articles, and chapters that followed, I continued to offer new interdisciplinary evidence that right brain emotional processes beneath conscious awareness are operative not only in early human development and psychotherapy but across the lifespan.

In 2009, the American Psychological Association invited me to present a plenary address, "The Paradigm Shift: The Right Brain and the Relational Unconscious" (Schore, 2009a). I suggested that psychoanalysis, clinical psychology, and psychotherapy were experiencing a paradigm shift in models of change in therapeutic action, from left hemisphere verbal conscious cognition, interpretations, and insight to right brain nonverbal unconscious emotional and relational functions. As Dowds (2021) later observed,

> Classical psychoanalysis claims to work with the unconscious of the client, but it is usually the left brain of the therapist analyzing the products (dreams, images, impulses, fantasies) of the client's right brain and translating them into left hemisphere interpretation: "where id was there ego shall be." The client's feelings and experiences or their reaching out towards relationships are subjected to the cold, detached and dissecting left hemisphere of the analyst. . . . Even when the interpretation is correct and the client feels understood, their own self-discovery has been hijacked. (p. 195)

Citing my work (Schore, 2011), Håvås et al. (2015) concluded, "Verbally attuned responses have little impact on outcomes if they do not go hand-in-hand with adequately attuned nonverbal responses. In other words, *verbal responses would fall on deaf ears if nonverbal attunement is not in place* [emphasis added]" (p. 13). Only psychobiologically attuned responses have access to the patient's right hemisphere, where they can be implicitly bidirectionally communicated and regulated in therapist–patient right-brain-to-right-brain nonverbal interactions. This is not possible if, in these therapeutic moments, the clinician remains up in his or her left hemisphere.

Note that classical psychoanalysis, like classical attachment theory (as well as CBT and other left brain techniques), focuses on the conscious left hemisphere, as opposed to neurobiologically informed modern attachment theory, neuropsychoanalysis, and interpersonal neurobiology that focus on the unconscious right hemisphere. Over the entire course of his career, Freud sat behind the patient, listening to the patient's voice with his left ear, a portal to his right hemisphere (you can find a picture of Freud's couch on the internet). Freud continued to place the couch as the primary and sole physical context of psychoanalysis and never advocated seeing the patient face-to-face. After his death, two socially and culturally oriented psychoanalysts, Erich Fromm, a social-psychological theorist, and the psychiatrist Harry Stack Sullivan, who developed a theory of psychiatry based on interpersonal relationships, opposed the rigid stance of using the couch and emphasized face-to-face contact with the patient.

At about that same time, the clinical psychologist Carl Rogers, the creator of psychotherapeutic empathy, also worked face-to-face. Starting in the 1970s with the self-psychology of Heinz Kohut, who incorporated empathy into psychoanalysis, and especially in the 1990s with the onset of a truly relational emotionally focused psychoanalysis, this trend continued. This paradigm-shifting transition from classical to relational psychoanalysis, from Freud's couch, which prevents eye-to-eye contact between the psychoanalyst and the patient, to the face-to-face context of right-brain-to-right-brain psychodynamic psychotherapy, represents a transformation from a one-person intrapsychic unconscious to a two-person interpersonal unconscious. In this manner, the goal of the clinical session shifts from a left brain reasoned narrative and cognitive insight to a right brain spontaneous emotionally laden conversation.

In 2018, my colleague Paul Valent published "Paradigm Shift in Psychiatry: What May It Involve?" Citing my work, this psychodynamic psychiatrist asserts that the right hemisphere, which is invisible to the left hemisphere, "emotes, relates, intuits, attunes, divines patterns, integrates, and creates" (p. 74). He observes,

> In retrospect it appears that the organic and psychoanalytic streams in psychiatry have reflected the chasm between the different perspectives of the right and left hemispheres of the brain and the unawareness of each hemisphere of the other. *A prospective paradigm shift would incorporate knowledge of the function of both hemispheres* [emphasis added]. It would recast organic and psychoanalytic psychiatry into a new stereoscopic perspective. (p. 75)

I would add that the impact of the current paradigm shift on psychiatry would be the reestablishment of a vitalizing connection between biological psychiatry and psychodynamic psychiatry.

Toward that end, I continue to offer an expanding body of neurobiological and clinical studies indicating that the functional and structural differences between the two brain hemispheres are profound (Schore, 2019a, 2019b). A massive body of brain laterality studies describes in extraordinary detail how each cerebral hemisphere has a distinct mode of attending to the world and creates coherent, utterly different and often incompatible versions of the world, with competing priorities and values. Due to current rapid advances in neuroscience, brain asymmetry, although once controversial, is now in agreement that different dual lateralized cortical-subcortical systems exist with unique structure-function relationships (e.g., rational brain vs. emotional brain; linguistic brain vs. social brain; analytical vs. intuitive brain; explicit vs. implicit self-system; conscious vs. unconscious mind).

In his classic volume *The Right Brain and the Unconscious: Discovering the Stranger Within*, the clinical neuropsychologist Rhawn Joseph (1992) observed,

> Just as we have a conscious and an unconscious mind, as well as a right and left brain, we also have two self-images. One is consciously maintained and the other is almost wholly unconscious. The *conscious self-image* is associated with the *left half of the brain* in most people. However, *this self-image is also subject to unconscious influences*. By

contrast, the *unconscious self-image* is maintained within the *right brain* [emphasis added] mental system and is tremendously influenced by current and past experiences. . . . The two self-images . . . interact. Indeed, sometimes the conscious self-image is fashioned in reaction to unconscious feelings, traumas, and feared inadequacies that the person does not want to possess, but that nevertheless, are unconsciously maintained.

Continuing this theme, the neurologist Guido Gainotti (2005) offered an article, "Emotions, Unconscious Processes and the Right Hemisphere," where he concluded, "The right hemisphere may subserve the lower 'schematic' level (where emotions are automatically generated and experienced as 'true emotions') and the left hemisphere the higher 'conceptual' level (where emotions are consciously analyzed and submitted to intentional control)."

More recently, the neuropsychiatrist Iain McGilchrist (2015) asserts,

If what one means by consciousness is the part of the mind that brings the world into focus, makes it explicit, allows it to be formulated in language, and is aware of its own awareness, it is reasonable to link the conscious mind to activity almost all of which lies ultimately in the left hemisphere. The right hemisphere both grounds our experience of the world at the bottom end, so to speak, and makes sense of it, at the top end. . . . This hemisphere is more in touch with both affect and the body. . . . Neurological evidence supports what is called the primacy of affect and the primacy of unconscious over conscious will.

Note that these right hemispheric emotional experiences emerge bottom-up from the bodily-based lower depths of the unconscious, the origin of human nature (see Figure 2.1). And yet the right hemisphere also contains the highest structures that make meaning out of this experience, in everyday life.

Another central area of my work is in neuropsychoanalysis, the science of unconscious processes, where I contend that the right brain is the psychobiological substrate of the human unconscious mind first described by Sigmund Freud. Authors are now describing a right hemispheric dominance in nonconscious processing, concluding, "The right hemisphere has an advantage in shaping behavior with implicit attention whereas the left hemisphere plays a greater role in expressing explicit knowledge" (Chen & Hsiao, 2014). Indeed, there is now agreement that implicit processing is equated with unconscious processing (see Schore, 2019a, 2019b; McGilchrist 2021a). Similarly, Gainotti (2020) offers evidence on "the unconscious aspects of right hemisphere functioning."

In 1994, I proposed that the right brain is dominant in maintaining an unconscious cohesive, continuous, and unified sense of self (Schore, 1994/2016). I further suggested that in two-person attachment dynamics the bodily-based subjective self intersubjectively communicates its emotional states nonverbally, right brain to right brain, with another subjective self. Just as the left brain communicates its states to other left brains via conscious linguistic behaviors, so the right nonverbally communicates its unconscious self-states to other right brains that are sensitively tuned to receive these salient intersubjective emotional communications. Following this up in my 2003 volumes, I stated that in contrast to a static, deeply buried storehouse of ancient memories silenced in "infantile amnesia," contemporary psychoanalysis now refers to a "relational unconscious," whereby one unconscious mind intersubjectively communicates with another unconscious mind (Schore, 2003a, 2003b).

This model harkened back to Freud's assertions at the beginning of the 20th century, "The analyst must turn his unconscious like a receptor organ towards the transmitting unconscious of the patient . . . so the doctor's unconscious is able, from the derivatives of the unconscious which are communicated to him, to reconstruct that unconscious" (1912/1958, pp. 115–116). Three years later he observed, "It is a very remarkable thing that the *Ucs* of one human being can react upon that of another, without passing through the *Cs*" (Freud, 1915/1957). It also acknowledges the pioneering work of the Hungarian psychoanalyst Sandor Ferenczi (1926/1980, 1932/1988), "the father of intersubjectivity," who first described his concept of an intersubjective dialogue between one unconscious and another unconscious. As an example, Ferenczi (1932/1988) described an unconscious communication of loss between the therapist and patient in an intersubjective third space where "the tears of the doctor and patient mingle in a sublimated communion" (p. 65).

Indeed, there is a long tradition in psychoanalysis that conceptualizes intersubjectivity as an unconscious interaction between the unconscious mind of the clinician and the unconscious mind of a patient (Stolorow et al., 1987). Ogden (1994a) described the intersubjective experience as "the analytic third," the jointly created unconscious life of the analytic pair. Over the course of her productive career, the relational psychoanalyst Jessica Benjamin (2017) has explored the reciprocal, mutually influencing quality of interaction between individuals, which she also termed "the analytic third." She documented that the ability to engage in this kind of relationship requires the therapist to surrender to the intersubjective process, a process of "letting go into being with" another. She states that in order for this to happen, the therapist must yield to the rhythm of the other in order to share aspects of the other's subjective state. Note the previous characterization of mutual surrender as a synchronized callosal shift from the conscious left mind into the unconscious right mind.

From a neuropsychoanalytic perspective, intersubjectivity represents an emotional interaction between two brains, a dyadic, reciprocal right-brain-to-right-brain unconscious communication system between two subjective self-systems cocreating a shared affectively energized dynamic electromagnetic intersubjective field. McGilchrist (2016) observes,

> Where the left hemisphere tends to see linear chains of cause and effect, the right hemisphere sees reverberative, responsive relations in which all exists in *"betweeness"*—not the space between two entities, but the new whole that is made by their *coming together*, in which each party and the "space" *between* is taken up into *something radically new* [emphasis added]. (pp. 202–203)

I suggest this represents an interpersonal neurobiological model of Ogden's and Benjamin's analytic third.

The interpersonal neurobiological construct of an emotion-communicating relational unconscious is the most radical transformation of Freud's psychoanalytic theory. Updated reformulations of the unconscious have shifted from an intrapsychic unconscious that expresses itself only in dreams at night to an interpersonal relational unconscious, in which the unconscious mind of one communicates and shares its affective states with the unconscious mind of another and is omnipresent in everyday life. In parallel writings to my own, my colleague Karlen Lyons-Ruth (1999) offered a "two-person unconscious," asserting, "Most relational transactions rely heavily on a substrate of affective cues that give an evaluative valence or direction to each relational communication. These occur at an implicit level of *rapid cueing and response* . . . too rapidly for simultaneous verbal transaction and conscious reflection." I would add that these right-brain-to-right-brain communications emerge in early infancy, shaping the structural and functional development of the unconscious mind's right brain survival functions. Indeed, implicit right-brain-to-right-brain intersubjective nonverbal communications are expressed in attachment dynamics at unconscious levels throughout life.

Right-Brain-to-Right-Brain Intersubjective Communications and Interpersonal Synchrony in Early Human Development

At the core of my developmental work on intersubjectivity and attachment is the central principle of interpersonal neurobiology: The self-organization of the developing brain occurs in the context of a relationship with another self, another brain (Schore, 2003a). Utilizing an interdisciplinary perspective, regulation theory models the underlying mechanisms by which the structure and function of the mind and brain are shaped by early experiences, especially emotional experiences, as well as the relational mechanisms by which communicating brains intersubjectively synchronize, align, and couple their neural activities with other brains. There is now agreement that the process of interpersonal synchrony acts as a primal social bonding mechanism, and that early synchronous shared social interactions are the foundation of the human experience (Schore, 1994/2016, 2012, 2019a).

In classic research, Colwyn Trevarthen (1993) documented the early origins of human intersubjectivity at two to three months, when infants are ready to engage in behavioral turn-taking and expect social contingency and predictable back-and-forth interactivity. He observed visual (mutual gaze), auditory, and tactile playful, affectionate emotional communications in which the intuitive mother and her infant, intently looking and listening to each other, bidirectionally synchronize and mutually regulate their emotional states (see Figure 7.1). The collaborative emotional transactions of these protoconversations trigger interpersonal resonance within the emotionally communicating dyad, thus generating the intercoordination of synchronized and thereby shared positive affective brain states. But his model also describes how the intrinsic regulators of human brain growth in a child are specifically adapted to be coupled, by emotional communication, to the regulators of adult brains.

In a recent article on the interpersonal neurobiology of intersubjectivity, I cited a body of brain asymmetry studies to argue that Trevarthen's synchronized intersubjective protoconversations represent rapid, reciprocal, bidirectional visual-facial, auditory-prosodic, and tactile-gestural right-brain-to-right-brain implicit nonverbal communications between the mother and her developing infant (Schore, 2021a). I emphasized the essential functions of the right TPJ in the posterior sensory areas of the developing right hemisphere sending, receiving, and integrating these emotionally charged imagistic nonverbal communications. The right TPJ, a central hub of the right-lateralized social brain, integrates input from visual, auditory, somesthetic, autonomic, and emotional limbic areas. For the rest of the lifespan, this system is a pivotal locus in self-functions: face and voice processing, perceptual awareness, collaborative social interactions, and the representation of subjective emotional experience.

Soon after, the neurologist Kaisa Hartikainen (2021), in "Emotion-Attention Interaction in the Right Hemisphere," stated,

> The right TPJ has been suggested to be a central hub for . . . non-verbal emotional communication and interaction between a caregiver and an infant (Schore, 2021a). This caregiver–infant pre-verbal prosodic, gestural, and facial emotional expression provides a basis for the development of attachment. . . . Successful emotional communication and downregulation of infant's negative emotions relies on right hemispheric functions of both the caregiver and infant.

She further states that the right TPJ is also involved in "emotional arousal linked with positive emotion" (Schore, 2021a) and in "the synchronization between the brains of two people."

In classic writings, John Bowlby (1969) proposed that attachment communications are accompanied by the strongest of feelings and emotions and, like Trevarthen, suggested they occur within a context of facial expression, tone of voice, and posture. A large body of research supports what de Heering and Rossion (2015) called "rapid categorization of natural face images in the infant right hemisphere." In an overview of research on the laterality of the "human social brain," Brancucci and colleagues (2009) concluded, "The neural substrates of the perception of voices, faces, gestures, smells, and pheromones, as evidenced by modern neuroimaging techniques, are characterized by a general right-hemispheric functional asymmetry."

Indeed, the essential task of the first two years of life is the cocreation of an intersubjective right-brain-to-right-brain attachment bond of emotional communication and interactive regulation between the infant and primary caregiver. Secure attachment occurs via the mother's attention and implicit background presence of synchronized attunement, recognition, and regulation, not of the infant's voluntary behavior, but with moment-to-moment alterations of right brain autonomic involuntary emotional arousal, the physiological dimension of the child's affective state. Hartikainen (2021) observes a central role of the right hemisphere in attention, emotion, and arousal.

The research of Manini et al.'s (2013) laboratory reports that synchronization of the mother's responses to infant signals in their dyadic interaction is a central aspect of sensitive parenting, because it directly relates to the promptness of the mother's response and her adaptation moment by moment to the child's emotional state. This embodied and prereflective sensitivity allows the mother to immediately recognize any shift in the child's emotional needs in a timely fashion, as well as to promptly soothe the child when distressed. These synchronized interactions enable the psychobiologically attuned mother and child to become sensitive to each other's physiology and behavior, and thereby cocreate the formation of a unique familiar bond between them. They conclude that the autonomic nervous system represents an elementary mechanism supporting emotional synchrony between mother and infant.

In support of this model, Wass et al. (2019) observed that parents mimic and influence their infant's autonomic activity through dynamic affective state matching (synchrony). They documented that alterations in infant arousal lead to autonomic changes in the parent, and that moments when the adult showed greater autonomic reactivity were associated with faster infant quieting. But the mother is not just downregulating negative states—she also is upregulating positive states. Killeen and Teti (2012) reported, the "greater relative right frontal activation in response to seeing one's own infant is related to maternal negative affect matching during times of infant distress, and greater perceived intensity of infant joy during times of joy." Secure attachment thus enhances the child's capacity to play.

That said, both research and clinical evidence indicate that the primary caregiver is not always attuned, that there are frequent moments of stressful misattunement in the dyad, ruptures of the attachment bond. A major attachment process is expressed in interactive repair following misattunement, in which the caregiver who induces a stress response in a timely fashion spontaneously reinvokes a reattunement and regulates the infant's negatively charged emotional arousal (Schore, 1994/2016, 2012). It has long been established that stress is defined as an asynchrony in an interactional sequence, and thus "a period of synchrony, following the period of stress, provides a 'recovery' period" (Chapple, 1970, p. 631). It also generates trust in the infant that the caregiver will be emotionally available at times of stress. With respect to the patient-therapist relationship, this repair has been described as "messy" (Tronick, 2004), an ongoing flow of missteps, matches, tries, retries, and matchups. Synchronized rupture and repair of the emotional attachment bond between the patient and therapist is an essential interpersonal neurobiological mechanism of the treatment (Schore, 1994/2016, 2003b, 2012, 2019b). Rupture repair is common in secure but not insecure avoidant, insecure resistant, or especially disorganized attachment mother–infant dyads.

In 2008 my wife Judith and I published an article, "Modern Attachment Theory," where we suggested a body of experimental and clinical data on how affective bodily-based processes are nonconsciously interactively regulated had shifted attachment theory to a regulation theory (Schore & Schore, 2008). Recall, I use the term *regulation theory* in order to explicitly denote that I am offering a theory, a systematic exposition of the general principles of a science. At the core of the theory, the developmental process of intersubjectivity represents the right-brain-to-right-brain communication of emotion, while attachment represents the right brain interactive regulation of states of affective arousal.

Thus, the evolutionary mechanism of attachment represents the regulation of biological synchrony between and within organisms. It is accessed by the secure mother to implicitly track and regulate the infant's emotional arousal in a conversation between limbic systems. A central tenet of the theory dictates that the structural organization of attachment circuits self-organizes in an early critical period of growth of the emotional right brain from the last trimester of pregnancy through the first and second until the beginning of the third year, and that the infant's anterior right orbitofrontal (ventromedial) cortex, the apex of the limbic system, matures over this period. This right-lateralized system acts as an attachment control system of effortless, implicit, subliminal affect regulation.

Recall, in previous chapters I cited extant research demonstrating that the right hemisphere shows an earlier maturation than the left and is in a critical period of growth over the prenatal and postnatal stages of human development (e.g., Schore, 1994/2016; Chiron et al., 1997; Matsuzawa et al., 2001; Gupta et al., 2005; Sun et al., 2005, Mento et al., 2010; Ratnarajah et al., 2013). Eight large-scale lateralization studies done around the world have now been published that directly support my model of the early structural and functional maturation of the right brain that I first proposed 30 years ago in my 1994 volume.

In Japan, Tanaka et al. (2012) offered an MRI study of the development of the frontal and temporal lobes beginning at one month to 25 years. With respect to "rapid and dynamic" early brain development over the first three years, they reported that both regions displayed "significant rightward asymmetry," regardless of sex. The right frontal and temporal lobes showed a greater increase in volume than the left for the first several years, with this tendency reversed at around six years of age. As compared to the right hemisphere, the peak age of left hemisphere volume occurred later by about 0.5–0.8 years for the frontal lobe and 1–2 years for the temporal lobe. These authors concluded, "Brain developmental trajectories differ depending on brain region, sex and brain hemisphere. Gender-related factors such as sex hormones and functional laterality may affect brain development" (p. 477). These findings are in accord with my own laterality studies, in which I documented more rapid development of the right hemisphere in females and slower maturation in males over the first three years (Schore, 2017a).

One year later in the United States, Lin et al. (2013) asserted that "understanding the evolution of regional hemispheric asymmetries in the early stages of life is essential to the advancement of developmental neuroscience" (p. 339). Using a near-infrared spectroscopy study to study oxygen metabolism in the temporal and parietal regions of premature and full-term newborns, they reported, "Most parameters were significantly greater in the right hemisphere than in the left" (p. 339). They showed that at birth, oxygen metabolism is highest in the temporal and parietal primary sensory regions, as opposed to a later increase in the frontal cortex between 6 and 12 months. Note that functional near-infrared spectroscopy (fNIRS) alone can rapidly identify markers of typical and atypical cortical development at birth (and throughout the lifespan) with good spatial localization, unlike any other neuroimaging technique.

In order to investigate right hemisphere communications within mutual gaze interactions in seven-month infants, in Japan Urakawa et al. (2015) reported an fNIRS study of social interactive play in the journal *Brain Topography*. During the recording, the infants sat on their mother's lap looking at a young woman who performed a "peek-a-boo" experiment, in which both visual and auditory infant-directed speech was presented (see Chapter 7). The results indicated that during direct gaze but not averted gaze the infant fixated on eye regions for a longer duration, and that a partner's direct gaze shifted an infant's attention to the partner's eyes for interactive communication. The noninvasive optical neuroimaging technique of fNIRS localized hemodynamic activity in the infant's medial prefrontal and right hemispheric prefrontal cortex. The authors pointed out that these data support other studies showing that the anterior part of the medial prefrontal cortex is activated when interpreting social signals and emotional processing (Parise & Csibra, 2013), while the right hemisphere is involved in eye gaze and facial expression, not only in adults (Tong et al., 2000) but also in infants (Grossmann et al., 2008; Nakato et al., 2009). These early right brain functions in mutual gaze thus serve as a primary foundation of the later development of social skills.

In 2018, Hakuno and her colleagues in Japan and the UK published a multinational study, "Optical Imaging During Toddlerhood: Brain Responses During Naturalistic Social Interactions" in the journal *Neurophotonics*. In order to investigate the early development of the social brain and the ability to interact and communicate with others, these authors used NIRS, "an ideal imaging technique for studying infants in more ecologically valid settings." They studied 12- to 14-month-old toddlers while they were interacting with adults in two naturalistic social scenarios—singing nursey rhymes with gestures or reading a picture book. In the interaction condition, the infants viewed a female experimenter singing infant-directed nursery rhymes, with accompanying gestures such as a "peek-a-boo" with direct gaze and a smiling, wide-eyed, positive emotional face. The custom-built lightweight fNIRS headgear consisted of an array over the infant's right hemispheric temporal lobe that delivers and detects near-infrared light into the infant's head, and thus measurements were restricted to the right hemisphere. During these real-life interactions, the researchers observed cortical activation in the right superior temporal sulcus (fusiform gyrus) and the right TPJ of the right-lateralized social brain, areas specialized in infants for processing social signals that are sensitive to communications with others.

Two years later in 2020, Lemaître and his colleagues in France published a neuroimaging MRI study of infant brain maturation over the first year in the journal *Cerebral Cortex*, where they reported:

> Our study shows for the first time the dynamics of local rest functional brain maturation throughout the first year of life using a noninvasive imaging method. Global rest cerebral blood flow increased significantly from 3 to 12 months of age and this increase was more pronounced in the right than in the left hemisphere. . . . This agrees with previous studies that showed greater right than left rest CBF for these regions at birth (Lin et al. 2013) and from 1 to 3 years old (Chiron et al. 1997), supporting the hypothesis that the right hemisphere functionally matures earlier than the left. (p. 1779)

A hyperscanning EEG study in *Scientific Advances* in 2021 from Feldman's lab in Israel documented right-lateralized interbrain synchronization in face-to-face communication and free interaction between mothers and their 7- to 12-month-old infants. They observed,

> Across . . . interacting partners, adult-infant brain-to-brain synchrony implicated the early-maturing right brain. . . . Neural synchrony connected regions in the right hemisphere in both the adult's and infant's brains. The right hemisphere in humans and other mammals sustains functions critical for survival, such as visuospatial attention, interpretation of social information, and emotional processes. The "right hemisphere hypothesis," proposed nearly 50 years ago (Gainotti, 1972), posits a general dominance of the right hemisphere for all emotions. . . . Because of its critical role in survival-related functions and nonverbal communication, right hemisphere dominance is thought to

have appeared early in animal evolution and to mature early in human ontogeny; right hemisphere dominance is found at birth and persists throughout the first 3 years of life. (Endevelt-Shapira et al., 2021, p. 6)

Recall that in Chapter 1, I pointed out that the current primary developmental neuroimaging research design is having the infant respond to a cognitive task presented by the experimenter, while the infant is sitting on the mother's lap, and thereby not in face-to-face interaction with her. In this hyperscanning study, the seven-month-old infant and mother were face-to-face (vs. back-to-back) and interacting, though not in physical contact. They documented an interbrain synchrony between the right central area of the mother and the right occipital temporal area of the infant, what I have termed a right-lateralized interbrain synchronization. The authors noted that "neural synchrony connected regions in the right hemisphere in both the adult's and infant's brains." They concluded that this mother–infant right-brain-to-right-brain synchronization may enhance the salience of social cues, increase the infant's social motivation, and externally regulate the infant's maturing brain and tune it to living in a social world (Endevelt-Shapira et al., 2021).

In the most comprehensive study to date on early right brain development, Bosch-Bayard and colleagues (2022) in Mexico offered a study in *NeuroImage*, "EEG Effective Connectivity During the First Year of Life Mirrors Brain Synaptogenesis, Myelination, and Early Right Hemisphere Predominance." These authors measured the connectivity of different areas of the infant brain at 2–3, 5–8, and 8–12 months, and showed an asymmetric lateralized increase in specifically the right and not left hemisphere. They concluded,

The right hemisphere develops first in the ontogenetic development of the brain. . . . The human brain is right hemisphere predominant during the preverbal epoch in infants . . . and lasts during the first three years of life (Schore, 2000b). The right hemisphere is understood as an executive regulatory system of the emotional brain involved in inhibitory control. In particular, the right orbital prefrontal region acts as an executive control for the entire right brain (Schore, 2000b). The right predominance starts shifting to the left hemisphere by the age of 3 years. (pp. 7–8)

I would add that until age three, the critical period of rapid exponential growth and lateralization of the infant/toddler's early-developing right hemisphere is dependent upon the implicit safe and trusting emotional interactions generated in the mother–infant attachment relationship (Schore, 2000b).

As opposed to optimal early development, infant brain research documents that infants born prematurely with low birth weight show deficits in specific brain areas that lead to psychosocial problems and difficulties in early socioemotional relations, including an inability to engage caregivers in attachment communications via eye contact, vocalizations, or facial expression, as well as later psychiatric disorders such as ADHD, conduct, and communication disorders (Weiss, 2005). The earliest prenatal intervention, the neonatal intensive care unit (NICU), is now seen as a context for positive maternal-infant interactions that can maximize neurodevelopmental outcomes in premature infants. In this context, nurses can empower mothers to overcome the stressors in the NICU, promote sensitive interactions between mothers and their vulnerable infants, facilitate the development of specifically their premature infant's right brains, and thereby the quality of the attachment and later capacities for emotion regulation. For much more on this, I refer the reader to the article of Weber et al. (2012) in the journal *Biological Research for Nursing*, "Schore's Regulation Theory: Maternal-Infant Interaction in the NICU as a Mechanism for Reducing the Effects of Allostatic Load on Neurodevelopment in Premature Infants."

Furthermore, the early postnatal intervention of skin-to-skin kangaroo mother care (KMC) with preterm infants has been shown to lower mortality (Conde-Agudelo et al., 2011). Bembich and his Italian colleagues (2022) reported a NIRS study of very preterm newborns (gestational age 24–32 weeks) receiving skin-to-skin KMC, where the newborn is placed on the maternal chest in an upright position. In the first 30 minutes of kangaroo care, a cortical activation lateralized to the right hemisphere is seen in the neonate's right motor and primary somatosensory cortex (see Figure 2.2). The authors concluded,

This hemisphere is dominant in human early development, and a biological control system, involved in the regulation of attachment function, was found to expand in the right hemisphere (Schore, 2000). The kangaroo maternal care experience, therefore, might activate such attachment control system, at least in its cortical sensorimotor portion, already before the gestational term. . . . The right hemisphere has also been associated with spatial processing of haptic information (Gonzalez et al., 2018). Such an aspect, in turn, may be associated with the sense of touch, which is an important part of the KMC experience. (p. 8)

These authors suggest that KMC improves the oxygen supply to regions of the right hemisphere and that it should be considered a neuromodulatory intervention in preterm infants between 30 and 36 weeks of gestation. Toward that end, they cite research showing KMC induces an accelerated neurophysiological maturation in the neonate brain (Kaffashi et al., 2013), that this increase is mediated by autonomic nervous system modulation (Sehgal et al., 2020), and that it has a protective effect on young adults born preterm (Charpak et al., 2022). It also sets the stage for optimal right-brain-to-right-brain intersubjective communications at two to three months. In other words, KMC is a powerful early intervention that optimally shapes the future development of the early-evolving right hemisphere and thereby improves the lives of countless individuals worldwide born preterm and low birth weight.

In total, these studies across a variety of Eastern and Western cultures, in addition to the earlier research cited in my previous chapters and books, definitively demonstrate the critical role of the right hemisphere in the first two years of human life that I first described in my 1994 volume. Early interventions optimizing right brain functions can prevent future suffering in more human beings. This laterality information needs to be incorporated into not only the mental health field but also mainstream developmental psychology, classical attachment theory, and pediatrics, as well as preventive psychiatry.

Recall that the mother–infant attachment relationship impacts the developing, malleable right brain, for better or worse. It can either facilitate a healthy resilience to stress or create a vulnerability to characterological affect dysregulation and deficits in social relationships, and thereby later psychopathology. In the former, interactively regulated attachment histories are imprinted into developing right cortical-subcortical circuits in implicit-procedural memory, thereby generating a secure internal working model of attachment that encodes efficient strategies of affect regulation that nonconsciously guide the individual through interpersonal relational contexts. These adaptive capacities are central to the dual processes of self-regulation: interactive regulation, the ability to flexibly regulate, communicate, and share a variety of positive and negative emotional states with other humans in interconnected contexts; and autoregulation, which occurs apart from other humans in autonomous contexts.

As opposed to a secure attachment, in an early right brain context of insecure attachments the primary caregiver frequently misattunes and fails to coordinate, synchronize, and repair the infant's emotional states. In essence, insecure avoidant deactivating attachment strategies can only autoregulate and not interactively regulate emotional stress, while insecure anxious hyperactivating strategies are biased to interactively regulate and not autoregulate emotional stress. Under stress, disorganized-disoriented attachments can do neither. In the latter, what I have termed relational trauma, chronic attachment trauma, during a right brain critical period that results from repeated and prolonged exposure to highly dysregulated early relational and emotional experiences without repair, induces disorganized-insecure attachments that imprint a physiological reactivity and susceptibility to early-developing disorders of affect regulation. Thus both secure and insecure preverbal attachment dynamics are imprinted in the early-developing emotional right brain, before left hemispheric maturation.

With respect to early-forming unconscious nonverbal right brain and later-forming left brain conscious verbal representations of the self, 50 years ago John Bowlby (1973), the creator of attachment theory, suggested,

> When multiple models of a single figure are operative they are likely to differ in regard to their origin, their dominance and the extent to which the subject is aware of them. In a person *suffering* from an emotional disturbance, it is common to find that the model that has had greatest influence on his feelings and behavior, is one developed during his early years and is constructed along fairly *primitive* lines, but that the person may be relatively unaware of while simultaneously there is operating within him a second, and perhaps radically incompatible model that developed later, that is much more sophisticated, and that the person is more clearly aware of and he may mistakenly assume to be dominant.

Modern attachment theory offers an unconscious right brain preverbal model of implicit "primitive" emotional attachment dynamics and the early origin of human nature, while classical, academic attachment theory describes the explicit conscious behavioral-cognitive functions of the later-forming verbal left brain. The *Oxford English Dictionary* defines *primitive* as "of or pertaining to the first age, period, or stage; early, ancient," and therefore to the evolutionary foundations of the human experience. Earlier I cited Freud's (1914-1916/1957) observation, "The primitive stages can always be re-established," and asserted that the right brain primitive mind represents the origin and depth of human nature. As every chapter in this book has shown, a deeper understanding of this "primitive" regulatory system directly bears upon my questions posed in the first paragraph of this book: How does prolonged psychobiological stress induce pain and suffering in human beings? Why do some of us suffer more than others? And how can we enhance our coping abilities, reduce this suffering, and increase the joy of living in more members of our communities?

Further Clinical Applications of the Right-Brain-to-Right-Brain Model in Psychotherapy

The right brain attachment dynamic is a central focus of regulation theory, and affect dysregulation plays a critical role in both the symptomatology and treatment of all psychiatric and personality disorders. In my studies, I offer interdisciplinary and clinical evidence indicating that the coconstructed psychotherapy relationship itself plays a major role in symptom-reducing and growth-promoting treatment, and that the right hemisphere is dominant in psychotherapy (Schore, 2012, 2019b). Effective clinical work with "primitive" nonverbal emotional attachment dynamics of the first foundational years of life focuses not on verbal cognitive insight but on the formation of a nonverbal emotion-communicating and regulating bond between the patient and the empathic clinician.

This conceptualization attends to two essential problems—how do we work directly with the patient's and our own emotions, and how do we access "primitive" nonverbal intersubjective emotional communications within the psychotherapy session? In any session, the empathic therapist is consciously, explicitly attending to the patient's verbalizations in order to objectively diagnose and rationalize his or her dysregulating symptomatology. However, the psychotherapist is also intersubjectively listening and interacting at another level, an experience-near subjective level, and implicitly tracking and synchronizing with the patient's moment-to-moment nonverbal bodily-based emotional communications at levels beneath the words.

It is well established that unconscious processing of emotional information is mainly subsumed by a right hemisphere subcortical route, and that unconscious emotional memories and motivations are stored in the right hemisphere. Neuroscientists are now describing "the left hemisphere's relatively limited capacity to understand human motivation and feeling," as opposed to the right hemisphere's "understanding the motivation of an action" (McGilchrist, 2021a, p. 210). Furthermore, Rotenberg and Weinberg (1999) described the limitations of left hemispheric words, especially in describing subjective affective experiences:

> Words can name emotions, but they cannot convey the essence of emotional experience in its wholeness and subtlety. The words fail. Emotions, incessantly, transform themselves into one another. This continuous transformation is the essence of personal experience. Only the right hemisphere, can sustain emotional experience in its uniqueness, inner complexity, and elusiveness.

In subsequent writings, Rotenberg (1995) concluded that "the left hemisphere constructs a convenient but simplified model of reality." According to Damasio (1999), "The left cerebral hemisphere of humans is prone to fabricating verbal narratives that do not necessarily accord with the truth."

Daniel Stern (1985) posed the essential question, "How can you get inside of other people's subjective experience and then let them know that you have arrived there, without using words?" (p. 138). Recall Freud's (1913/1958) dictum, "The therapist must surrender himself to his own unconscious." In order for this to happen, the empathic psychotherapist must have access to a psychotherapeutic process that can shift out of the left and surrender to the right hemisphere in order to receive the patient's intersubjective affective and motivational states, including the patient's unconscious implicit-procedural autobiographical memories of early attachment experiences stored in the right temporal lobe. This allows receiving and sending right-brain-to-right-brain subjective emotional communications, and thereby sharing an emotional state, especially in transference-countertransference interactions.

This process, an unconscious communication that allows the clinician to know the patient "from the inside out" (Bromberg, 1991), represents a transient reversal of dominance from the later-developing conscious left mind to the early-developing unconscious right mind. Relational psychoanalysts are now asserting that regression, the process of returning or a tendency to return to an earlier stage of development, enables "the emergence of the patient's inner world and his or her way of being in the world" (Grossmark, 2012). He states that in this regression, the clinician offers "the very deepest engagement that is humanly possible" (p. 634).

Ghent (1990) asserts that the clinician "surrenders" or "lets go" into the adaptive regression. This is a spontaneous and not a voluntary activity, and it does not necessarily require another person's presence, "except possibly as a guide." Indeed, it allows for a context in which left hemispheric "secondary processes have receded from consciousness," thereby facilitating an experience of being 'in the moment' and 'totally in the present'" (p. 111). Furthermore, the callosal shift of hemisphericity, of surrendering out the left and into the right, instantiates a regression, described as a "letting down of defensive barriers" that potentially allows for "a liberation and expansion of the self" (Ghent, 1990, p. 108).

In his book *The Neuroscience of Psychotherapy: Healing the Social Brain*, my colleague Lou Cozolino (2010) asserts, "The therapist's ability to traverse the callosal bridge between his or her own right and left hemispheres serves as a model and guide for the client" (pp. 110–111). As a result of this topographic shift, the clinician can now act as a guide in the mutual therapeutic journey into the patient's right-lateralized unconscious mind. Dan Hill (2024) offers an evocative clinical description of the clinician acting as an implicit guide of the patient's right hemispheric internal world in the burgeoning therapeutic relationship:

> I can assume the role of guide once the patient has begun to speak their mind spontaneously. . . . Once spontaneous speaking starts, I speak less and less. I listen in as attuned a way as possible, sharing the patient's subjective experience. The attunement generates a flow that I think twice about interrupting. This is not to say I don't communicate, but that the communication is implicit-non-verbal. I convey intense interest. The felt resonances and sense of closeness coming from the attunement mark that I am sharing my patients' consciousness, that I recognize and

have entered their subjective world. . . . I believe that my ongoing affect attunement induces spontaneous speech.

Working with adults, Gnaulati (2021) describes this clinical surrender and regression into right brain unconscious communications:

Empathically immersed psychotherapists *give themselves over to the organically unfolding interaction* [emphasis added], unconsciously and preconsciously adapting their responses to make them assimilable for a given client. Synchronized, well-timed nods, frowns, grunts, grimaces, leg folds, and chin rubs emotionally lubricate and embolden client disclosures. Optimally, there is abundant barely conscious facial dialoguing that leaves the client feeling the therapist is quietly familiar with what is being revealed, inviting further disclosure. Sometimes empathic responses by the psychotherapist encompass short phrases or poignant idiomatic offerings inserted into the client's flow of speech to pithily sum up what the client feels. (p. 595)

In describing his use of regression in treating disturbances from the earliest years, Rentoul (2010) suggests,

On the part of the therapee, regression happens spontaneously. On the part of the therapist, I do not know whether the ability to allow it can be learned, or whether it depends on having a particular personality. I certainly found that I was drawn into it by my own individual background, and that I was able to understand and tolerate the more extensive extreme demands that the work put upon me by the fact that in the other person's behavior I could recognize my own. (p. 64)

According to Frayn (1990), regressive transferences can be observed on an intermittent or attenuated basis in every course of intensive, deep psychotherapy.

The processes of surrender and regression into the unconscious are essential in not only adult but also child psychotherapy. Children, like all humans, have an unconscious mind located in the right brain, as well as unconscious defenses that blot out painful, dysregulating affective self-states. A cardinal therapeutic principle states that therapy should match the developmental level of the patient. The empathic child therapist's inter-personal synchrony allows the clinician to meet the child at his or her emotional relational level in order to form an optimal working alliance. The synchronized left-right shift of surrender in a mutual regression in turn enables the child worker to make emotional contact with the patient's moment-to-moment changes in right brain affective self-states and also to access her own right brain creativity and imagination during joint regressions of mutual play.

Frankel (1998) observes that in this therapeutic context,

> The therapist's willingness to regress along with the child—to let new and surprising areas of himself into the play—and especially his willingness and ability to let the child largely control the pace and content of the mutual regression, help the child to feel safe to open areas of himself to the therapist. The particular aspects of himself that the therapist brings to the play are used by the child as a pivot to help the child engage new areas of himself. . . . Each self-state that is expressed by each of us is highly responsive to self-states of the other. The emergence and articulation of self-states in each of us is constantly regulated by both of us in a continuous, nonverbal process of negotiation. (p. 178)

An adaptive clinical mutual regression thus involves a playful synchronized surrender of the child patient along with the therapist, who is acting as an implicit guide into the deeper early unconscious realm, where both are nonverbally communicating gestures, facial expressions, and prosodic vocal expressions, right brain to right brain.

Another renowned child psychotherapist, Kenneth Barish (2020), writes on the essential role of play in contemporary child psychotherapy:

> We play with children for many reasons—to establish rapport and engage a child in treatment, to facilitate the expressions of feelings, and to promote children's ego development and social maturity. Our enthusiastic play also supports a child's willingness to participate in collaborative plans to arrest vicious cycles of negative family interactions. Together these therapeutic processes help restore and strengthen affirming responsiveness between parents and children, an essential

condition for a *child's emotional health* and, arguably, *the most lasting benefit of all our therapeutic efforts* [emphasis added]. (p. 156)

We now know that emotional health involves implicit, subliminal affect regulation, which occurs in rapid bidirectional right-brain-to-right-brain nonverbal communications, created in human infancy and continuing in the next stages of emotional development, childhood, and then adolescence. Directly alluding to these the master child clinician Graham Music (2023) offers case material in working with these latter two clinical populations. Citing my work (Schore, 1994/2016) and McGilchrist's (2009, 2021a, 2021b) on the right brain, he asserts, "I increasingly have felt the need for a receptivity to messages sent out by our own and others' nervous systems, something I have termed *'nervous system whispering.'* Nervous systems talk to each other, albeit out of consciousness, and *the body can be considered another royal road to the unconscious* [emphasis added]" (p. 6). He states that when mothers and babies, children, and adolescents enjoy each other, their brain waves and heartbeats are "in sync" and that this healthy "electrical connection" is seen in good therapist–patient and teacher–pupil relationships.

Music (2023) emphasizes the importance of both psyche and soma, mind and body in contemporary child psychotherapy. As a supervisor of child therapists, he emphasizes an enhanced awareness of the bodily aspect of the clinician's somatic countertransference and provides an illustration of the interaction through physically acting the part of the patient. He notes, "This came about because too often I heard case descriptions which conveyed little sense of the tone of voice or gestural feel, and without these I found it much harder to make sense of those sessions" (p. 11). Furthermore, he underscores the heightened affective meaning of moments in the session when the child lets herself into what Balint (1968) and Guntrip (1969) described as a regression.

Toward that end, Winnicott's understanding of early development was based on his extensive pediatric work, especially his experience with "severely regressed patients" and soul-searching of his own personal condition (Rodman, 2003). In 1955 he stressed the clinical importance of a regression to the point of environmental failure so that emotion could be (re)experienced and not defended against (Winnicott, 1955). Offering case material, Music (2023) observes moments of "mutual resonance and synchrony." In this therapeutic context, "When we feel safe and held . . . we can let go into what Winnicott calls 'going-on-being,' an experience of deep ease and relaxation, which is very different from the edgy over-alert 'doing' and active 'thinking' so common in today's world" (p. 1). Note the description of a left-to-right shift, in both the child and the therapist, especially as the child lets go of defenses enough to bear feelings she had been avoiding, that leads to safety and trust in exploring dark, difficult places.

Furthermore, in all cases—child, adolescent, and adult—this left-right hemispheric shift allows the empathic clinician to perceptually receive what is outside conscious awareness into what is being nonverbally emotionally communicated, right brain to right brain, between them. In order to perceptually (and not cognitively) receive and synchronize with these nonverbal communications, the empathic clinician intuitively transitions into the right hemisphere, which is "more perceptually intelligent than the left" (Corballis, 2003, p. 168). In this open, receptive state of mind, the therapist listens with right brain wide-ranging attention, reverie, and intuition directly to the implicit changes in emotional state of the patient's bodily-based right brain. In this manner, relational, affectively focused infant, child, adolescent, and adult psychotherapy can positively facilitate the intrinsic plasticity of the right brain.

As opposed to the classical approach of listening to the patient's verbal outputs, more and more emotionally focused clinicians are now following the affect, wherever it may lead, and listening and interacting with the preverbal physiological expressions of the earliest unconscious levels of the personality. This type of deep psychobiological listening to the early bodily-based unconscious requires a regression from the therapist's left mind to his or her right mind (for more on regression, see Chapters 3 and 4 in Schore, 2019b). The clinician's adaptive regression from left brain explicit verbal communication to right brain implicit nonverbal communication lies at the core of my therapeutic model of how a shift from the analytical left to the intuitive right brain allows listening and responding to the emotional psychophysiology of the patient's unconscious.

Note the commonality of affect regulation psychotherapy in child, adolescent, and adult treatment. In all, the receptive clinician enters a listening state of evenly suspended attention. In this quiet alert state of autonomic balance, the clinician can subjectively attend to barely perceptible cues that signal a change in state in both the patient and herself, and to intersubjectively detect the patient's nonverbal behaviors and shifts in affects. As I have described in previous chapters, the synchronized matching of the musical rhythmic crescendos and decrescendos of changes in the patient's affective arousal enables the empathic psychobiologically attuned therapist to enter into and share the patient's subjective, bodily-based feeling state.

Hess (2019) offers a brief characterization of this synchronized dynamic intersubjective context:

> Neuropsychologist Allan Schore (2014) describes psychotherapy as a dance, a synchronicity of mind and body that occurs between therapist and client. His description of the psychobiologically attuned clinician recognizes the intricacy and inextricable entanglement between human biological processes, unique experience, and mental life. Schore paints an evocative image of psychotherapy as an arena for intimate authentic, and unique encounter between the client and the therapist. However, Schore's dance metaphor is not merely a romantic notion; the assertions contained within are truisms supported by a larger scientific body of evidence.

This interpersonal neurobiological mechanism allows the clinician to synchronize with and thereby emotionally recognize, intersubjectively share, and interactively regulate the patient, which in turn enables the patient's right brain subjective self to emotionally experience feeling felt by the therapist (Schore, 1994/2016, 2012, 2019a). This "feeling felt" subjective experience is evidence that a right-brain-to-right-brain intersubjective connection has been made between the patient and empathic therapist. As a result of this moment-by-moment state matching, both partners increase their degree of engagement. In this manner, the emergent therapeutic intersubjective conversation between two aligned, coupled right hemispheres initiates a right-lateralized interbrain synchronization between the patient's and the therapist's nonverbal systems.

In his pioneering volume *Reaching the Affect*, Emmanuel Hammer (1990) describes a therapeutic synchronized mutual regression:

> My mental posture, like my physical posture, is not one of leaning forward to catch the clues, but of leaning back to let the mood, the

atmosphere, come to me—to hear the meaning between the lines, to *listen for the music behind the words*. As one *gives oneself to being carried along* by the affective cadence of the patient's session, one may sense its *tone* and subtleties. By being more *open* in this manner, to resonating to the patient, I find pictures forming in my *creative* zones; an *image* crystallizes, reflecting the patient's experience. I have had the sense, at such times, that at the moments when I would pick up some image of the patient's experience, he was particularly ripe for receiving my perceptions, just as I was for receiving his. An empathic channel appeared to be established which carried his state or emotion my way via a kind of *affective "wireless." This channel, in turn, carried my image back* to him, as he stood *open in a special kind of receptivity* [emphasis added]. (pp. 99–100)

Note that the right-brain-to-right-brain communication is bidirectional, reciprocal, and synchronized, and that right brain activity is expressed in imagery (Gabel, 1988). This image may be negatively or positively valenced, such as falling into an abyss (hopelessness and depression) or soaring, or seeing a sunrise (hopeful). In this reciprocal affective communication, the empathic clinician intuitively perceives the patient's bodily-based affects and voice tone, and both members of the therapeutic dyad are synchronously sharing an unconscious communication of an implicit creative perceptual state of "openness to experience" (McCrae & Costa, 1997).

In this intersubjective dialogue, the psychobiologically attuned, intuitive clinician, from the first point of contact in the first session is learning the nonverbal moment-to-moment rhythmic structures of the client's internal states and is relatively flexibly and fluidly modifying her own behavior to synchronize with that structure, thereby cocreating a growth-facilitating context for the organization of a right-brain-to-right-brain emotional communication system. Within the burgeoning therapeutic alliance, the emotional attachment bond between the therapist and client is strengthened over time. Across the treatment, the sensitive, empathic clinician's monitoring of unconscious process rather than verbal content calls for right brain attention to her synchronizing and matching the patient's implicit self-states of affective arousal.

According to Bromberg (2011), "Self-states are highly individualized modules of being, each configured by its own organization of cognitions, beliefs, dominant affect, and mood, access to memory, skills, behaviors, values, action, and regulatory physiology" (p. 73). In this interactive matrix, both partners match the dynamic contours of different emotional-motivational self-states (e.g., fear, aggression, shame, joy) and simultaneously synchronize and adjust their social attention, stimulation, and accelerating or decelerating arousal in response to the partner's signals. Rapid communications between the right-lateralized emotional brain of each member of the therapeutic alliance allows for here-and-now, moment-to-moment, right-brain-to-right-brain self-state sharing, a cocreated, organized, dynamically changing dialogue of mutual influence. This includes the sharing of painful emotional states with the empathic clinician, who then can act as an interactive regulator of the patient's psychobiological states. Ultimately, effective psychotherapeutic treatment of early-evolving self-pathologies facilitates increases in complexity of the patient's right hemispheric unconscious system. These changes are expressed in the therapeutic context, as the goal of a session moves from a left brain reasoned narrative and cognitive insight to a right brain spontaneous, improvised, emotionally laden conversation.

In a clinical article, "Relational Healing in Psychotherapy," Gnaulati (2021) observes,

> When psychotherapy is "rolling along" the therapist fluidly tracks and matches the client's shifting emotions with vocal expressions, head nods, well co-ordinated facial expressions, and pithy or elaborative verbal statements rooted to the client's level of receptivity. . . . Summing this up Schore (2003) writes, for a working alliance to be created, the therapist must be experienced as being in a state of vitalizing attunement to the patient; that is, the crescendos and decrescendos of the therapist's affective state must be in resonance with similar states of crescendo and decrescendos of the patient. (p. 594)

In a clinical case study, Kykyri and colleagues (2017) report that interaction synchrony, usually in the middle of a session, lasts only a few seconds and occurs in a silent moment of the session, when the therapist intuitively lowers the pitch of her voice to soft prosody and is thereby "soothing and friendly." They observe, "Affective attunement between two or more persons is assumed to happen, below conscious monitoring" and report the ensuing therapeutic change occurs in a time frame of 90 seconds (see the Sands vignette in Chapter 5). Note the temporal dimensions of a synchronized and thereby well-timed right-brain-to-right-brain connection. Chan and his colleagues observe, "Small inputs may result in large changes within a single session. The type and timing of an intervention may be just as important as their delivery and relevance" (2022, p. 1). Synchrony is thus the psychobiological mechanism beneath optimal clinical timing.

In such a "heightened affective moment" of a session, the empathic therapist transiently callosally shifts out of the left brain into a right brain state of "free floating," "wide ranging" attention in order to "follow the patient's affect" (Schore, 1994/2016, 2012, 2019b). In this bodily-based therapeutic interaction, the sensitive clinician intuitively and fluidly tracks and synchronously matches the patient's rhythmic moment-to-moment crescendos and decrescendos of emotional arousal and metabolic changes in the patient's affective states. Recall, neuroscientists assert that the most basic level of regulatory processes is the regulation of arousal (Tucker et al., 1995), and that the right brain is dominant for the regulation of arousal (Heilman & van den Abell, 1979; Levy et al., 1983; Schore, 1994/2016, 2012; Hartikainen, 2021). In 1994 I suggested that, as in the secure mother's attachment relationship, in therapy the empathic clinician's right orbitofrontal cortex implicitly follows the affect and thereby intersubjectively and interoceptively monitors and regulates the patient's dynamically changing positive and painful negative emotional arousal associated with human suffering (Schore, 1994/2016).

A very large body of neuroscience studies has now established that the orbitofrontal cortex plays a central role in emotional experience (Rolls & Grabenhorst, 2008), including signaling emotions. Recall that the orbitofrontal cortex is fundamentally involved in "emotion-related learning" (Rolls et al., 1994). This prefrontal system operates as a hub within an emotional salience network that is activated by the anticipation of stressful negative, aversive experiences (Grupe et al., 2013). The forward-looking functions of the "orbitofrontal oracle" (Rudebeck & Murray, 2014) predict imagined future outcomes (Takahashi et al., 2013) and are centrally involved in interoception, the integration of sensory and bodily signals that guide behavior (Damasio, 1996). Toward that end, the orbitofrontal cortex rapidly tracks and decodes subjective decision-making (Rich

& Wallis, 2016), acts as "gateway to subjective conscious experience" (Kringelbach, 2005, p. 699), and mediates changes in subjective experience (Fox et al., 2018).

Recent groundbreaking studies are focusing on perhaps the most intense form of subjective emotional suffering, the highly aversive state of chronic pain, an enduring stressful asynchronized state of negatively valenced dysregulated sympathetic autonomic hyperarousal and neuroinflammation. Basic neurological research on pain demonstrates that the orbitofrontal cortex and its reciprocal connections with the anterior cingulate, insula, amygdala, and ventral striatum involved in emotional regulation represent a functional pain network (Shirvalkar et al., 2023). These authors observe that acute pain decoding is associated with anterior cingulate activity, while chronic pain, with a larger affective component, relies on orbitofrontal activity, which tracks the subjective perception, decoding, and severity of chronic intense pain. They note, orbitofrontal cortex "circuits may integrate pain expectation and context-dependent predictions that influence subjective pain evaluation, which may include rumination or engagement of coping mechanisms," specifically mentioning ventromedial prefrontal areas involved in individual variability in brain representations of pain and negative affect (Kohoutova et al., 2022; Ceko et al., 2022). Recall that the amygdala, insula, anterior cingulate, and orbitofrontal limbic areas all have direct reciprocal connections with the autonomic nervous system.

On the other hand, research with romantic partners demonstrates that synchronized brain-to-brain coupling during handholding is associated with right hemisphere activation in the pain observer and pain reduction in the pain receiver (Goldstein et al., 2018). I suggest this intimate context is specifically the intersubjective relational and emotional context in which both chronic and especially acute emotional pain, a common focus of psychotherapy, can be tracked by the empathic therapist. They conclude, "As the adaptive value of pain may be to alert the organism to impending tissue damage, arousal effects may be a fundamental component of the complex subjective perception of pain itself."

In 2012, Goodkind and colleagues published "Tracking Emotional Valence: The Role of the Orbitofrontal Cortex" in *Human Brain Mapping*. These researchers observed that the right orbitofrontal cortex is involved in continuously tracking dynamically changing emotions, "enabling us to understand the emotions expressed by others in real time, follow them as they unfold and change, and adjust our behavior in ways that are appropriate." Their data support my assertion that the psychobiologically attuned therapist, at levels beneath awareness, follows the affect by implicitly tracking metabolic changes in not only the patient's but her own limbic emotional and autonomic arousal. This allows the decoding of bodily-based nonverbal communications of the patient's right brain by interoceptive actual felt emotional reactions, and thereby a form of empathic responding. Craig (2003) defines interoception as the sense of the physiological condition of the body. The intuitive clinician is implicitly learning the rhythmic structures of the patient's bodily-based internal states and modifying her behavior to synchronize and couple with that structure, right brain to right brain. Writing in the *Journal of Counseling Psychology*, Lee and his colleagues (2023) reported, "The advocation of right brain-to-right brain psychotherapy in recent years showcases how neural coupling in the right hemisphere (involving emotions) of the therapists and clients enable[s] clients to experience 'feeling felt' by empathic therapists" (Schore, 2014, 2018, 2019, 2022). This includes the patient's feeling that his or her emotional pain has been felt by the empathic clinician.

In "Physiological Synchrony in Psychotherapy Sessions," Tschacher and Meier (2019) state that synchrony between therapist and patient is expressed in their central and autonomic nervous systems moving in a synchronized way over time. I have suggested that the patient's right-lateralized psychobiological system intersubjectively synchronizes and couples with another "emotional" right brain that is "attuned" and "on the same wavelength." Recall the earlier discussion of Greenberg's (2014) therapeutic presence, which according to Tschacher and his colleagues (2018) "denotes a therapist's being attuned and 'present' in the session. The concept includes being receptively open to a client, and extending the therapist's inward experience to make *contact* with the patient." In this receptive state, the synchronized clinician can share an emotional connection between his or her right brain unconscious and the patient's right brain unconscious. Gotti (2024), a psychoanalyst, gives a clinical example of an intersubjective synchronized physiological regression at the point of disconnection of the therapeutic relationship, the end of a psychotherapy session:

> Towards the end of the session, a reciprocal behavior developed in a spontaneous and initially unremarked and unpremeditated way, one

which later produced a sort of rituality. We noticed, only in a later moment, that we both gathered our hands, on our abdomens, in an almost *synchronous* manner, at the end of the hour—a ritual that prepared and contained separation. (p. 238)

Recall Decety and Chaminade's (2003) observation, "Mental states that are in essence private to the self may be *shared* between individuals. . . . Self-awareness, empathy, identification with others, and more generally intersubjective processes, are largely dependent upon . . . right hemisphere resources, which are the first to develop." More recently, McGilchrist (2021b, p. 876) writes, "The social and empathic self, and the continuous sense of self, with '*depth*' of existence over time, is more dependent on the right hemisphere," concluding, "Without a self, there is no capacity for intersubjectivity, for the experience of shared time and shared space."

The neuropsychologist Julian Keenan and colleagues (2005) state, "The right hemisphere, in fact, truly interprets the mental state not only of its own brain, but the brains (and minds) of others." In my 2012 volume *The Science of the Art of Psychotherapy*, I suggested that across disciplines we were witnessing a paradigm shift from a one-person intrapsychic to a two-person relational psychology, a shift in perspective from within a brain to an intersubjective relationship between brains, in the right-brain-to-right-brain therapist–patient psychotherapy relationship, and thereby in the coconstructed therapeutic alliance.

Clinical and Neuroscientific Research on Right-Brain-to-Right-Brain Communications Within the Therapeutic Alliance

In a comprehensive overview of studies of the psychotherapy relationship, Norcross and Lambert (2018) assert,

Decades of research evidence and clinical experience converge: *the psychotherapy relationship makes substantial and consistent contributions to outcome independent of the treatment* [emphasis added]. . . . We need to proclaim publicly what decades of research have discovered and what hundreds of thousands of practitioners have witnessed: The relationship can heal. . . . What does not work are poor alliances in adult, adolescent, child, couple, and family psychotherapy as well as low levels of cohesion in group psychotherapy. Paucity of collaboration, consensus, empathy, and positive regard predict treatment dropout and failure.

They conclude, "Efforts to promulgate best practices or evidence-based practices without including the relationship are seriously incomplete and potentially misleading" (p. 308). Indeed, almost five decades of research confirm that the patient-therapist relationship consistently predicts a stronger treatment outcome than actual treatment type (e.g., Doran, 2016; Fluckiger et al., 2018). In fact research does not support the superiority of any one type of psychotherapy over another (Sparks et al., 2008). On the other hand a large body of studies supports the school-independent relational principle that the therapeutic relationship acts as a "foundational pan-theoretical change agent" (Markin, 2014).

Psychotherapy research is now focusing on the critical role of common factors, qualities of effective therapists associated with successful treatment outcomes, such as collaboration, empathy, conveyed respect, acceptance, genuineness, maintaining a warm emotional bond with the patient, and a capacity for building the therapeutic alliance (Lambert, 2013; Wampold et al., 2017; Hess, 2019). More than left brain semantics, each of these essential functions is expressed in the clinician's nonverbal right brain. Hess (2019) concludes common factors are responsible for the majority of change outcomes that occur from therapy. I suggest common factors represent right brain change mechanisms embedded in the therapeutic alliance that can be accessed in all forms of psychotherapeutic treatment.

In 1936 Rosenzweig first suggested that nonspecific common factors operating as implicit unverbalized aspects of the therapeutic relationship underlied the success of psychotherapy. An essential source of the common factors literature is the seminal work of Bordin (1979) on the generalizability of the psychodynamic concept of the working alliance:

I propose that the working alliance between the person who seeks change and the one who offers to be a change agent is one of the keys, if not the key, to the change process. . . . A working alliance between a person seeking change and a change agent can occur in many places besides the locale of psychotherapy. The working alliance can be defined and elaborated in terms which make it universally applicable. (p. 25)

Updating Bordin's common factor model, Wampold (2015, p. 272) cites research demonstrating "more effective therapists were able to form a strong alliance across a range of patients" and that "patients with poor attachment histories and chaotic interpersonal relationships may well benefit from a therapist who is able to form alliances with difficult patients."

Overviewing the central role of the alliance in mental health, Wampold and Fluckiger (2023) now assert,

> Psychotherapy research has shown that the age, ethnicity, gender, profession of therapist, therapist's theoretical orientation . . . do not differentiate more effective from less effective therapists. The strongest predictor of effectiveness is a set of interpersonal skills of the therapists displayed in interpersonally challenging situations. (p. 30)

In light of the fact that stressful ruptures of the therapeutic alliance are a primal example of such challenging moments, these authors cite research evidence that "repairing ruptures" and affect dysregulation in psychotherapy are associated with better psychotherapy outcomes.

At the end of their recent article, these authors echo the central themes of regulation theory and right brain psychotherapy discussed in these chapters:

> [The] patient's emotional dysregulation negatively affects mental and physical health, and consequently several mental health treatments are focused on reducing this dysregulation. . . . There is evidence that emotion regulation is an unconscious dyadic process, in that the presence of an intimate other can attenuate arousal and distress through a process that is referred to as co-regulation, social regulation, or interpersonal emotion regulation. . . . In psychotherapy, interpersonal co-regulation has been detected in moment-to-moment emotional states of the patient and therapist. (Wampold & Fluckiger, 2023, p. 37)

The authors conclude, "Relational psychodynamic approaches to psychotherapy consider the alliance a specific effect, in that the development of the alliance over the course of therapy is therapeutic in and of itself" (p. 38).

Toward that end, an extensive body of research supports the essential tenets and practice of psychodynamic psychotherapy in working with implicit relational processes (e.g., Leichsenring et al., 2015; Luyten et al., 2015). In fact, there is a growing body of data on the efficacy of psychodynamic psychotherapy. Compared to cognitive behavioral and dialectical behavior therapy, its effects are longer lasting and increase with time. According to Shedler, in contrast to cognitive therapies, "psychodynamic therapy sets in motion psychological processes that lead to ongoing change, even after therapy has ended" (2010, p. 101). Shedler concluded that beyond symptom remission, "psychodynamic therapy may foster inner resources and capacities that allow richer, freer, and more fulfilling lives" (p. 107).

Contemporary relational psychodynamic models citing my right brain work (Schore, 2021a, 2022) are now calling for a shift to a personalized therapy based on a holistic view of the patient's unique needs, preference, and interpersonal styles (Levendosky et al., 2022). It thereby fosters a uniquely individualized and attuned treatment (Zilcha-Mano, 2021) that is more responsive to both the personal and cultural contexts of any patient (Tummula-Narra et al., 2018). Especially in psychodynamic therapy, the therapeutic alliance is seen as the primary agent for the early development of mechanisms of change that predict treatment outcome (Zilcha-Mano & Errazuriz, 2017).

This approach highlights the importance of the clinician collaborating with the patient in forming an effective therapeutic alliance in the initial stages of the treatment, one that strengthens the alliance and reduces premature termination and dropout (Spencer et al., 2019). Low nonverbal synchrony in early therapy sessions is reflective of a mismatch between the patient and therapist in the therapeutic alliance and predicts a premature termination (Schoenherr et al., 2019). These latter authors suggest that therapists should now be trained in how their own and their patients' nonverbal communications are subjectively perceived, which allows for awareness of unconscious nonverbal behavior.

Over the last three decades, I have continued to offer brain laterality research and clinical data on working right brain to right brain in the evolving therapeutic alliance. Beginning in the first session, the therapist intuitively follows the affect and tracks metabolic changes of arousal in the patient's emotional states, beneath the words. These synchronized, spontaneous nonverbal communications of regulated and dysregulated emotional self-states take place in the present moment, a time frame of thousandths of a second to 2 to 3 seconds. My colleague Russell Meares (2012) referred to a form of therapeutic conversation that can be conceived as a dynamic interplay between two right hemispheres. Philip Bromberg (2011) a pioneer in relational psychoanalysis observed, "Allan Schore writes about a right brain-to-right brain channel of affective communication—a channel that he sees as an organized dialogue comprised of dynamically fluctuating moment-to-moment state sharing. I believe it to be this process of state sharing that allows a good psychoanalytic match." Note the direct allusion to the therapist and patient being in sync.

According to the classical theory of emotional contagion, another's state may be perceived and shared through mimicry or synchronization, and this capacity, which occurs without conscious intent or awareness, allows individuals to empathically mirror other minds (Hatfield et al., 1994). Indeed, the right hemisphere is dominant for mutual gaze, "the process during which two persons have the feeling of a brief link between their two minds" (Wicker et al., 1998). Koole and Tschacher (2016) assert that interpersonal synchrony establishes interbrain coupling that provides "patient and therapist with access to another's internal states, which facilitates common understanding and emotional sharing." Writing on brain-to-brain coupling as a mechanism for creating and sharing a social world, Hasson et al. (2012) suggests, "Brain-to-brain coupling is analogous to a wireless communication system in which two brains are coupled via the transmission of a physical signal (light, sound, pressure or chemical compound) through the shared physical environment."

Note the direct correspondence of these descriptions to my right-brain-to-right-brain nonverbal communications in every chapter in this book, including Buck's spontaneous emotional communications as a "conversation between limbic systems" in Chapter 1; Freud's unconscious acting as a receptor organ turned toward the "transmitting unconscious" of the patient, Dorpat's primary-process communications, Mandal and Ambady's assertion that human beings rely on nonverbal channels of communication in their day-to-day emotional and interpersonal exchanges in which the face is centrally involved in signaling affective information, and Buchanan's "secret signals" rapidly transmitted between two individuals in Chapter 2; Rigas's (2008) "silent dialogues" of primitive nonverbal communication in Chapter 3; Hammer's "affective wireless" between the empathic therapist and patient, and Beebe and Steele's mother–infant "subterranean rapid communications that are not perceptible in real time" in Chapter 7; and Music's "whispering nervous systems" and Trevarthen's nonverbal emotional protoconversations and emotional sharing that occur beneath verbal conversations in this chapter. To this I would add the hyperscanning studies of this chapter showing a rapid right-lateralized interbrain synchronization within right-brain-to-right-brain face-to-face interactions between the mother and infant.

With relevance to the lateralization of the face-to-face therapeutic alliance, basic research on face processing indicates that at levels beneath awareness, humans, regardless of handedness, tend to display a right hemispheric unconscious "left gaze bias," whereby they direct their initial visual gaze to the left side of the other's face, and look longer exploring the left side, which is more expressive (Salva et al., 2012). These researchers document that face-sensitive neurons in the right temporal cortex respond more rapidly to a face than those on the left, which respond much later. Other studies report that when normal individuals are presented faces in the left visual field of the right hemisphere, they recognize them faster and more accurately than for the right visual field controlled by the left hemisphere (Demaree et al., 2005). The dominance of the left visual field for face recognition has been shown to correlate with the activation of the right fusiform face area (Forrester et al., 2018). These latter authors observe that humans express facial emotions earlier on the left side of the face, which is controlled by the right motor cortex. This means in a face-to-face right-brain-to-right-brain emotional interaction, both the empathic clinician and the patient are unconsciously receiving and sending facial emotions in their left visual fields, reflecting joint activation of their synchronizing right hemispheres.

More specifically, during direct eye contact, especially close, intensive moments of mutual gaze, beneath awareness the patient and therapist (like the infant and mother) engage in the two-person process of "pupil mimicry" (Kret et al., 2015). In this dyadic process, pupil sizes synchronize between partners, where the pupils of one dilate or constrict in synchrony with the dilation and constriction of the pupils of another, leading to respectively synchronized arousal increases and decreases in the

amygdala. These researchers demonstrate that individuals trusted partners with sympathetically dilating pupils and withheld trust from partners
with parasympathetically constricted pupils, and that their pupils implicitly mimicked changes in their partner's pupils. They conclude, "Precisely
because pupil changes are unconscious, they provide an honest reflection
of the person's inner state" (p. 1402).

Synchronized autonomic mimicry, centrally involved in right-lateralized

FIGURE 8.1
Lateral view of the neurological mechanisms of
unconscious autonomic mimicry

*Sender on the left: (1) Sender's stress response is initiated by hypothalamus-pituitary-
adrenal axis activation. (2) Adrenal gland secretes adrenocorticotropic hormone (ACTH),
increasing the level of corticotropin-releasing hormone (CRH) in the bloodstream. (3) These
neuroendocrinological reactions are accompanied by cardiovascular changes, muscle tension,
pupil dilation, and sweating. Receiver on the right: (4) The affective information is implicitly
registered by the receiver's senses and passes through (5) the superior colliculus (CS) pulvinar
(Pulv) pathway to the amygdala (AMG). (6) The amygdala and locus coeruleus (LC) activate
the hypothalamic-pituitary-adrenal axis. (7) The amygdala and LC project to higher cortical
networks such as the orbitofrontal cortex (OFC) and anterior cingulate (ACC), influencing
social decisions. (8) Sender and receiver emotionally converge on physiological (lower
gray) levels. For clinical purposes, think of the sender as patient, receiver as therapist.*

Reprinted from Neuroscience & Biobehavioral Reviews, Vol 80, Eliska Prochazkova &
Mariska E. Kret, "Connecting minds and sharing emotions through mimicry: A neurocognitive
model of emotional contagion," Pages 99–114, © 2017, with permission from Elsevier.

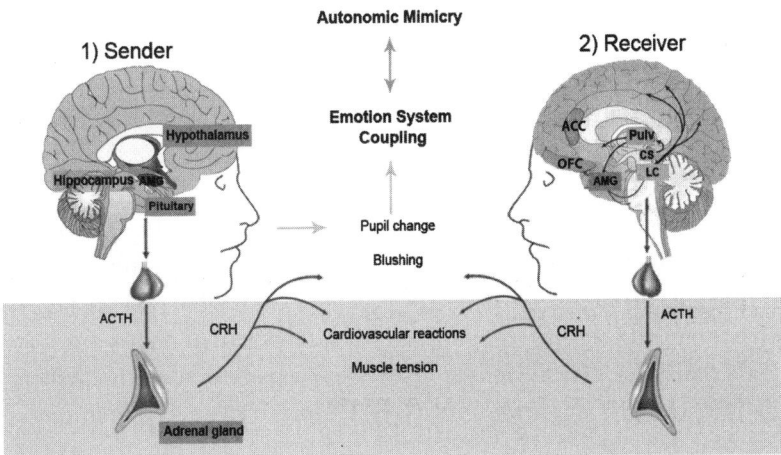

trust, emotional contagion, social bonds, and empathy, underlies the implicit intersubjective nonverbal communication and sharing of positive states of affiliation as well as stressful, negatively valenced limbic-autonomic emotional states. For the latter, see the lateral view of unconscious autonomic mimicry in Figure 8.1, from Prochazkova and Kret (2017), "Connecting Minds and Sharing Emotions Through Mimicry." According to these authors, autonomic mimicry relies on an unconscious signaling system that is controlled by the ANS.

These researchers cite studies showing that the right temporoparietal junction, anterior cingulate, and medial prefrontal and inferior frontal cortex play significant roles in empathy (Carr et al., 2003; Decety & Lamm, 2007; Shamay-Tsoory et al., 2009). I would add that in an interaction between the stressed sender's right TPJ and the empathic receiver's right TPJ, the communications of these face-to-face emotional signals are bidirectional.

Using hyperscanning research to study real-time eye-to-eye interaction contact, Noah and his colleagues (2020) show increased activity in the right TPJ in both partners viewing each other in a live (and not video) face-to-face context, a neural mechanism of a dynamic social interaction in which facial cues are reciprocally exchanged (see Figure 8.2). These researchers assert that during social face-to-face interactions of reciprocal eye contact, people automatically align with and mimic their interactors' facial expressions, vocalizations, postures, and bodily states, and that this unconscious mimicry is implicated in empathic emotional contagion and is impaired in several pathologies. Utilizing NIRS hyperscanning, they show that compared to eye-to-eye contact with a real partner, increased activity is seen in the right temporoparietal cortex in the live condition and not in the video condition. They conclude,

> Live interaction between individuals engages neural functions not engaged during similar tasks performed alone, i.e., without interactions. The increased activity in the right TPJ during the real eye task is consistent with sensitivity to social interactions in that region and suggests that these neural circuits reflect ecologically valid social activity highlighting the importance of two-person paradigms. (Noah et al., 2020, p. 6)

FIGURE 8.2

Live real-time eye-to-eye contact compared to gaze-at-face video responses

The black circle on the right hemisphere diagrammatically represents the tight TPJ. The top row shows responses of the right TPJ for the real face-to-face task, and the bottom row responses for the video-gaze task. Increased right TPJ activity is seen in the live but not the video condition.

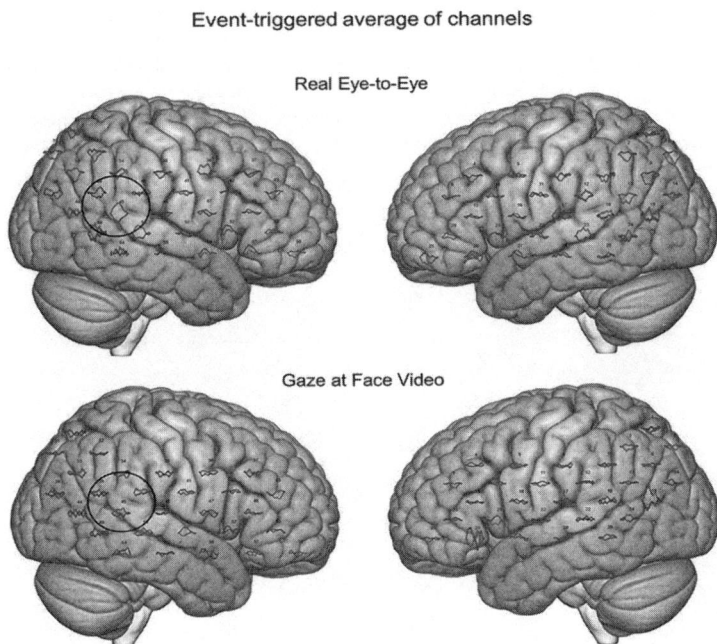

Event-triggered average of channels

Real Eye-to-Eye

Gaze at Face Video

A schematic of interpersonal neurobiological research on adult face-to-face communication by Bradley (2010) is seen in Figure 8.3. Note an essential change from Figure 7.2. In addition to the synchronized nonverbal communications of face, voice, and gesture of their central nervous systems in the top half of the figure, the bottom half depicts the shared physiological synchrony and resonance between their bodily-based autonomic nervous systems, a synchronized heart-brain entrainment in both.

According to Bradley, this implicit electromagnetic intersubjective field of social connection between them results in an energetic resonance with

FIGURE 8.3
Lateral view of multiple channels of face-to-face implicit communication

Speaking and listening, visual reading of facial expression, hand gestures, body posture, and involuntary movements that signal emotional states, along with psychophysiological patterns (heart rhythm patterns and resonant autonomic system activity), while depicted as arrows in the figure, are actually wave forms of energy oscillations that encode emotional information communicated between individuals. Note the synchronized two-way reciprocal heart-brain connections.

Figure 1-Multiple channels of face-to-face communication. From R.T. Bradley, "Detecting the Identity Signature of Secret Social Groups: Holographic Processes and the Communication of Member Affiliation," World Futures (66:124–162, 2010). Adapted and redrawn from "Figure 8.1. Chapters of face-to-face communication in protoconversation, and three phases in the cycles of expressions between mother and baby," C. Trevarthen, "The self born in intersubjectivity." In Ulric Neisser (Ed.), The Perceived Self, pp. 121–173. New York: © Cambridge University Press 1993, reproduced with permission of Cambridge University Press through PLSclear.

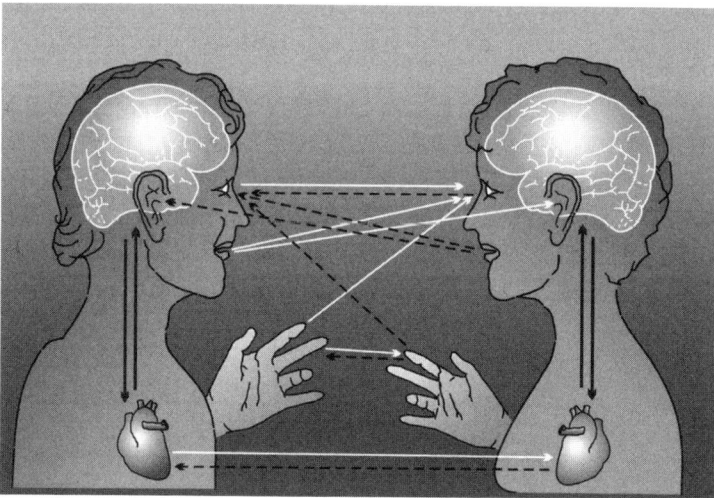

each member's psychophysiological systems—the brain, the heart, and the body as a whole. He states that this channel of coherent interaction that cocreates an embodied emotional experience is generated unconsciously between two persons at a deeper level of psychosocial connection than that of the phonemic level of language. Bradley cites the work of McCraty (2004), "The Energetic Heart: Bioelectromagnetic Communication Within and Between People," where he suggests that magnetic fields produced by the heart carry information that is detectable *by other persons or animals.*

McCraty observes that the heart's magnetic field induces a cardiac entrainment when the R-waves of one person's electrocardiogram become precisely synchronized with the onset of electroencephalogram alpha waves of another at a distance of up to five feet. These data suggest that the synchronized mutual entrainment of the limbic brains and autonomic cardiovascular systems of two interacting individuals is involved in the processing and coregulation of a shared emotional response.

In accord with this model, recall Porges's (2011) observation that "the right hemisphere—including the right cortical and subcortical structures—would promote the efficient regulation of autonomic functions via the source nuclei in the brainstem." He also suggests that "the right vagus and, thus, cardiac vagal tone are associated with processes involving the expression and regulation of emotion, and communication." The right vagus has pathways to and from the right insular cortex, a limbic-autonomic structure deep in the right temporal lobe that generates heart-focused interoception (Schultz, 2016), the perceptual processing and integration of sensory and bodily signals of visceral sensations.

Earlier I described how the right insula is a "hub of a salience network" that is activated in visceral sensations, body movement, emotions, vocalizations, pain, and consciousness. Interoception, the sense of the physiological condition of the body, thus allows for the detection of what Gallese (2007) calls the beating heart of bodily-based intersubjective processes. The right brain process of interoception, the sense of the internal body state, is activated in moments when suddenly you can consciously feel accelerating or decelerating changes in your heartbeat and breath in response to emotion. This subjective awareness of bodily (and not mental) states acts as a portal into the energy-expending sympathetic and energy-conserving parasympathetic branches of the involuntary autonomic nervous system. In turn, this subjective awareness of inner-body feelings, visceral and autonomic functions, generates a "sentient self" (Craig, 2010). In the clinical context, the right insula mediates countertransference dynamics that are appraised by the therapist's interoceptive observations of her own bodily-based visceral responses to the patient's transferential unconscious emotional communications.

With respect to Figure 8.3, my own studies indicate that two other right brain cortical systems of the subjective self can be added to the image. The right TPJ in the posterior area of the right hemisphere is centrally involved in the communication of emotional states, while the orbitofrontal cortex in the anterior portion of the right hemisphere acts as a regulator of emotional states. Both of these right brain functions lie at the core of the face-to-face right brain nonverbal communications within the interaction between the empathic therapist and patient.

Applying the above neurobiological data to the two-person therapeutic alliance, a relational psychodynamic model of a face-to-face interaction facilitates the experience of "being seen" (Ünsalver et al., 2021). Citing my work (Schore, 2012), these authors show that eye-to-eye contact is essential to forming an object relationship of a self and other, an internal representation of a regulated self affectively interacting with a psychobiologically attuned other. This implicit face-to-face interaction indicates that during mutual gaze synchronization, "when the therapist and client face each other unconscious and involuntary pupil mimicry may occur, and the autonomic nervous systems of the client and the therapist may resonate through the mutual gaze" (Ünsalver et al., 2021). They assert that this eye-to-eye autonomic "pupillary contagion" (Harrison et al., 2006) builds trust between two people via joint oxytocin release in the amygdala and sends the nonverbal message "I am present with you." I suggest that this unconscious message is nonverbally transmitted in a positive affectively charged right-brain-to-right-brain communication. Ünsalver and his colleagues (2021) contend that we understand information about the inner state of another through unconscious and involuntary pupil mimicry between two people. Autonomic pupillary contagion is regulated by the medial prefrontal cortex (Wang et al., 2011) and the amygdala, and this dynamic pupillary exchange is linked to empathy (Harrison et al., 2006).

Due to the cumulative effects of interactive regulation over time, especially after numerous regulated negatively charged rupture-repair transactions and positively charged mutual play transactions, increases in trust and safety within the therapeutic alliance result from coregulated oxytocin releases that are resonantly amplified by the therapeutic dyad. This hypothalamic neuropeptide is a key modulator of complex socioaffective responses such as attachment stress, anxiety, social approach, and affiliation (Meyer-Lindenberg, 2008), and synchronized oxytocin levels occur during early parent-infant bonding (Szymanska et al., 2017; Scatliffe et al., 2019). Over the lifespan, oxytocin heightens awareness of social cues (Bartz & Hollander, 2006), enhances social learning and emotional empathy

(Hurlemann et al., 2010), and regulates complex social behavior like affiliation and trust (Donaldson and Young, 2004), all of which are right brain functions. Parasympathetic oxytocin counteracts the effects of stress by inhibiting the secretion of the major stress hormone corticotropzin-releasing factor (Boeck et al., 2018) and thereby reducing activity in the sympathetic branch of the autonomic nervous system (Uvnas-Moberg, 1996). In this manner oxytocin interacts with social support to suppress cortisol and subjective responses to psychosocial stress (Heinrichs et al., 2003).

This regulatory neuropeptide also facilitates a sense of connection and empathy with others. In adults (including those in psychotherapy), oxytocin broadly enhances interpersonal synchronization (Mu et al., 2016) and facilitates reciprocity in social communication (Spengler et al., 2017), thereby contributing to its prosocial effects on social bonding (Gebauer et al., 2014) and its association with human trustworthiness (Zak et al., 2005). Indeed, oxytocin and synchrony are psychobiological markers of resilience (Priel et al., 2019). Studies document that oxytocin synchrony and "alliance rupture repair" (Eubanks et al., 2018), a recoupling between the patient and the empathic therapist, are associated with better psychotherapy outcomes (Zilcha-Mano et al., 2020). Synchronized regulated rupture and repair of the dynamic right-lateralized emotional attachment bond between the patient and therapist is thus a major interpersonal neurobiological change mechanism of the treatment (Schore, 1994/2016, 2003b, 2012, 2019b).

In every chapter of this book, I have described my right-brain-to-right-brain model of facial, prosodic, and gestural emotion communication of attachment dynamics at levels beneath awareness of both partners, as well the unconscious dynamics between the clinician and patient in psychotherapy. Indeed, throughout these pages I refer to face-to-face synchronized implicit visual (light), auditory (sound), and tactile (pressure) nonverbal emotional communications intersubjectively transmitted between two coupled right brains at ultrarapid rates, and thereby "hidden in plain sight" and invisible to the left hemisphere.

Neurobiological research indicates that the social perception and complex processing of the smallest change within a human face occurs rapidly, within 100 milliseconds (Lehky, 2000), and that such facially expressed state changes are mirrored (Dimberg & Ohman, 1996) and synchronously matched by an observer's right hemisphere within 300–400 milliseconds, at levels beneath awareness (Stenberg et al., 1998). Recall that the right hemisphere perceptually recognizes an emotion from a visually presented facial expression and then generates a somatosensory, bodily-based representation of how another feels when displaying that facial expression at levels beneath conscious awareness (Adolphs et al., 2000). This rapid and therefore invisible empathic response in turn allows for the right brain expression of the adaptive function of dyadic subliminal affect regulation (Koole & Jostmann, 2004).

In discussing the regulation of social behavior and perception, Todd and Anderson (2009, p. 1217) refer to "invisible social force fields that regulate close physical proximity." Brain laterality research now documents that the right amygdala initiates an ultrarapid high-speed detection of unconscious stimuli (Costafreda et al., 2008) and is associated with "subjective emotionality" (Ally et al., 2013). Other studies demonstrate the right occipital-temporal cortex, which is connected to the right amygdala, generates a holistic face representation in only 170 milliseconds, beneath conscious awareness (Yovel, 2016).

Both research and clinical data indicate that states shared between two individuals in both development and psychotherapy and indeed in everyday life occur via interpersonal synchrony, and that this fundamental developmental mechanism underlies emotion transmission, affective reciprocal exchange, physiological linkage, and empathy, all right brain relational functions beneath conscious awareness. Recall that people are commonly unaware of becoming synchronized (Tschacher et al., 2023). Furthermore, synchrony is associated with a "we-mode" of cognition (Gallotti & Frith, 2013), a blurring of self-other boundaries (Paladino et al., 2010), and a self-other merging in which the interacting partner is perceived as part of oneself, with thereby an enhanced feeling of closeness.

Kaiser and Butler (2021) assert that in relational systems, successful engagement is expressed in automatic and implicit sharing of social content, including emotions, where two or more persons understand the world "more or less as one":

> The implicit sharing process is temporal and bidirectional between . . . people. . . . A mutual dynamic process is occurring, whereby partners make micro-adjustments over time driven by implicit information

from high-resolution perceptions of the others' states and intentions (Schore, 1994/2016). Mutual interaction . . . involves a complex fitting-together of the individuals involved, producing a resonance between two attuned systems and feelings of psychological closeness. (Schore, 1994/2016)

This fitting together of an emotional engagement between people, what Erich Fromm (1956) called "becoming one with another" and Amid (2024) terms "at-one-ment," is the outcome of a synchronized, intersubjective, nonverbal interaction embedded in an intimate right-brain-to-right-brain emotional bond between close individuals, including those in the therapeutic alliance.

In describing a heightened affective moment of a session when the therapist and patient are in sync, Langer (2024) observes,

Most of us who have made psychotherapy our careers have experienced therapy sessions when everything is "clicking." When it feels like we and our client can virtually anticipate what each other is about to say. When time speeds up and the hour is over almost before you know it. When you feel so close to each other that you almost forget what you are doing. When you do not have to think about what you are going to say next. There is a feeling of pure joy, a kind of an altered state of consciousness. Often, there is shared laughter, sometimes inside jokes. This is what it feels like to relate right brain-to-right brain, to play together. (p. 6)

Meares (2012) describes this "heightened affective moment" of a shared positively valenced connection between two right brains:

An interplay between two right brains provides a structure for the therapeutic engagement. . . . The language is emotionally expressive. As a consequence, the phonology is salient, the toning and inflections of the voice have a powerful communicative effect that is combined with facial expressions and the movements of the body. . . . This kind of language creates the feeling of "being with" in a way that is greater than a logical, completely syntactical left-hemisphere utterance, which sets up a different kind of relatedness.

A central theme running through this chapter is that these moments of emotional engagement occur in an intersubjective context of a therapeutic mutual regression, a synchronized shift from the patient's and clinician's analytic rational left brains into their intuitive socioemotional right brains. This allows both members of the therapeutic dyad to experience and share affects, from pleasure to pain, *together.*

Recall, in these emotionally charged moments of the session the clinician must be "safe but not too safe," enabling both members of the therapeutic dyad to synchronously lower defenses and take more risk. In describing the role of safety in this change-promoting relational context Podolan and Gelo (2024) assert,

> [T]he safety of the therapist, the client, and the relationship must be neither perfect, steady, or static, but rather *safe enough, adaptive, and dynamic* [emphasis added], leaving space not only for self-discovery and self-awareness but also for the co-regulation of tolerable frustration, disappointments, and insecurities that facilitate the client's resilience and adaptation. (p. 403)

In support of my idea that these heightened affective moments of shared affectively charged right brain emotional connections significantly generate change in the patient, Grafanaki et al. (2007) offer the observation,

> Clients and counselors often described their experience during peak (extremely helpful and memorable) moments of therapy as flowing or being in a flow. . . . Such moments captured high levels of connection with one's experience and high level of connection with the other person in the interaction that was usually perceived as a trusting and safe presence. Those moments in therapy that clients and or counselors described as flowing promoted important therapeutic outcomes and helped clients increase their sense of mastery, hope and understanding of important life issues. (p. 242)

In *The American Journal of Psychoanalysis,* Amid (2024) discusses Bion's (1970) classic construct of *at-one-ment,* a knowing not through rational understanding but by a primal, intuitive unconscious nonverbal mode of knowing and communicating, or a knowing of the other from the inside that allows one to experience the other's experience as one's own, rather than like one's own. Within the therapeutic alliance, this primitive communication (Bion, 1970), a "dialogue of oneness," is entered through a temporary eclipse of rational knowing via "surrender" (Ehrenzweig, 1957; Ghent, 1990, 1995). This in turn allows for "being with" the patient (Reis, 2018) and what Amid terms "new forms of knowing, communicating and being." In discussing the neurobiological basis for this capacity of nonverbal communication, Amid observes,

This understanding of at-one-ment as a formless, "embryonic" kind of unconscious communication which, paradoxically, allows one to know the other without knowing (i.e., unconsciously) coincides with developmental research indicating an innate capacity to apprehend the intentional and emotional cues of others and a primal non-verbal mode of communication that the fetus uses *in utero*. . . . This understanding also coincides with Schore's (2009) argument that, until recently, all conceptualizations of the process of psychotherapeutic change have been dominated by models of cognition, frequently highlighting verbal, conscious cognition. The conceptual evidence goes against the grain of increasing evidence that it is unconscious and nonverbal therapist–patient communication—also known as "right brain-to-right brain communication" (Schore, 2014, 2019; Marcus, 1997)—that is the actual neuropsychological foundation of psychotherapeutic change (Schore, 2009). . . . The actual transferring or sharing of information as well as the particular level at which it is understood do not necessarily depend on intention or conscious awareness. In this respect, psychotherapy is not the "talking cure" but the "affect communicating and regulating cure" (Schore, 2005). (Amid, 2024)

Applying this right brain nonverbal communication model to the clinical context, Amid describes the importance of a moment of "becoming at-one with the patient," which commonly occurs at a turning point of the therapy:

Intersubjective work is not defined by what the therapist intelligibly *does* for the patient or *says* to her [left brain focus]. Rather, as Schore (2009) argues, "the key mechanism is *how to be with the patient* [right brain focus], especially during affectively stressful moments." . . . When the therapist refrains from intelligibly understanding the patient's thoughts and feelings, and instead, unconsciously surrenders to *experiencing* the thinker of these thoughts (as it inadvertently happens in at-one-ment), when the analytic pair moves from talking together about the suffering towards suffering together—then, sometimes, what seems like a failure to understand is, in fact, the precursor to true understanding. The eclipse may sometimes usher in the sunrise.

Chapter 9

Scientific Updates of Right-Brain-to-Right-Brain Communications: Hyperscanning the Therapeutic Relationship

In 1994 my right-brain-to-right-brain communication model was based on theoretical principles, clinical explorations, and extant neuroscience research. Even more direct evidence of the two-person, two-brain model awaited an emergent technology that could simultaneously measure two brains interacting face-to-face in real time. Over the last decade, hyperscanning methodologies utilizing functional near-infrared spectroscopy (fNIRS), electroencephalography (EEG), functional magnetic resonance imaging (fMRI), and magneto-encephalography, providing simultaneous measurements of two individuals, are now available. This technological advance allows for the study of two brains in real-time social interactions with each other.

Hyperscanning Synchrony and Brain Laterality: A Paradigm Shift in Psychotherapy and Psychopathology Research

Inspired by the classic, developmental psychoanalytic research of Beebe, Tronick, Feldman, and especially Trevarthen on intersubjective nonverbal synchronization and communication between a mother and her infant (see Figure 7.1), Dumas and his colleagues (2010) offered a now-classic dual

EEG hyperscanning study of a spontaneous nonverbal social interaction between two individuals, characterized by reciprocal communication and turn-taking. This two-brain, two-body methodology allows for a simultaneous measurement of brain activities of each member of a face-to-face dyad during a two-way intersubjective nonverbal communication, where "both participants are continuously active, each modifying their own actions in response to the continuously changing actions of their partner" (Dumas et al., 2010).

These researchers report changes in both brains in this relational context, where both share attention and compare cues of self and other. Furthermore, they document an interbrain synchronization, on a time scale of milliseconds, of right centroparietal regions, a neuromarker of social coordination in both interacting partners, as well as a synchronization between the posterior right temporoparietal junction (right TPJ) of one partner and right TPJ of the other. They cite studies showing that outside conscious awareness, the right-lateralized TPJ is activated in social interactions (Decety & Lamm, 2007), in allocating attention to self and other representations (Santiestaban et al., 2012), and in making sense of another mind (Saxe & Wexler, 2005). To this I would add the documented involvement of the right TPJ in "subjective judgements of humanness" (Dumas et al., 2020). Note the last function directly pertains to the theme of this book, *The Right Brain and the Origin of Human Nature.*

The top-down view in Figure 9.1 shows this right-lateralized interbrain synchronization of an emotionally communicating dyad, rapidly sending and receiving nonverbal attachment signals of face, voice, and gesture. These data document what I have termed a right-brain-to-right-brain interaction between one subjective self and another subjective self, whereby one unconscious mind intersubjectively communicates with another unconscious mind across an affectively energized electromagnetic intersubjective field. Note this top-down view of a right brain interaction is the same as the lateral views of a right brain communication in Figures 7.1, 7.2, 8.1, and 8.3.

The right-brain-to-right-brain synchronized communication model is also supported in a hyperscanning study by Stolk and his colleagues (2014). These authors generated fMRI brain images on each participant of a communicating dyad, where "both partners mutually learned to adjust to each other" (a fundamental mechanism of an evolving relationship between two interacting brains). Simultaneously measuring cerebral activities in pairs

FIGURE 9.1

Top-down view of a hyperscanned, right-lateralized
interbrain synchronization of a spontaneous bidirectional
nonverbal communication of face, voice, and gesture

© 2011 Guillaume Dumas, taken from "Towards a two-body neuroscience,"
Communicative & Integrative Biology, reprinted by permission of Informa UK
Limited, trading as Taylor & Francis Group https://www.tandfonline.com

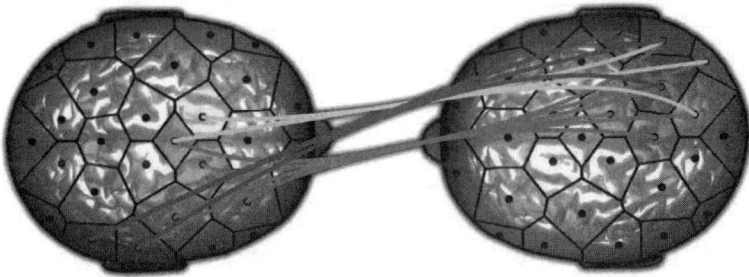

of communicators, these researchers reported that establishing mutual understanding of novel signals synchronizes cerebral dynamics across both communicators' right temporal lobes. Importantly, interpersonal synchronization occurred only in pairs with a shared communicative history. These researchers documented that in this nonverbal intersubjective communication, the processing of novelty and meaning is generated in the right (and not left) hemisphere.

Shortly after, Bilek and her colleagues (2015) published a dual fMRI hyperscanning study of "interacting dyads, the simplest and most fundamental form of human interaction" (p. 5207). Noting that human social interactions shape brain evolution and are essential to development, health, and society, this work investigates "a social interaction that is used by humans to *coordinate and communicate* [emphasis added] intentions as well as guiding others in nonverbal ways, especially through eye gaze" (p. 5208). In order to study "the information flow *between* brains of human dyads during real-time social interaction," they hyperscanned both brains during a nonverbal interaction. This two-person methodology allowed for audiovisual interactions between two subjects in linked fMRI scanners, enabling them to see and hear each other, and to monitor changes in eye gaze and facial expressions.

The authors report a "cross-brain" connectivity pattern unique to interacting individuals, identifying an interbrain information flow between the sender's and receiver's right TPJs. They state that this "synchronization of the sender's and receiver's right TPJ" was unique to interacting subjects, and that this coupling of their TPJs represents a "real world measure of social behavior" and is related to "social expertise." These researchers also observe that the right TPJ is coupled with the orbitofrontal cortex and the medial prefrontal cortex. Bilek's group describes the right TPJ as a central component of the human social brain network, a supramodal association area that integrates input from visual, auditory, somesthetic, and limbic areas (see Figure 9.2).

Underscoring the uniquely human existence of this right-TPJ-to-right-TPJ coupling, they conclude, "Our findings support a central role of human-specific cortical areas in the brain dynamics of dyadic interactions" (Bilek et al., 2015, p. 5207). Note that this right temporoparietal "cross-brain" interaction is identical to Dumas's right-lateralized interbrain synchronization (Figure 9.1). I suggest this "information flow between two interacting brains" is the flow of nonverbal information between two coupled right

FIGURE 9.2

Lateral view of neural coupling sites within the right temporoparietal junction in nonverbally interacting subjects

Note location in the posterior cortical areas of the right hemisphere.

Bilek, E., Ruf, M., Schäfer, A., Akdeniz, C., Calhoun, V. D., Schmahl, C., Demanuele, C., Tost, H., Kirsch, P., & Meyer-Lindenberg, A. (2015). Information flow between interacting human brains: Identification, validation, and relationship to social expertise. Proceedings of the National Academy of Sciences, 112(16), 5207–5212. https://doi.org/10.1073/pnas.1421831112 Cropped from original.

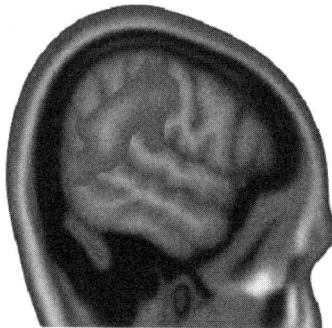

brains, a right-brain-to-right-brain communication system. This information flow is bidirectional. Note that this system, which I earlier identified with Freud's unconscious ego that emerges at about two to three months, is unique to our species and thereby lies at the core foundation of the origin of human nature.

Bilek's laboratory followed up this research with a dual fMRI hyperscanning study of cross-brain information flow in borderline personality disorders, known to experience early childhood neglect and trauma and later show affect dysregulation, social deficits, unstable interpersonal relationships, and reduced interpersonal synchrony (Bilek et al., 2017). They report reduced interbrain synchrony in the right TPJ during social interactions with patients currently diagnosed as borderline compared to healthy controls. Interestingly, they document that individuals with borderline personality disorder in remission showed the same synchrony as healthy controls, due to interbrain plasticity within psychotherapy. Recall that effective psychotherapy with these patients involves the empathic therapist's ability to implicitly synchronize, communicate, and regulate the borderline's dysregulated affective states.

Hyperscanning studies also document reduced interpersonal synchrony in another early-appearing developmental disturbance, autistic spectrum disorders (McNaughton & Redcay, 2020), specifically in the temporoparietal junction, during a conversation compared to typically developing individuals (Quinones-Camacho et al., 2021). Kanner (1943), the pioneer of autism studies, observed that these individuals make less eye contact, while later laboratories reported abnormal asynchronized gaze and a focus more on the mouth when viewing faces (Neumann et al., 2006) as well as a deficit in interoception (Dubois et al., 2016), an inability to read their own bodily states, especially under stress. Indeed, fMRI research demonstrates that the brains of high-functioning autistic individuals do not synchronize with others', indicating their minds "do not 'tick together' with others while perceiving identical dynamic social interaction" (Salmi et al., 2013, p. 489).

In a 2014 article in the *Journal of Infant, Child, and Adolescent Psychotherapy*, I offered a body of research and clinical data indicating that although both the analytic left hemisphere and holistic right hemisphere are affected by a common neuropathological process that begins in utero, at the core, autism, which shows a higher incidence in males, represents a severe impairment of the right-lateralized cortical-subcortical

limbic-autonomic self-system that acts implicitly beneath levels of conscious awareness (Schore, 2014a). Citing studies observing a deviance of
fetal growth in autistic spectrum disorder (Abel et al., 2013), I suggested
that alterations of the right amygdala occur prenatally due to untoward
intrauterine influences, and that autistic disorders reflect altered connectivity and "developmental derangement" of the right brain. This underdevelopment of the social emotional right brain is commonly associated with an
overdeveloped left brain. Autistic spectrum disorders show a hemispheric
asymmetry: a compensatory strong left over a weak right hemisphere (see
Chapter 4).

In support of this hemispheric asymmetry model, researchers are now
concluding that autism is not principally a cognitive or intellectual deficit,
but fundamentally a nonverbal communication deficit of the developing
networks in the right hemisphere (Leisman et al., 2023). In a review article
in *Brain Research Bulletin*, these authors cite my work on the right brain
(Schore, 2005) and assert,

> The core issue related to autistic spectrum disorders and its repetitive
> stereotypical behaviors, verbal and nonverbal deficits and especially
> socialization and attachment deficits are primarily related to a defi-
> cit of development of right hemisphere networks that underlie these
> issues. . . . This bottom-up interference impacts right brain development
> which commences in utero and continues over the first three years of
> life. (Leisman et al., 2023, p. 73)

These researchers conclude that autistic disorders are fundamentally an
underdevelopment of right hemispheric networks, wherein various prefrontal regions are not effectively synchronized with each other. This socioemotional deficit is expressed in "less nonverbal reflexive communication and
reciprocation with parents and caregivers, a lack of eye contact, and lesser
emotional responsivity to facial expressions" (Leisman et al., 2023, p. 71).

It is important to note that a substantial overlap exists between autism,
first discussed by Kanner in 1943, and Asperger's syndrome, first explored
in 1944. Both share a common prenatal and perinatal etiology and a deficit
in social interaction, nonverbal communication, and empathy, with ASD
focusing on alterations in the early developing social right hemisphere
and Asperger's focusing on unusual speech and obsessive interests of the

later developing left hemisphere. I suggest that an essential component of any effective treatment model with both of these patients is the therapist's implicit ability to cocreate a right-lateralized interbrain synchronization that underlies a nonverbal right-brain-to-right-brain therapeutic relationship. This work involves working with subliminal affect regulation, as I have discussed in these chapters.

Schizophrenia involves both positive symptoms, left hemispheric language deficits, and negative symptoms, right hemispheric relational and emotional deficits (McGilchrist, 2021a). With respect to the latter, negative symptoms of impaired emotional expression and reduced motivation for social contact, schizophrenics show communication deficits in nonverbal synchrony in social interactions (Kupper et al., 2015). In an article in *Schizophrenia Research*, Basavaraju et al. (2023) report that individuals at high risk for later psychosis show increased prenatal gyrification of the right lateral parieto-occipital area, which develops earliest in utero. This abnormal right-lateralized gyrification includes the early-developing right inferior prefrontal, insula, and superior temporal areas that show impairments in early neurodevelopmental processes. They conclude,

> The right-sided brain is shown to develop earlier than the left and infants under the age of 2 years are predominantly right brained (Matsuzawa et al., 2001). The neural circuitry stress-coupling strategies and adaptive regulation of affect is proposed to be located in the rostral regions of the early developing right hemisphere (Schore, 2002). This finding of increased gyrification in the fronto-insular-temporal areas may reflect cortical folding abnormalities in early prenatal development that might potentially be an anatomical marker for vulnerability to stress and affect dysregulation that are proposed to play a major role in onset of psychosis. (Basavaraju et al., 2023, p. 252)

Yet another study reports that schizophrenic patients increase interactional synchrony after body-oriented psychotherapy (Galbusera et al., 2018). The key to any form of psychotherapy is the clinician's ability to synchronize with these schizophrenic patients and cocreate a stronger nonverbal therapeutic alliance.

With regard to other psychiatric disorders, research on the developmental attachment origin of depression shows that maternal depression symptoms disrupt left-sided cradling (Pileggi et al., 2020), and that moth-ers with a history of depression are less synchronized in interactions with their infants during the regulation of their infant's negative and positive emotions (Woody et al., 2016; Granat et al., 2017). In addition, research on the negative impact of maternal postpartum depression on mother-to-infant bonding and attachment reports, "Women with depressive symp-toms showed less closeness, warmth, and sensitivity and a significantly lower level of mutual attunement (with regard to emotional availability) and experienced more difficulties in their relationship with their child during the first year" (Slomian et al., 2019, p. 24). Other studies document a disturbed processing of negative emotion in depressed females, expressed as an implicit deficit in automatically and unconsciously orienting attention to the negative social information of a sad face (Yang et al., 2011).

Furthermore, major depressive disorder in adults is associated with reduced facial synchrony in clinical interviews (Altmann et al., 2021). Rotenberg (2004) offers a brain asymmetry model of depression as a func-tional insufficiency of the right hemisphere. Regulation theory dictates that the early asynchronous dysregulated emotional and relational etiology of depression and its treatment by right brain psychotherapy contrasts sig-nificantly with that of cognitive-based classical attachment theory, which relates left hemispheric harmful thinking patterns to depressive symptoms and completely overlooks right brain emotional attachment dynamics. In order to effectively reduce this symptomatology, the clinician must shift out of the left brain and into the right in order to access the patient's dysregu-lated implicit attachment dynamics, cocreate a right-lateralized interbrain synchronization, and regulate the negative and positive affects associated with the depression disorder.

In clinical research on synchrony and hemispheric asymmetry, Zhang and her colleagues (2018) published in *Psychiatry Research Neuroimaging* the first hyperscanning study of simultaneous recordings of a patient's brain interacting with a therapist's brain during a face-to-face psychotherapy session in the laboratory. In a noninvasive functional near-infrared spec-troscopy (fNIRS) investigation titled, "Interpersonal Brain Synchronization Associated With Working Alliance During Psychological Counseling," col-lege students (mostly female) presented with both problems in emotions and interpersonal relationships. The researchers reported that clinicians focused empathically on the patient's "emotional states," and in this "reciprocal communication both members observed each other's nonverbal cues, facial expressions and gestures," in other words, attachment communications. Therapists reported being attentive to "moment to moment cues" of "emotional expression and body posture," and offered emotional feedback.

During the 40-minute first counseling session, the researchers observed increases in cortical blood flow (hemoglobin oxygenation) and interpersonal brain synchronization of the right TPJ in both the clinician's and patient's brains. This increased right-lateralized interbrain synchronization was specifically related to subjective ratings of the affective bond or positive personal attachments between dyads. They reported that this interbrain synchrony was higher in the treatment sessions than in day-to-day encounters, in line with my ideas about the enduring impact of heightened affective moments of a session. The authors interpreted these findings as showing that the clinician and client form an interbrain synchronization that plays an essential role in building a working alliance and a positive therapeutic relationship, and that this brain-to-brain coupling facilitates the development of an emotional bond in the therapeutic alliance in the first session. They concluded that this important nonverbal skill improves the working alliance, and that training should now focus on how to effectively synchronize with patients. Recall that the right TPJ is a central hub for interpersonal synchronization.

In a subsequent publication, this laboratory offered another fNIRS study, "Experience-Dependent Counselor-Client Brain Synchronization During Psychological Counseling" (Zhang et al., 2020). Here they use fNIRS hyperscanning of the patient and therapist to study the role of the counselor's clinical experience in building an alliance with clients. Working with a similar clinical population as before, during the first counseling session the therapeutic dyad in a face-to-face context focused on each other's nonverbal cues and on bodily-based emotional states (see Figure 9.3 for this "naturalistic psychological context" in the laboratory).

Note the distance between the two faces and bodies in Figure 9.3, one similar to the typical clinical psychotherapy context. In this reciprocal communication, both members observed each other's nonverbal cues, facial expressions, and gestures (attachment signals). Zhang et al. (2020) reported that experienced therapists (psychologists) with 600–4,000 hours of clinical experience utilized an "integrative" clinical approach, focusing on empathizing and offering emotional feedback to the client. These expert

FIGURE 9.3

Experimental design of hyperscanning fNIRS study of right-lateralized interbrain synchronization between client and experienced therapist during a counseling session

Notice that the optic probes were placed only over the patient's and therapist's right hemispheres.

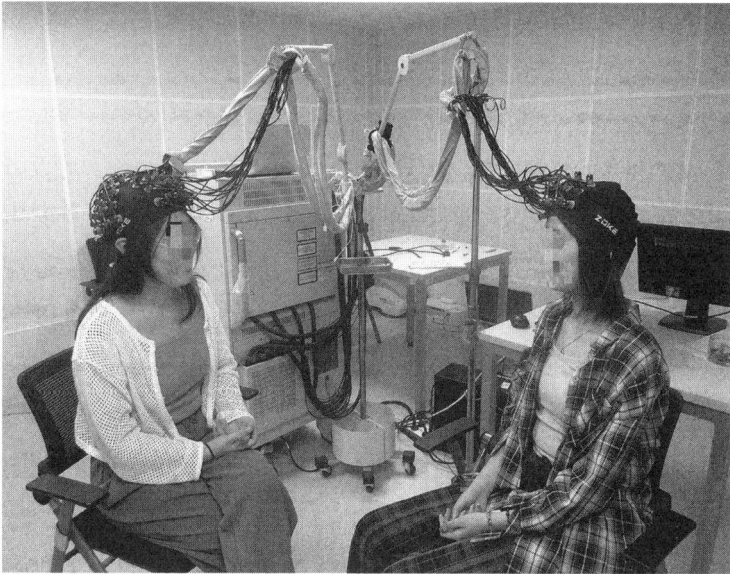

clinicians used "moment-to-moment cues (e.g., emotional expression, body posture) and tried to be attentive to their clients' reactions."

In Figure 9.4, the probes of the optic tomography system collecting the fNIRS data were placed over the right TPJ of the client and the therapist. I suggest that in this clinical emotional context, the emitter of the emotional signal is the client and the receiver is the regulatory clinician, which then shifts to the emitter being the clinician and the client being the receiver. This is in line with the idea that the right TPJ sends and receives bidirectional right-brain-to-right-brain communications between two individuals.

Hyperscanning the patient and therapist, this laboratory again documented a therapy-induced right-lateralized interpersonal synchronization,

FIGURE 9.4
fNIRS probe of the emitter and the sender in the posterior right TPJ

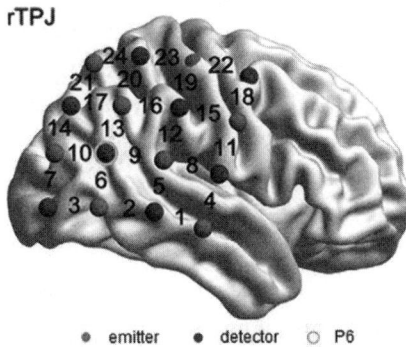

a right-TPJ-to-right-TPJ alignment that was especially evident with clinicians who had more psychotherapy experience. The researchers showed that in the first session the clinician's ability to specifically focus on the client's emotional states and to interpersonally synchronize with her or him is an expression of therapeutic expertise. Zhang et al. (2020) concluded that increased right-lateralized interbrain synchronization over the session is associated with tighter interpersonal closeness or connectedness and better alliance or emotional interaction, and that this study confirms an interpersonal synchrony model of psychotherapy which dictates that "the more tightly the client and counselor's brains are coupled, the better the alliance" (Koole & Tschacher, 2016).

In both Zhang studies, during the session synchronous brain activity is seen in a synchronized alignment of the action potential and physiological metabolic activity in the right TPJ of both members of the therapeutic dyad. This therapist–patient right-lateralized brain synchronization is the same as Dumas's two-body nonverbal intersubjective communication (see Figure 9.1), as well as Bilek's social information flow between interacting human right brains. As in those intersubjective contexts, the right TPJ cortex of the expert empathic clinician is interpersonally synchronized with the right TPJ cortex of the patient, thus cocreating a rapid emotional right-brain-to-right-brain nonverbal communication system that operates between the therapist's and patient's minds and bodies (Schore 1994/2016, 2003b, 2019b). Note that functional near infrared spectroscopy allows imaging of the right cerebral *cortical* hemisphere but not *subcortical* regions of the emotional right brain.

That said, in this conversation between limbic systems, invisible right-brain-to-right-brain communication is now portrayed in a visual representation. These hyperscanning data directly validate my 1994 right-brain-to-right-brain model that runs throughout this book, as well as my emotion-tracking and -synchronizing models of the psychotherapy and attachment relationships outlined in previous chapters. They also are represented on the cover of one of my recent books, *Right Brain Psychotherapy* (see Figure 9.5).

Neuroscientists now assert, "Synchrony is generally defined as the social coupling of two (or more) individuals in the here-and-now of a communication context that emerges alongside, and in addition to, their verbal exchanges" (Tschacher & Meier, 2019). The spatial positional reference in Figure 9.5 describes the nonverbal right hemisphere alongside the verbal left hemisphere, and coupled right brains. Note the shift of hemispheric dominance in the nonverbal emotional interaction and the lack of activity in the left TPJ of the brains of the therapist and patient. In contrast to the right TPJ's involvement in implicit emotional engagement, the left TPJ is involved

FIGURE 9.5

Top-down view of a right-lateralized interbrain synchronization and right-brain-to-right-brain nonverbal communication of emotion in psychotherapy

Based on Dumas et al. (2011) and Zhang et al. (2018, 2020).

Illustration by Beth Schore

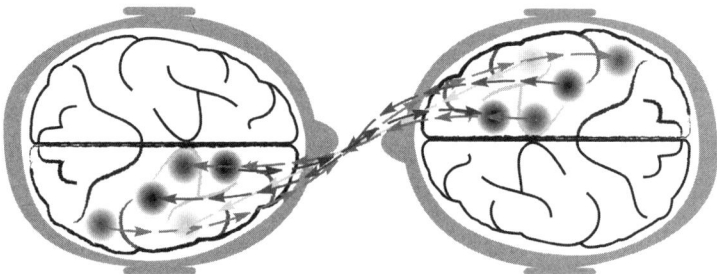

in the cognitive processes associated with the inference of someone else's conscious belief (Samson et al., 2004). As opposed to the right TPJ's involvement in implicit emotional engagement, the left TPJ is involved in high-level mentalizing (Jiang et al., 2015), as well as in the cognitive processes associated with the inference of someone else's conscious belief and in voluntary emotional distancing and cognitive control. This distancing is a central mechanism of the cognitive reappraisal of cognitive behavioral therapy.

While administering cognitive behavioral therapy, the therapist stays up left and focuses on the patient's conscious negative thoughts and verbal communication, and thereby neglects right hemisphere unconscious affective and relational nonverbal communication. I suggest that right-lateralized interbrain synchronization within the coconstructed therapeutic alliance would not be expressed in the hyperscanning of left brain technique-driven cognitive behavioral therapy or mentalization. Mentalization, the ability to understand the mental state of oneself and others (Euler et al., 2021), is shown by Fonagy and colleagues to reflect left hemispheric activation (Nolte et al., 2010). In left brain mentalization, self and other are explicitly and cognitively represented as autonomous individuals with their own separate left minds, in contrast to right brain implicit representations where self and other synchronously share emotions between two linked right minds and coupled right brains.

These hyperscanning studies directly support the clinical principles that the establishment of an effective relationship is the most important criterion for measuring therapeutic expertise, and that expertise is expressed in the clinical ability to establish an affective relationship with various types of patients, just as I have described in these chapters. Both of these involve the cocreation of a right-brain-to-right-brain emotional communication system within the therapeutic alliance. In neuroimaging research on affective processing in psychotherapy, Tschacher, Schildt, and Sander (2010) report that "activation of structures in the right hemisphere (the 'emotional' hemisphere) preceded activation of left-hemispheric structures." They state these findings are in accordance with a leading role of right-hemispheric structures in the processing of affective stimuli and conclude, "Psychotherapy research is no longer concerned with efficacy but rather with how effective change occurs." In an overview of synchrony in psychotherapy titled, "In Sync With Your Shrink: Grounding Psychotherapy in Interpersonal Synchrony," Koole et al. (2020) show that a high level of synchrony is associated with the formation of a strong working alliance between the patient and the therapist, as well as greater effectiveness of the treatment.

In a more recent article on hyperscanning interbrain synchrony, the coupling of brain activity between people interacting with each other, Sened and colleagues (2022) extensively describe the Zhang psychotherapy research and the synchronized right-TPJ-to-right-TPJ finding. Building upon the Zhang studies, they offer a clinical model of therapeutic change in which they suggest,

> . . . therapy improves patients' ability to achieve such synchrony through inter-brain plasticity—a process by which recurring exposure to high interbrain synchrony leads to lasting change in a person's overall ability to synchronize. Therapeutic sessions provide repeated situations with high inter-brain synchrony. This can lead to a long-term increase in the ability to synchronize, first with the therapist, then generalized to other interpersonal relationships, ultimately leading to symptom reduction. (Sened et al., 2022, p. 1)

This interbrain plasticity occurs in mutually synchronized social interactions, in which "brains that fire together wire together" (Shamay-Tsoory, 2022), that is, the coupling of the emotional energies of right brains. Recall that neuroplasticity is dependent upon energy.

Further Thoughts on Right-Brain-to-Right-Brain Unconscious Communication

The coupling of two right brains occurs in what the child psychiatrist Daniel Stern (2004) describes as an affectively charged, well-fitted "moment of meeting":

> Moment of meeting is a present moment between two participants that potentially . . . reshapes the intersubjective field and alters the relationship. It is called forth as an emergent property . . . and must be exquisitely sensitive to this context. . . . It cannot be a general technical response but must be a specific authentic one that carries the therapist's personal signature, so to speak. This is necessary because there is an

interpersonal sharing in this moment that alters the intersubjective field between the two. The affectively charged sharing expands the intersubjective field so that their relationship as mutually sensed is suddenly different from what it was before the moment of meeting. This change in the intersubjective field does not require verbalization or narration to be effective and lasting. (Stern, 2004)

In interpersonal neurobiological terms, during a synchronized face-to-face intersubjective dialogue, a therapeutic emotional bond and an interpersonal relational connection is (re)established. In "heightened affective moments" of high interbrain synchrony of a session, two coupled right brains are unconsciously bidirectionally communicating emotions across an affectively energized and expanded intersubjective field (see Figures 8.1, 9.1, 9.5, and especially 8.3, showing Bradley's [2010] bidirectional energy oscillations that encode emotional information communicated between individuals). The shared psychodynamic electromagnetic intersubjective field of emotional energy is a major source of neuroplasticity.

Hosseini (2021) offers evidence that brain-to-brain communication involves similar patterns of action potentials in the cortex of two individuals, and that this synchronized activity of neurons generates membrane depolarizations, oscillations, a stronger electromagnetic field, and synaptic activity in limbic and subconscious centers. McFadden (2002) discusses how synchronized activity of a large number of neuronal action potentials can give rise to large oscillations, generating a strong electromagnetic field that produces an image of the information in the neurons and impacts brain function. The concept of a field is derived from physics and refers to a spatially distributed nonmaterial element that is able to impart a force upon an object within it (Rubik et al., 2015). Resilience, a construct also taken from physics, is defined as the capacity of matter to absorb energy when it is deformed and then release that energy and come back to a normal state.

According to Naviaux (2019), energy-generating mitochondria are involved in the "metabolic features and regulation of the healing cycle." He asserts that the first stage of the healing cycle that leads to adaptation and recovery is regular cycling between wakeful activity and restorative sleep, a parasympathetic-dominant autonomic state that restores cell damage and normal cell-cell communication. Naviaux cites data indicating that healing involves recovery of energy in mitochondrial oxidative phosphorylation throughout the organism.

I suggest that this recovery also occurs in the mitochondria of right brain limbic-autonomic circuits that provide energy utilized in the emotion communication and regulation healing processes of psychotherapeutic change, including metabolic changes in an energized intersubjective field as well as in subsequent new neuroplasticity and synaptogenesis. In turn, this therapeutic relational context promotes structural and functional regulatory changes within the patient's right brain, the emotional brain, and thereby symptom reduction. Acting at implicit levels beneath awareness, the right brain, the social brain, is thus the psychobiological source of social support, a well-documented major factor in the recovery from both psychological disorders and physical disease.

Overviewing hyperscanning and multibrain neuroimaging, Ray and his colleagues (2017) assert that among all forms of interbrain communications, the communication of emotion is the most important process for mental health, confirming another central theme of this volume. With respect to psychopathology, they argue that the interpersonal perspective of between-brain functional connectivity can allow for a deeper understanding of the relational deficits of depression, autism spectrum disorders, schizophrenia, personality disorders, social anxiety disorder, somatic symptom disorder, eating disorders, sexual dysfunctions, and suicide. Furthermore, they see the direct application of this paradigm shift in interbrain neuroimaging to the therapeutic alliance, defined as the collaborative bond between patient and therapist.

In offering the same hyperscanning image of coupled, synchronized right brains in Figure 9.1, Ray et al. (2017) point out that all mental disorders unfold in an interpersonal context, and that in most social settings, the human brain works in interaction with other brains establishing a coupling between themselves. They conclude, "At present functional neuroimaging is on the brink of a *paradigm shift*, quantifying the *brain interactions between individuals transcending the boundary of the skull*" (see Figures 8.1 and 9.1, and the distance between the faces and right-lateralized interbrain synchronization in the cocreated energized electromagnetic intersubjective field). Recall my earlier assertion that we are now experiencing a paradigm shift in psychotherapy from a one-person intrapsychic to a two-person interpersonal perspective (and thus ultimately an integrated model of both).

As I have described throughout these chapters, interbrain synchrony provides a therapeutic context for a face-to-face dialogue of two nonverbal emotional right brains engaged in a rapid, reciprocal, bidirectional right-brain-to-right-brain communication system, beneath conscious awareness. A very recent article reports that the human sensory systems gather data at ~10^9 bits/second (gigabits) as opposed to the slowness of human behavior and cognition at only 10 bits/second (Zheng & Meister, 2024). The authors state that this vast gulf from processing bits of thoughts to gigabits of sensory data reflects the difference between the rapid and parallel processing in the peripheral nervous system (ANS) and the slow and serial processing of cognition in the central nervous system. The authors note that the "glacially slow pace" of human thought and behavior at 10 bits/s "only takes into account things that we can consciously experience and access, so that we can talk about them," and is "ridiculously small compared with any information we encounter in daily life." Note the well-documented differences between the slow processing of the linear left hemisphere and the rapid parallel processing of the right hemisphere, which is specialized to represent multiple sensory information channels in parallel (Bradshaw & Nettleton, 1981).

In "The Neurobiology of Human Super-communication," Hoffmann (2021) asserts,

> The more rapidly an organism can assess the environment, the more effective its coping skills and survival are. Our communication heritage evolved to include a penta-sensory input system and a multimodal output communication proficiency. . . . This system utilizes facial micro expressions, body postures, leg movements and scents. . . . The five human sensory systems together acquire about 11 million bits of information every second, whereas the conscious mind is only able to process 16–50 bits per second. . . . Many survival aspects and important decisions occur without our conscious awareness. (p. 288)

Hoffmann refers to "our evolutionary fine-tuned survival features of rapid subconscious reflexes. . . . To benefit from our non-conscious processing capability, about each other, for optimum communication between us, we have to be in each other's company, that is, face-to-face!" (p. 289).

Authors are now suggesting a "two-body approach" that captures face-to-face interbrain synchronization and unconscious mutual attunement, and that the dynamic exchange between individuals represents the "dark matter" of live social interaction (Ayache et al., 2021). Indeed, the right hemisphere has literally been described as "the dark side of consciousness" (Keenan et al., 2005), and thereby the origin of human nature. Freud (1916–1917/1963) speculated that the feared unknown *"dark continent* of psychological inquiry" was his self-proclaimed inability to understand the female mind (in 1937 the psychoanalyst Karen Horney, a Norton author, challenged Freud's view of female psychology, arguing that his theories were male-centric and did not reflect social and cultural factors). Freud's developmental psychoanalytic model focuses on the central role of power and aggression in masculine oedipal dynamics between a son and father. This contrasts with his disinterest and neglect of the earlier preoedipal stage, where the mother is the central figure in the psychic development of both sexes, which therefore became terra incognita, the dark continent. For a recent neurobiologically informed model of the feminine mind and body I refer the reader to my Jungian colleague Tina Stromsted's (2025) remarkable volume, *Soul's body: Active imagination, authentic movement, and embodiment in psychotherapy.*

Indeed, as opposed to Freud, Carl Jung offered gendered images of the polarities and variations of the paternal and maternal functions:

> Maternal function, suggesting femininity, is represented as feeding, nurturing, containing—or as suffocating and engulfing. Paternal function, suggesting masculinity, is represented in terms of structure, discipline, authority, prohibition, and boundary setting—or as the misuse of power expressed through harshness, domination, and abuse. (Woodhead, 2004, p. 78)

Neurobiologically, these regulating and dysregulating gender differences are represented in, respectively, the early-maturing nonverbal right and later-maturing verbal left hemispheres. I suggest that the right brain is the neurobiological locus of Jung's anima, the source of the feminine component of the personality, while the left brain is the locus of Jung's animus, the masculine component of the personality.

Earlier I discussed Hecht (2014), who cites a large body of brain laterality studies indicating that the right hemisphere mediates affiliation motivation, the left hemisphere power motivation. This human need for affiliation—being connected with and accepted by other people—motivates people to seek warm, stable, and intimate interpersonal relationships, form friendships, and affiliate with specific groups. Also recall Kuhl and Kazen's (2008) characterization of two different basic social needs in humans, affiliation and power, and a basic link between affiliation and right hemispheric processing and power and left hemispheric processing. They point out that the right hemispheric affiliation system is associated with a "holistic and intuitive" style and is involved in "intimacy and affective sharing in close relationships." The *OED* defines *intimate* as "involving very close connection or union." These brain laterality data indicate that the dark continent also includes the human capacity for love, a cardinal right brain expression of the origin of human nature.

Informed by developmental psychoanalytic data, Rosenbaum (2011) suggests that the dark continent female receptive space intuitively processes experience, holds and waits, yet also interacts. This inner space, which the mother shares with the child, is filled with sensation, arousal, and symbolic meaning, and is "unseen." She characterizes the dark continent as the realm of "unconscious, nonverbal communication and attunement, and mental states residing at the far reaches of a continuum of empathy and intuition" (p. 58). Citing my work, she asserts, "It appears to share common ground with aspects of the therapeutic bond, transference and countertransference, the intersubjective field, and integration of conscious and unconscious processes" (p. 57). I suggest that dark continents interact with each other through unconscious right-brain-to-right-brain communications and that the early-developing right brain represents the dark continent of human psychology.

Thirty years ago, in the last chapter of *Affect Regulation and the Origin of the Self*, I cited the philosopher of science and mathematician Jacob Bronowski (1972), whose words ring true today:

> So science takes its coherence, its intellectual and imaginative strength together from the concepts at which its line cross, like knots in a mesh. Gravitation, mass and energy, evolution, enzymes, the gene and *the unconscious*—these are the bold creations of science, the strong *invisible* [emphasis added] skeleton on which it articulates the movements of the world.

As the chapters of this book show, I would now amend this description to include an omnipresent relational unconscious in everyday life, an ultra-rapid right-brain-to-right-brain nonverbal communication and regulation system within a cocreated dynamic electromagnetic intersubjective field that is hidden in plain sight and invisible to the left hemispheric conscious mind. Myron Hofer (1984) showed that relationships act as "hidden regulators." The right prefrontal system is the anatomical locus of "the hidden observer," described as a preconscious system "that the person had registered and stored in memory without being aware that the information had been processed" (Hilgard, 1984, p. 248). This unconscious system also acts as a "participant observer" (Sullivan, 1953) of not only another self's external behavior but also internal subjective states.

Recall that the deeper strata of this right mind is the locus of the subcortical right amygdala, the deep unconscious, which "senses the *invisible* [emphasis added]" and is centrally involved in "invisible social force fields that regulate close physical proximity." In basic social psychological research, "Getting in Under the Radar: A Dyadic View of Invisible Support," Howland and Simpson (2010) suggested, "Invisible support is a dyadic phenomenon, one that requires both skillful support by providers and relative lack of awareness by recipients to yield maximal benefit" (p. 1879). They observed that invisible support is skillfully delivered less overtly and noticed less by recipients, and that it is enacted in spontaneous interactions and unstructured conversations. Clearly, invisible social support is provided by implicit, subliminal interactive affect regulation.

In another publication, "Reading Minds and Being Invisible: The Role of Empathic Accuracy in Invisible Support Provision," Howland (2016) reports that implicit invisible social support that takes place "between the lines" is superior to explicit visible social support in improving relationship quality (Maisel & Gable, 2009) and in reducing stress (Bolger & Amarel, 2007). These latter authors posit that "skillful" support is rooted in "the everyday fabric of relationships" that is "delivered so smoothly" that the other does not consciously notice it. They also propose that the absence of explicit support is associated with the strength of a close relationship. Indeed they document that visible-support social behavior is viewed by recipients as inappropriate or insulting. I would add, this is especially so in left-dominant avoidant patients.

From a clinical perspective, I suggest that these studies on invisible social support are describing the therapist's rapid and thereby unconscious subliminal interactive affect regulation of the patient's emotional states and attachment dynamics. This omnipresent mechanism is embedded in the empathic clinician's implicit receiving, sending, and regulating the unconscious nonverbal communications of the patient's emotional right brain via the therapist's right social brain, under the radar of consciousness, beneath the words.

This work highlights a central theme of these chapters—the fundamental differences between right brain implicit and left brain explicit affect regulation. As I have discussed, these two regulatory processes are respectively located in the unconscious right and conscious left hemispheres. Only implicit emotion regulation is associated with the patient stating at the end of a therapy session "*I feel better but I don't know why*" (Koole & Rothermund 2011; Koole, Webb, & Sheeran, 2015). In contrast to "I understand," this spontaneous expression of the patient indicates that he or she has experienced an unconscious right brain-to-right brain interactive affect regulation.

In total, the brain laterality and hemispheric asymmetry research I've cited throughout this book strongly validates and expands my work on a relational unconscious, an omnipresent ultrarapid and thereby invisible face-to-face right-brain-to-right-brain communication system in the psychotherapeutic relationship, and on an affectively focused model of psychotherapy, including not only psychodynamic psychotherapy but all forms of treatment. In my article in the *Annals of General Psychiatry*, I proposed that psychiatry should consider expanding its clinical models from exclusively focusing on conscious left brain verbal anxiety and depression symptomatology to also include unconscious emotional and relational deficits of the right brain (Schore, 2022). The ability to cocreate a right-brain-to-right-brain relationship with different clinical populations directly impacts the psychologist's or psychiatrist's skill in forming a bond of safety and trust with a variety of patients, in reducing treatment dropout, and in facilitating stronger drug compliance.

In 2014 I published an article in *Psychotherapy*, the flagship journal of the American Psychological Association Division of Psychotherapy, "The Right Brain Is Dominant in Psychotherapy," wherein I offered interdisciplinary evidence indicating that psychotherapy, "a relationship of care," can alter more than the patient's left-lateralized conscious mind. It also directly influences the growth and development of the unconscious "right mind" (Schore, 2014b). Note only a right and not left brain therapeutic approach can change the patient's unconscious self-image and unconscious internal working model of attachment.

In more recent clinical applications of regulation theory, I have focused on autistic spectrum disorders (Schore, 2014a), group psychotherapy (Schore, 2020), working with pathological dissociation (Schore, 2022), therapeutic mutual regressions in clinical reenactments of early attachment trauma (Schore, 2021b), and applications to psychiatry (Schore, 2022). In all my writings, I continue to explore the critical role of right brain emotional and relational processes in psychotherapy and psychoanalysis, asserting that the right brain is dominant in short-term symptom-reducing and long-term growth-promoting deep psychotherapy. In both, the psychotherapist's relational and emotional expertise in working in psychotherapeutic relationships with a wide variety of patients, more than a mastery of techniques, lies at the core of the art of psychotherapy.

Chapter 10

Applications to Current U.S. Culture: Related Right Brain Studies and Future Directions

Looking backward, I'd like to return to the introduction where I discussed the 30th anniversary of *Affect Regulation and the Origin of the Self: The Neurobiology of Emotional Development,* the foundation of my scientific and clinical investigations of the right brain, dominant for the unconscious processing of attachment, emotion, intersubjectivity, bodily-based nonverbal communications between human minds, and indeed, the depths of human nature. Everything I've written since that book has used the interpersonal neurobiological lens of regulation theory to investigate certain fundamental aspects of the human experience that operate beneath conscious awareness. The previous contents and descriptions of the chapters of this book are examples of the wide range of heuristic scientific questions about human nature first explored in that pioneering work. Then I'll look back in another sense—briefly discussing a number of other publications in areas I have not covered in the preceding chapters. Then I'll look forward and give some thoughts on what I see as essential areas of scientific research for the mental health field, and on the implications of my work for current U.S. culture.

The *Affect Regulation* volume laid out the foundation of a modern scientific approach to the problems of human development and human emotion. It was the first articulation of the groundbreaking fields of interpersonal neurobiology and of neuropsychoanalysis, the science of unconscious processes. In the very first sentence of that volume, I boldly asserted,

The understanding of early development is one of the fundamental objectives of science. The beginnings of living systems set the stage for every aspect of an organism's internal and external functioning throughout the lifespan. . . . Of special importance are the incipient interactions the infant has with the most important object in the early environment—the primary caregiver. Events that occur during infancy, especially transactions with the social environment, are indelibly imprinted into the structures that are maturing in the first years of life. The child's first relationship, the one with the mother, acts as a template, as it permanently shapes the individual's capacities to enter into all later emotional relationships. These early experiences shape the development of a unique personality, its adaptive capacities as well as its vulnerabilities to and resistances against particular forms of future pathologies. Indeed, they profoundly influence the emergent organization of an integrated system that is both stable and adaptable, and thereby the formation of the self. (Schore, 1994/2016, p. 1)

In the subsequent pages of this 1994 volume, I articulated for the first time a number of fundamental scientific questions about early human emotional and social development to be addressed by regulation theory:

1. What part do early social-affective experiences play in the postnatal maturation of the human brain?
2. How does the infant's early social environment influence the growth of structural systems involved in emotional functioning that are maturing in infancy?
3. How does the earliest relationship with a specific human being, the attachment to the primary caregiver, permanently influence the individual's capacities to enter into all later relationships?
4. What psychobiological mechanisms underlie the attachment process?
5. What is the role of emotional communications in the child's continuing dialectic between himself and the social environment?
6. How does the child respond to the changes in the social environment that occur over the stages of infancy, and how do these changes affect the course of socioemotional development?

7. How does the developing child retain continuity and self-regulate as he traverses these changes?
8. What factors facilitate or inhibit the emergence of the adaptive capacity for self-regulation?
9. What is the relationship among failures of development, impairments of adaptive capacities, and psychopathology?
10. How can an elucidation of the events of infancy, especially early socioemotional transactions, lead to a deeper understanding of adult normal and abnormal phenomena?
11. How can developmental knowledge be utilized to formulate heuristic strategies toward the treatment of psychological developmental disorders?
12. How does the self evolve?
13. How do early events influence the development of consciousness?

These questions, first proposed 30 years ago, would be addressed by myself and subsequently thousands of other researchers and clinicians over the ensuing three decades.

In terms of the breadth and depth of this body of work over three decades, my professional activities have spanned from generating developmental psychoanalytic conceptions of the early origins of the human unconscious mind to a large body of brain laterality research that underlies interpersonal neurobiological models of the enduring impact of early emotional attachment experiences on right brain development, to neuroscience and psychiatric research on trauma and borderline personality disorder, to biological studies of trauma in wild elephants, to studies of the neurobiology of PTSD, to the early diagnosis of attachment and autistic spectrum disorders, to clinical models of individual and group psychotherapy, to my practice of psychotherapy over the last five decades, and more. Over this time period, I've led study groups in right brain psychotherapy in Los Angeles, Berkeley, Boulder, Portland, Seattle-Vancouver, and Melbourne. I've offered many hundreds of lectures in 22 countries in North and South America, Europe, Asia, and Australia, and have given over 400 scientific presentations and more than 650 group clinical consultations (see Dr. Allan N. Schore, https://www.allanschore.com/). I've acted as past editor of the acclaimed Norton Series on Interpersonal

Neurobiology and as a reviewer or on the editorial staff of more than 50 journals.

As I stated earlier, my studies have now generated over 36,000 Google Scholar citations across a broad range of scientific and clinical disciplines. Their positive impact is also reflected in the fact that along the course of my professional career I have received a number of major awards:

Sapienza University of Rome Lifetime Achievement
   Award in Recognition of Outstanding Contributions
   to Psychotherapy and Neuroscience, 2022
Reiss-Davis Child Study Center, Los Angeles, CA,
   Lifetime Achievement Award, 2022
Sigma Xi, the Scientific Research Honor Society (https://
   www.sigmaxi.org/about), induction, 2021
Sanville Institute for Social Work and Psychotherapy,
   Honorary Degree, Doctor of Humane Letters, 2016
University of California–Davis, Department of Psychiatry and
   Behavioral Sciences, Thomas L. Morrison Endowment
   for Excellence in Psychotherapy Education, 2015
Family Law Meets Attachment Science: Making Better
   Decisions for Children, Honored Speaker, Portcullis
   House, British House of Parliament, Westminster, 2014
American Psychoanalytic Association Honorary Membership, in
   Recognition of Achievements in Integrating the Psychological
   and Biological and for Outstanding Contributions to
   Psychoanalytic and Neuropsychoanalytic Studies, 2014
UCLA Lifespan Learning Interpersonal Neurobiology Conference,
   Celebrating 20 Years of Outstanding Innovations in Affect
   Regulation Theory and Neuroscience Scholarship, 2014
American Psychological Association Division of Trauma
   Psychology, Distinguished Practice Award for Outstanding
   Contributions to Practice in Trauma Psychology, 2013
American Psychological Association, Division of
   Psychoanalysis, Scientific Award in Recognition of
   Outstanding Contributions to the Research, Theory and
   Practice of Neuroscience and Psychoanalysis, 2008

Group Psychotherapy Association of Southern California, in
  Appreciation and Recognition of Groundbreaking Contributions
  to the Fields of Affective Neuroscience, Psychoanalysis,
  Psychotherapy, and Group Psychotherapy, 2007
Reiss-Davis Child Study Center, Los Angeles, Edna-Reiss-Sophie
  Greenberg Chair, Recognizing Outstanding Professionals
  in the Field of Child/Adolescent Mental Health, 2005
Australian and New Zealand Journal of Psychiatry,
  Most Outstanding Article of the Year, 2002

Looking Back and Looking Forward: Other Areas of Study and Implications for the Future

Now I'll look back in another sense—other areas of exploration of regulation theory in a number of publications apart from the preceding chapters. As the reader will note, each of these illuminates and generates highly relevant yet controversial implications for both the individual and human culture.

In 2005, my colleague Gay Bradshaw and I joined with internationally renowned elephant researchers to coauthor an article in *Nature*, "Elephant Breakdown. Social Trauma: Early Disruption of Attachment Can Affect the Physiology, Behaviour and Culture of Animals and Humans Over Generations" (Bradshaw et al., 2005). This study in elephant ethology began with an emotionally powerful visualization of attachment trauma:

The air explodes with the sound of high-powered rifles and the startled infant watches his family fall to the ground, the image seared into his memory. He and other orphans are then transported to distant locales to start new lives. Ten years later, the teenaged orphans begin a killing rampage, leaving more than a hundred victims. A scene describing posttraumatic stress disorder in Kosovo or Rwanda? The similarities are striking—but here, the teenagers are young elephants and the victims, rhinoceroses. In the past, animal studies have been used to make inferences about human behavior. Now, studies of human PTSD can be instructive in understanding how violence also affects elephant culture.

Bowlby's attachment theory was originally grounded in ethology. Integrating behavioral biology with neurobiology, the article cites my *Affect Dysregulation* volume (Schore, 2003a), which shows that studies in both animals and humans indicate that trauma early in life has lasting psychophysiological effects on brain and behavior. Indeed, elephant society in Africa has been decimated by mass deaths and social breakdown from poaching, culls, and habitat loss. Elephants are social animals and are renowned for their close relationships. Young elephants are reared in a matriarchal society, embedded in complex layers of extended family. Culls and illegal poaching have fragmented these patterns of social attachment by eliminating the supportive stratum of the matriarch and older female caretakers (allomothers).

Elephant calves witnessing culls and those raised by young, inexperienced mothers are high-risk candidates for later disorders, including an inability to regulate stress-reactive aggressive states. Even the fetuses of young pregnant females can be affected by prenatal stress during culls. The rhinoceros-killing males may have been particularly vulnerable to the effects of pre- and postnatal stress for two reasons. Studies on a variety of species indicate that male mammalian brains develop at a slower rate relative to females and are more vulnerable, but also that male elephants require a second distinct phase of socialization, adolescence.

The article discussed how wild elephants are displaying symptoms associated with human PTSD: abnormal startle response, depression, unpredictable asocial behavior, and hyperaggression. Under normal conditions, early mother–infant interactions facilitate the development of self-regulatory structures located in the corticolimbic region of the right hemisphere. But with early developmental trauma, an enduring right-brain dysfunction can develop, creating a vulnerability to PTSD and a predisposition to violence in adulthood. Profound disruptions to the attachment bonding process, such as extensive maternal separation, deprivation, or trauma can impair psychobiological and neurochemical regulation in the developing brain. Beyond the individual, trauma can define a culture. Elephant sociality is both a strength and a weakness. As with humans, an intact, functioning social order helps buffer trauma. However, as human populations increase, more elephants are likely to live in environments characterized by severe anthropogenic disturbance. The human species is thus a major source of trauma and PTSD in another species, elephants (Bradshaw et al., 2005).

It is now twenty years since the *Nature* article was published and the practice of culling has stopped. Yet at this point in time the African elephant population has rapidly diminished to 415,000, down from 1.3 million in 1979. There is a now general agreement that *the biggest threat to elephants is human poaching.* This population reduction and highly stressful anthropogenic disturbance within the species is a major contributing factor to the fact that the African elephant is now technically considered "critically endangered."

All mammals share a ubiquitous developmental attachment mechanism and a common stress-regulating neurophysiology. A wealth of human-animal studies and the experiences of human victims of violence are now available to help large-brained intelligent elephants survive. Indeed, this groundbreaking research has been highly cited and incorporated into the field of conservation biology. In 2007 Gay Bradshaw and I expanded this model in the journal *Ethology*, where we asserted that as the dominant species on Earth we have a moral obligation to protect the survival of other species with whom we share the planet.

In another article in *Infant Mental Health Journal*, "All Our Sons: The Developmental Neurobiology and Neuroendocrinology of Boys at Risk" (Schore, 2017a), I described significant gender differences between male and female social and emotional functions in the earliest stages of human development (see Chapter 1). I offered both neurobiological and neuro-endocrinological evidence to show that these result from not only differences in sex hormones and social experiences but also in rates of male and female brain maturation, specifically in the early-developing right brain. Interdisciplinary research indicates that the stress-regulating circuits of the male brain mature more slowly than those of the female in the prenatal, perinatal, and postnatal critical periods, and that this differential structural maturation is reflected in normal gender differences in right brain emotional functions. At the same time, due to this maturational delay, developing males also are more vulnerable over a longer period of time to stressors in the social environment (attachment trauma) and toxins in the physical environment (neurotoxic endocrine disruptors).

In 1962, Rachel Carson published the groundbreaking and transformational volume *Silent Spring*, which triggered a national debate on the worldwide unrestricted proliferation of environmental toxins (chemical pesticides such as DDT) as well as on the role of the responsibilities of science, the chemical industry, and the government. She also questioned the wisdom of the government in allowing toxic chemicals to be so massively discharged into the environment before knowing the long-term consequences. In this forward-looking work, Carson proposed that one detrimental consequence of these toxins was the alteration of the proper balance between male androgenic and female estrogenic hormones in the endocrine system that would lead to an excessive accumulation of either, a foreshadowing of the later-discovered developmental toxicity of endocrine-disrupting chemicals, another aspect of human-induced climate change.

Human exposure to these environmental disruptors is ubiquitous and universal, in the air, water, and earth—herbicides, fungicides, insecticides, and plasticizers. It is important to note that endocrine disruptors such as bisphenol (Symeonides et al., 2024) are environmental toxins that don't break down, and that these "forever chemicals" are found in the human placenta, amniotic fluid, and breast milk (Schore, 2017a). During critical periods of fetal and postnatal development, children are more sensitive to low doses of neurotoxic hormones than adult tissues, and thereby during these "critical windows of exposure" developing infants are highly vulnerable to endocrine disruption. Indeed, a large body of research demonstrates that endocrine disruptors interfere with the organizational functions of the sex hormones, such as the androgenic testosterone system, which in early infancy is involved in programming brain development.

In my 2017 article I offered interdisciplinary evidence showing these neurotoxins specifically interfere with the early development of the right brain and are therefore implicated in the psychopathogenesis of certain early-evolving psychiatric disorders, especially in males. Indeed, this developmental neuroendocrinological mechanism has been posited by a number of authors to be directly involved in the increased vulnerability of males to early-onset schizophrenia, conduct disorder, autism, and ADHD, all of which are showing recent widespread increases in U.S. culture. I suggest these ubiquitous endocrine disruptors are also a major factor in the documented decrease in reading skills in the majority of children in the U.S. At the time of this writing the current administration has eviscerated the Environmental Protection Agency, which monitors and regulates these neurotoxins.

Three years after I wrote about the enduring impact of environmental toxins on early brain development, Robert Naviaux (2020) described the "mitochondrial cell danger response" (see Chapter 3), an ancient, universal stress response to environmental threat or injury, including not only psychological trauma, neglect, and absence of healthy play but also ubiquitous "manmade pollutants" that are "invisible to human eyes, tasteless, and odorless" that we "sense . . . through subconscious cellular responses":

> Over 7,000 chemicals are now made or imported to the U.S. for industrial, agricultural, and personal care use in amounts ranging from 25,000 to over 1 million pounds each year, and plastic waste now exceeds 83 billion pounds/year. This chemical load creates a rising tide of manmade pollutants in the oceans, air, water, and food chain. Fewer than 5% of these chemicals have been tested for developmental toxicity. In the 1980s, 5–10% of children lived with a chronic illness. As of 2018, *40% of children, 50% of teens, 60% of adults under age 65, and 90% of adults over 65 live with chronic illness* [emphasis added]. Several studies now report the presence of dozens to hundreds of manmade chemicals and pollutants in placenta, umbilical cord blood, and newborn blood spots. (p. 40)

Naviaux (2020) suggests that children are more susceptible to these toxins because the cells in their metabolism, brain, and endocrine system are growing rapidly, and therefore more sensitive to disruption. He notes these ubiquitous manmade chemicals strike children in periods of rapid growth in the womb and the first few years of life, laying the groundwork for chronic medical illnesses such as asthma, irritable bowel syndrome, chronic fatigue syndrome, and fibromyalgia, as well as psychiatric disorders like autism, ADHD, PTSD, suicidal depression, and bipolar disorder, the prevalence of which have all increased significantly in recent years. One example is that the United States has the highest prevalence of postpartum depression in developed countries (Norhayati et al., 2014). Another is autism, which has risen from 1 in 150 in 2000 to 1 in 31 today.

The cell danger response produces signs and symptoms of these disorders, including withdrawal from social contact. These chemical toxins, like social adversity, can thereby trigger structural changes in brain growth and permanently alter the trajectory of not only child development but the individual's mental and physical health over the lifespan. Naviaux (2019) states, "Learning and development emerge from both conscious stresses and subconscious chemical senses encountered throughout life" (p. 2). He offers a sober warning: "The toxic chemicals passed on to our children will soon have *more devastating effects on human health than any mutation in DNA*, leading to escalating infertility rates, miscarriages, childhood and adult chronic disease" (Naviaux, 2020, p. 42).

On the matter of early social stressors, I'd like to discuss another important problem I pointed out in 1994 that still is not being directly addressed in the United States. Now that the early roots of resilience and psychopathogenesis are being understood in terms of interpersonal neurobiology and developmental neuroscience, interventions, both preventive and therapeutic, need to take place during the critical periods of their origins in the earlier stages of human life, starting in pregnancy. In other words, the field of infant mental health is poised to actively move toward the goal of not only treating but also potentially preventing psychiatric illnesses and personality disorders. The new information that science is providing on attachment, trauma, emotions, and right brain development is directly relevant to the creation of more effective early intervention and prevention programs. My own work in this area describes a clinical model for assessing and diagnosing not only autistic spectrum disorders but attachment disorders in the early months of the first year (Schore, 2014a; Schore & Newton, 2012).

These advances in scientific knowledge have practical value in generating more complex models of human development that can potentially facilitate the optimization of brain maturation and human potential. This is especially true for emotional development in the critical period of the brain growth spurt in infancy, a temporal interval of right brain dominance. The timing of these interventions to periods of enhanced brain plasticity is essential: We can maximize the short- and long-term effects of our interventions by concentrating on the period of the brain growth spurt—the last trimester of pregnancy through the second year. Whether or not our government will fund such sorely needed efforts is highly doubtful. The current administration is the most antiscientific in history.

In a recent UNICEF report on child well-being in 38 rich countries (Gromada et al., 2020), the United States placed at the bottom, 32 in mental well-being, 38 in physical health, and 32 in academic and social skills. In most of these countries, both maternal and paternal leave are provided by the culture, and day care usually begins at the end of the first year. Even more disturbing is the fact that of all the industrialized nations, the United States is the only one that does not have a national maternal and paternal leave policy, with the effect that many mothers experience stressful isolation, devaluation, neglect, and lack of support from American culture, and that large numbers of infants enter early day care, much of which is substandard, at six weeks of age.

As I stated in Chapter 7, eight weeks is the time of an essential advance in human development—the infant's rapidly growing right brain begins to play its central role in the foundations of human intersubjectivity, play, and love. It also represents a critical period in the development of the right-lateralized autonomic nervous system. In each of these adaptive functions, the infant's right hemisphere needs to engage in sustained and consistent synchronized interactions with the right hemisphere of an intimate primary attachment figure. Recall that neuroscience is now demonstrating that the first expression of love, the one between a mother and her infant, represents "one of the most powerful and evolutionarily preserved forms of positive affect in the emotional landscape of human behavior," that "the phylogenetically ancient role of maternal care . . . appears to be underpinned by evolutionarily ancient structures," and that maternal love for the infant is "a biologically essential mechanism for the preservation of the human species."

In other words, early intimate intersubjective experiences shared with a loving mother positively shape the right brain depths of human nature. Early day care interferes with the very origin of human nature, the formation of the burgeoning mother–infant attachment relationship and the foundation of the human personality, in that at this very time many mothers return to the workforce. These infants are left in day care well before they have formed the bonds of healthy attachment, the foundation of their emotional security in life. Recall my earlier assertion that individual development arises out of the relationship between the brain/mind/body of both infant and caregiver held within a culture and environment that either supports, inhibits, or even threatens it.

With respect to the latter, entry into early day care cannot provide an interpersonal emotional environment for optimal development of the infant's right brain, and it represents a lack of cultural scaffolding of the infant and mother in this earliest period of human development. As I have shown, six weeks represents a critical period of growth for the maturation of the right amygdala, right insula, and right cingulate, the foundational structures of the evolving personality. This accelerated right brain growth is experience-dependent, and it cannot be provided by early day care that usually operates on a 1-to-5 or 1-to-10 ratio of day care workers to infants. In addition, early day care cannot provide increased interventions on a societal basis in the growth-promoting evolutionary mechanisms of left-sided cradling and kangaroo maternal care.

Not one neurobiological or neuropsychological study has been done on the short- and long-term effects of early day care here in the United States. I propose that the lack of legislated temporal protection for the establishment of the early maternal-infant relationship has long-term effects on the emotional health of the culture, in both females and especially males, whose right brains mature more slowly than those of females, making them more vulnerable to early relational stressors and susceptible to developmental disorders and externalizing psychopathologies that are associated with increased aggression (Schore, 2012b, 2017a, 2019a).

In 1994, I reported studies showing early day care was specifically associated with an increase in avoidant (dismissive) attachment (Schore, 1994/2016). Where does the increase in this insecure attachment typology show up 30 years later? Indeed, the continuity of attachment styles over the lifespan has been an essential area of study in child development, attachment theory, and interpersonal neurobiology. A study of 10,000 Adult Attachment Interviews documented dismissing attachment in 35% of nonclinical adolescents, compared with only 23% of adults of the prior generation (Bakermans-Kranenburg & van IJzendoorn, 2009). Research with more than 25,000 American college students by Konrath and colleagues (2014) reported that between 1988 and 2011, secure attachment decreased from 49% to 42%, while insecure attachment increased from 51% to 58%, with the largest rise (56%) in dismissing attachments, which in previous chapters I have associated with increased grandiose narcissism and decreased empathy and intimacy.

In a study of more than 75,000 American high school and college students from 1938 to 2007, Twenge and her colleagues (2010) documented that the current generation of young adolescents report significantly higher symptoms of psychopathology on the Minnesota Multiphasic Personality Inventory (MMPI). In order to understand the underlying mechanism for this significant cultural change, they proposed that "large changes over relatively short periods of time cannot be attributed to genetics" (p. 152), and that "there are also strong cultural influences on psychiatric symptoms—that is, an environmental influence outside of the individual family" (p. 153).

In agreement with Konrath and Twenge, I suggest that the ongoing significant changes in insecure attachment status and reduced socio-emotional health of our children are in part due to epigenetic cultural social stressors associated with early day care, which usually begins at six to eight weeks, due to our unique lack, among wealthy countries, of a national parental leave policy. This culturally sanctioned premature separation of the early-developing brain from the primary caregiver occurs even before the attachment system is fully formed, thereby generating enduring future deficits in right brain social, emotional, and stress-regulating functions.

In my writings I have also discussed further expansions of my right brain developmental models and their relevance to a number of other societal problems. Our cultural conceptions of both mental and physical health as well as the aims of all levels of child development and education continue to narrowly over-stress left brain rational, logical, analytic thinking over right brain intuitive, holistic, bodily-based, emotional, and relational functions that are essential to homeostasis and survival. In a study titled "What Predicts a Successful Life? A Life-Course Model of Well-Being" at the London School of Economics, Layard and his colleagues (2014) concluded, "The most important childhood predictor of adult life-satisfaction is the child's emotional health, followed by the child's conduct. The least powerful predictor is the child's intellectual development" (p. F720). The differences in brain laterality alluded to in this statement are grounded in a long history of hemispheric asymmetry research. Recall that Luys (1879) first suggested the existence of an "emotion" center in the early-developing right hemisphere, as opposed to the "intellectual" center in the later-maturing left hemisphere.

Throughout these chapters, I have described a critical period of growth and development of the human brain in the first two years of life, as well as the 270 days preceding birth, known as "the first 1,000 days." Experiences occurring during this most important developmental window of life affect the ability to "grow, learn, work, succeed and, by extension, the long-term health, stability and prosperity of the society in which that child lives" (Thurow, 2016). This author concludes,

If we want to shape the future, to truly improve the world, we have 1,000 days to do it, mother by mother, child by child. For what happens in those 1,000 days through pregnancy to the second birthday determines to a large extent the course of a child's life.

Consonant with this time span and a large body of neurobiological data, I suggest that the United States should now legislate and implement the strategies currently operative in other industrialized nations: paid maternal leave of six months and paternal leave of two months. In addition, we must seriously address the problem of upgrading the training, quality, and pay of childcare workers. *Science-informed policies can change culture.*

Interventions need to pay more attention to the early foundations of the human personality and not later-forming verbal executive functions. It is ironic that at a time when clinicians and researchers are making significant breakthroughs not only in right brain social-emotional models of optimal development but also in the treatment of a wide range of psychopathologies, strong economic and political inhibitory restraints and cutbacks are being experienced in early-intervention and prevention programs. Silver and Singer (2014) described the wider economic implications of early brain research for the development of not only the individual, but also the culture:

> Recent advances in neuroscience indicate the importance of healthy brain development in the early years to human capital formation. . . . Investing in child development is the foundation for improved health, economic, and social outcomes. Not getting the early years "right" is linked to violent behavior, depression, higher rates of noncommunicable disease, and lower wages, and it negatively affects a nation's gross domestic product. (p. 120)

In my 2003 volume *Affect Dysregulation and Disorders of the Self*, I wrote a chapter, "Effect of Early Relational Trauma on Affect Regulation: The Development of Borderline and Antisocial Personality Disorders and a Predisposition to Violence" (Schore, 2003a). I discussed how in the introduction to Robin Karr-Morse and Meredith Riley's 1997 landmark book on the early roots of violence, *Ghosts From the Nursery*, the late renowned pediatrician Berry Brazelton stated, "Experiences in infancy which result in the child's inability to regulate strong emotions are too often the overlooked source of violence in children and adults." I suggested that when a child or adolescent commits a violent act, it means that their developmental trajectory has gone seriously askew so very early in the lifespan. The fact that they can't even make it through the next developmental stage (much less the later challenges of adulthood) is a direct outcome of a severe growth-inhibiting environment in their very beginnings, in their first relationship, the one in the nursery.

In classic research on the intergenerational transmission of traumatic attachment, Selma Fraiberg, a creator of the field of infant mental health, described "ghosts in the nursery," that are "visitors from the unremembered past of the parents" and that "the baby in these families is burdened by the oppressive past of his parents from the moment he enters the world" (Fraiberg et al., 1975). Fraiberg, a psychoanalyst, posited that these ghosts originate in a "subterranean dwelling place," which I suggest is located in the depths of the unconscious right brain. More recent research and clinical studies are documenting that the intergenerational transmission of trauma occurs across three generations (Lev-Wiesel, 2007; Mucci, 2013).

The interpersonal aspect of violence is highlighted in its definition as "aggression that has extreme harm as its goal (e.g., death)" and in the intrapersonal aspect in its association with aggressive personalities. In my chapter I cited a large body of studies in neurobiology indicating that an impairment of the right orbitofrontal cortex is a central mechanism in the behavioral expression of violence (Schore, 2003a). I suggested that during the right brain critical period, neurobiological trauma embedded in early abuse and neglect can produce an impaired orbitofrontal system and a later predisposition to violence. The "ghosts from the nursery" that are associated with the early roots of violence are in essence the enduring right brain imprints of the nonconscious intergenerational transmission of relational trauma.

Violence is aggression that has extreme harm as its goal, and when somebody commits a violent act, it means that his or her right brain development (if not also the left) has been severely impaired. Despite overall decreases in violent crimes in the United States, juvenile and adolescent homicide rates have increased, so we have to look at early childhood for the causes. We know that early relational trauma leads to the dysregulation of emotions such as fear and pain. I suggest that rage and aggression can also become dysregulated by early relational trauma. Under relational stress, a developmentally impaired right orbitofrontal cortex can't regulate the amygdala's response to threatening stimuli, thus it is easy to overreact with dysregulated rage or violence to what is subjectively perceived to be a threatening and humiliating stance in another.

All of this is processed very rapidly, beneath levels of conscious awareness, especially in the right mind of dysregulating young males. Furthermore, the severe disturbances in affect regulation and impulse control of borderline personality disorders and antisocial personality disorders are manifestations of right hemispheric aggression dysregulation, specifically of affective, impulsive, reactive, hot-blooded aggression. On the other hand, instrumental, predatory, stalking, cold-blooded left hemispheric aggression characterizes psychopaths (Schore, 2003a). Thus, right brain reactive aggression is more impulsive and stress related, while left brain instrumental aggression is premeditated and cold, without emotion. At present we are seeing increases in both.

High levels of testosterone are associated with aggressive behavior in men (Dabbs & Morris, 1990) and women (Dabbs et al., 1988). Researchers report that low levels of the stress hormone cortisol are also associated with aggression, and that elevated levels of testosterone combined with low levels of cortisol are activated in social aggression, especially in the most violent individuals, where it downregulates the conscious experience of fear (Terburg et al., 2009). These authors also suggest that testosterone impairs communication between the orbitofrontal cortex and the amygdala. The excessively impulsive, undermodulated subjective state of testosterone-infused blind rage is described as "not thinking, all feeling. He wants to demolish and destroy persons who frustrate him. He is not aware of ever loving or even faintly liking the object. He has no awareness that his rage is a passion that will decline. He believes that he will hate the object forever" (Horowitz, 1992, p. 80).

The fundamental question of why certain humans can in certain interpersonal contexts commit the most inhuman of acts must include practical solutions to how we can provide optimal early socioemotional experiences for larger and larger numbers of our infants, the most recent embodiments of our expression of hope for the future of humanity. The mental health field must move from late intervention to early prevention in order to address the problem of violence in children and adolescents, a growing concern of a number of societies. As I wrote at the beginning of this century, "In these tragic cases the seemingly *invisible* 'ghosts from the nursery' reappear in horrifyingly sharp outline during the ensuing stages of childhood, where they haunt and destroy not only individual lives but negatively impact entire communities and societies" (Schore, 2003b).

Indeed, 20 years after I wrote these words, we are now seeing on a daily basis horrifying television images, both massive destruction of cities and highly populated areas where drones and missiles rain down from above as well as public acts of violence. The latter are all too frequently associated with easily available automatic assault weapons that can indiscriminately kill large groups of people. Here in America, we are dismally failing in providing an essential moral obligation of a culture—keeping our citizens and particularly our children safe. Shame on us. I wholeheartedly add my voice to the vast majority of us who are calling for truly effective legislation on gun control and regulating the much too easy availability of military-style weapons and homemade rapid-fire ghost guns.

Further Applications of Neuroscience and Brain Laterality Research to Current U.S. Culture

Next, I want to offer some thoughts about the fundamental problem of the dominance of the left hemisphere over the right in current Western culture, and how this imbalance is culturally expressed in the United States, which is now undergoing stressful rapid, accelerated, and seemingly unpredictable, uncontrollable changes. Recall that in his seminal volume *The Master and His Emissary* Iain McGilchrist (2009) used brain laterality research on the right and left hemispheres to understand changes in Western culture. An essential tenet of his volume is expressed in its title: The right hemisphere is the master and the left the emissary, which is willfull, believes itself superior, and sometimes betrays the master, bringing harm to them both. Offering interdisciplinary evidence that spans the sciences and the arts, he convincingly argues that the left hemisphere is increasingly taking precedence in the modern world, with potentially disastrous consequences.

Listen to McGilchrist's description in 2009 of what the world would look like if the left hemisphere became so dominant that it managed more or less to suppress the right hemisphere's internal world altogether. He imagines that this left-brained world would lead to an increasing specialization and technicalizing of knowledge, as well as increased bureaucratization, inability to see the big picture, focus on quantity and efficiency at the expense of quality, valuing technology over human interaction, and devaluing of the unique, the personal, and the individual. Even more specifically,

> Knowledge that came through experience, and the practical acquisition of embodied skill, would become suspect, appearing either a threat or simply incomprehensible. . . . The concepts of skill and judgment, once considered the summit of human experience, but which come only slowly and silently with the business of living, would be discarded in favor of quantifiable and repeatable processes. . . . Skills themselves would be reduced to algorithmic procedures which could be drawn up, and even if necessary regulated, by administrators, since without that the mistrustful tendencies of the left hemisphere could not be certain that these nebulous "skills" were being evenly and "correctly" applied. . . . Fewer people would find themselves doing work involving contact with anything in the real, "lived" world, rather than with plans, strategies, paperwork, management and bureaucratic procedures. . . . Technology would flourish, as an expression of the left hemisphere's desire to manipulate and control the world for its own pleasure, but it would be accompanied by a vast expansion of bureaucracy, systems of abstraction and control. (McGilchrist, 2009, p. 429)

I suggest that this imagined left brain worldview now dominates not only our culture but the current mental health field in the form of a shift of psychotherapy from a profession to a business, an overemphasis on psychopharmacology over psychotherapy, an undue bureaucratic influence of the insurance industry on defining normative and acceptable forms of treatment, a trend toward "manualization" of therapy, an overidealization of evidence-based practice, a training model that focuses on the learning of techniques rather than on expanding relational and emotional skills, and an underappreciation of the large body of studies on the effectiveness of the therapeutic alliance. Importantly, due to the COVID-19 pandemic of 2020–2023 there has been a significant interest in online Zoom sessions in lieu of face-to-face psychotherapy. In the following, I offer very recent international research and clinical studies on teletherapy versus in-person face-to-face psychotherapy. I also offer some thoughts about artificial intelligence and its possible use in psychotherapy.

At the beginning of the COVID-19 pandemic, my Los Angeles colleague Terry Marks-Tarlow (2021) offered personal experiences conducting tele-therapy versus face-to-face psychotherapy. In dialogues with other therapists, she reports that nearly all preferred in-person over virtual sessions and that they experienced the latter as "less intimate and deep, plus much more tiring, and likely to induce screen fatigue." In discussing these trade-offs, she observes,

> The work can also be more tiring, less intimate, less private, and less conducive to dipping under the surface of everyday life. The increases in exhaustion, distraction, and difficulty achieving flow might arise from technological factors. . . . Many of these factors are at least partially the outcome of reduced interpersonal synchrony. Not only do we lack visual cues about body and body movements, but we are also deprived of smells, pheromones, and other in-person sensory information that helps us to align our breathing and heart rate alongside other forms of physiological synchrony. By residing in different environments, we also lose the synchrony of orienting to a common external context. . . . If interpersonal synchrony truly forms the foundation of the therapeutic alliance, as Koole and Tschacher (2016) suggest, then future research should ascertain whether there are significant differences in interpersonal synchrony between live and virtual platforms. It would be fascinating indeed to compare hyperscanning studies of the psychotherapeutic process in face-to-face versus virtual platforms. (p. 287)

On this last matter, recent hyperscanning EEG research in the journal *NeuroImage* directly compares face-to-face communication versus remote "technologically-assisted communication" such as Zoom or Skype (Schwartz et al., 2022). While the former increases right-brain-to-right-brain connectivity during live social moments that communicate affective signals, Zoom or Skype attenuates the level of synchronized interbrain coordination produced by naturalistic social interactions. These researchers from Ruth Feldman's lab in Israel observe that only during the live interaction did significant associations emerge, including shared gaze and empathic engagement. They conclude, "The facilitatory role of shared gaze may be limited to moments of co-present interactions and not to conditions of technological communication" and that "the gains to social development, empathic abilities, and brain maturation afforded by face-to-face interactions may not translate to technological encounters." These authors also describe the price we pay for technology—reduced right-brain-to-right-brain neural linkage—may increase cognitive load and "Zoom fatigue," a physical tiredness associated with virtual communication. This results from the additional conscious effort to interpret nonverbal cues such as body language and facial expressions that are not fully functionally expressed or perceived during remote contact.

I propose that in Zoom fatigue the explicit cognitive left hemisphere is effortfully expending energy trying to monitor what the implicit emotional right hemisphere does effortlessly. Although the right hemisphere is dominant for the spontaneous, unconscious, involuntary expression of emotions, the left hemisphere is dominant for the conscious, voluntary, posed/controlled expression of emotions (Gainotti, 2019). I also suggest that Zoom is characterized by a technological inability to access right-lateralized implicit bodily-based emotional empathy and a reliance on left-lateralized explicit cognitive empathy. Computer-mediated psychotherapy strongly favors the cognitive left hemispheric surface mind and cannot decipher the rapid, spontaneous face-to-face nonverbal right-brain-to-right-brain autonomic and limbic communications of the deeper emotional right mind which operate beneath conscious awareness that I have discussed in every chapter of this book. Recall Hoffmann's (2021) assertion about "human super-communication": "To benefit from our non-conscious processing capability, about each other, for optimum communication between us, we have to be in each other's company, that is, face-to-face!"

Indeed, Zhao and her colleagues (2023) in China, London, and the United States present hyperscanning evidence indicating separable pathways for processing live faces presented in person versus the same face presented on Zoom, and conclude that detection of salient facial micromovements may be reduced with the online format. Using near-infrared spectroscopy research (see Figure 10.1), they observe,

> The typically off-center video camera gives a distorted view of the partner's eyes in the virtual condition that may reduce activity in interactive and social processing streams. Face-to-face encounters that occur naturally are direct line-of-sight eye contacts, but this is not supported by current webcam technology. . . . *It is not possible for an individual*

to directly reciprocate eye contact when looking at a partner's face on the screen [emphasis added]. (p. 13)

In line with a large body of studies showing that during live interactions, dynamic facial cues and their spontaneous reciprocity are critical to the establishment of social skills, social bonds, and regulating social communications, Zhao's group shows that in-person as opposed to virtual media generates eye-tracking and longer dwell times on the face, larger pupil diameters, and increased arousal within both partners of a dyadic interaction. Peak activation for the real face and right-lateralized cross-brain synchrony was found only in the in-person condition. Other studies indicate that Zoom reduces conversational turn-taking behavior and interbrain coherence (Balters et al., 2023).

Note that these authors confirm Marks-Tarlow's (2021) finding of reduced interpersonal synchrony in teletherapy compared to face-to-face psychotherapy. These research and clinical data indicate that essential

FIGURE 10.1

The real-time in-person face viewing between two people occurred across a "smart glass" that was transparent in the in-person condition

In the virtual condition, the smart glass was replaced by a monitor that displayed the face of the partner in a Zoom-like condition. Note the 140 cm distance between them is about 4½ feet, a typical face-to-face distance for patients and therapists.

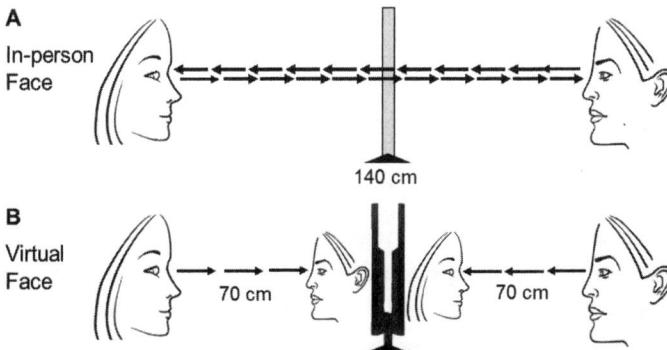

A
In-person Face

140 cm

B
Virtual Face

70 cm   70 cm

clinical processes of face-to-face therapy are attenuated by Zoom. Lower levels or loss of synchrony would impede the online development of the therapeutic alliance with all patients, making it more difficult for them to "get in sync with their shrink." But this would be especially problematic with early-forming right brain psychopathologies such as borderline, narcissistic personality, autistic spectrum disorders, and schizophrenic patients. A reduction of interpersonal synchrony would generate a weaker emotional bond between the patient and therapist in the online as opposed to the face-to-face context. This alteration of psychobiological dynamics impairs the therapist's ability to emotionally couple and relationally connect with new patients. I predict research will show higher dropout rates in video-mediated over in-person psychotherapies of all kinds.

Recall that in Chapter 7 I asserted that synchrony is the right brain interpersonal neurobiological mechanism that mediates affective reciprocal interchange, emotion transmission, physiological linkage, and coregulation, each of which would be reduced in the online therapeutic relationship. Zoom, a verbal cortical top-down intervention, has poor access to nonverbal bottom-up subcortical change processes and the foundation of the personality. This disembodied methodology increases left brain cognitive functions and attenuates the right brain emotional mechanisms of attunement, rupture, and repair, and therefore during stressful sessions there will be more psychobiological unrepaired misattunements in the online therapeutic dyad. From the perspective of the therapist's subjectivity, reduced access to interpersonal synchrony diminishes the clinician's capacity for empathic intuitively timed therapeutic interventions, and for following the patient's affect on a dynamic moment-to-moment basis and implicitly regulating the patient's state. In terms of the patient, the reduced physiological synchrony of online therapy would generate significantly lower levels of oxytocin than face-to-face contexts.

The Italian psychoanalyst Mabel Gotti (2024) offers an important recent contribution evaluating the shift from in-person to remote psychotherapy since the pandemic. She analyzes the methodology of online therapy from the perspective of updated psychoanalytic models grounded in infant research, interpersonal neurobiology, and affective neuroscience in order to describe the importance of bottom-up unconscious processes. These advances have generated more effective approaches to developmental trauma and early-forming personality disorders. She argues that contemporary psychodynamic models of "the fundamental structures of the functioning of the unconscious" can be used to understand the potential and limitations of online treatment. Gotti notes that her initial own personal experiences with Zoom were based on interiorized implicit bodily-based procedural knowledge derived from her in-person work. That said, she reports her own personal responses with online therapy:

> My first experience was that of a sort of flattening of analytical reflexivity beneath an objectifying weight. I felt constrained to *stay on the surface of the relationship and the communication*, homologating meanings that tended towards the concrete and were less reflective. In short, *I became dispossessed of the voice of the unconscious* [emphasis added]. (p. 230)

Note her intuitive self-awareness of an inability to send, receive, and process rapid bodily-based right-brain-to-right-brain nonverbal communications, the voice of the unconscious right mind.

Discussing the body in the online versus the in-person relationship, Gotti cites the work of Russell (2015), *Screen Relations: The Limits of Computer-Mediated Psychoanalysis and Psychotherapy*, who describes an absence of embodied copresence in online treatment that restricts therapy to states of mind over states of being. Gotti suggests that as opposed to the "in-person meeting of two bodies in the same room," the online context is characterized as "disembodiment," and that the body of the other is mainly accessed by the auditory sensory channel (prosody?) more so than the visual sensory channel. In describing the limitation of visual contact in the online therapeutic context, she observes,

> Until our mind registers the precise perception of being looked at in the eye, the person with whom we are connected has to look directly into the camera, something which is not done, and, if it were so, the person, in any case, would lose contact with our face and eyes. *Looking at each other in the eye from the screen causes a misalignment, no matter how small* [emphasis added]. (p. 239)

Note the allusion to asynchrony of dyadic visual processing in the online context. Gotti states that this limitation of sensory perceptual and bodily-based information in the online context is not on a par with the intense sensorial immersion of face, voice, and gesture of the live context. She concludes, "In the online setting, the sensorial contact of the analytic couple is physically different than what may be expected in the in-person setting" (p. 242).

Gotti cites a webinar of Stephen Porges (2020) on the critical sensory and regulatory functions of the autonomic nervous system's ventral vagal social engagement system:

> The system of co-regulation is fueled by facial observation, the perception of the tone of voice, and in the unconscious capturing of micro-expressions, but it is necessary to develop a setting that receives sets of abilities in order to be *interactive* to a greater degree, and *it is not possible to transpose the in-person setting online*. . . . In online therapy we forget that the motor signals that are naturally received, simply by being in-person, must be sought after instead. . . . For the mind and for our neuroceptive system, online therapy can be very tiring. . . . Our mind works continuously along a double track. . . . Therefore, for us, it is necessary to tirelessly work to remind ourselves that we are actually present. This requires a series of mental transformations that can be strenuous for the nervous system. . . . The online session brings with it the *loss of being with* [emphasis added], the loss of the effectiveness of the receptivity of our important signals to help the other in co-regulation. We are trying too hard, and trying is work. This means that our bodies are in a state of defense, and this is transmitted. . . . What happens when intentionality takes over is that spontaneity gets lost.

Note the ultrarapid subcortical activity of the bottom-up, right-lateralized, implicit spontaneous, involuntary, bodily-based autonomic nervous system is not directly accessed by the top-down cortical explicit left-lateralized online context (see Figure 2.1). Porges's model also supports the concept of Zoom fatigue and the compensatory activities of the conscious left mind's excessive utilization of explicit over implicit affect regulation. I suggest this limitation in detecting the unconscious implicit-procedural transmission of bodily-based autonomic signals is a serious limitation of Zoom psychotherapy.

Gotti (2024) asserts that in contrast to online therapy that has limited access to implicit procedural processes, the in-person face-to-face context is essential to implicitly work with deep unconscious processes in therapy, the central focus of clinical psychoanalysis and psychodynamic theory:

> They are the product of two mind/body unities working in tandem to maximize their own cohesion, understood as the product of a dynamic of co-regulation of different implicit psycho-biological states, which move and alternate in a process of disconnection, self-regulation, and reconnection (Schore, 2003). . . . These are aspects that do not so much refer to a subject of thought, but to a subject of feeling.

She concludes that seeing online therapy as a mere variation of in-person therapy can lead the clinician to mistake an online connection for a deep connection.

Presenting both clinical and neurobiological data, here in the United States, Leora Trub (2024) offers a cautionary discussion of online psychotherapy, "The Elephant in the Zoom: Will Psychoanalysis Survive the Screen?" She observes that the psychoanalytic clinical approach fundamentally relies on the establishment of a safe, intimate, and quiet space in which interior processes such as emotion can be contacted and fully experienced. Citing my work and Dan Hill's studies on affect regulation theory, she states that the interpersonal neurobiological process of affect attunement is essential to the cocreation of this therapeutic space. In this interdisciplinary work, Trub offers clinical and physiological data showing that computer-mediated communication breaks into and distorts affect attunement and the implicit felt sense of an intersubjective connection between both members of the therapeutic alliance. As opposed to the face-to-face context, this limitation of Zoom and Skype screen-mediated technology is critical, because in therapy "affect attunement can mitigate painful experience and fuel exploration of stressful thoughts and feelings (Schore, 2012, 2019)" (Trub, 2024).

Trub describes this essential limitation of teletherapy from the perspective of relational psychoanalysis and affective neuroscience:

> Affect regulation theory posits that the co-ordination of micro-interactions between the right brains of analyst and patient generates experiences that are encoded as implicit memories. The internalization of these experiences is the basis of changes in the patient's capacity to

regulate their affect and leans heavily on implicit interactional synchrony shaped by the reality of being bodies together. *Computer-mediated communication involves a delay, measured in microseconds, that likely interferes with the implicit communication of affect* [emphasis added]. I refer to affect communicated via facial expressions, the prosody of speech (rhythm, pitch, volume, speed, intonation, etc.), and gestures. To the extent that delay disrupts affect attunement and interactive affect regulation, it may undermine the very foundation of our work. Given our increased reliance on talking in the absence of physical co-presence, an increase on left-brain activity may shift our work away from the critical right brain functioning. And to the extent that central analytic tools—particularly intuition and reveries—are associated with right-brain activity, computer-mediated sessions may exclude an essential element of the clinical process.

Trub gives her own and others' observations about clinically working on Zoom. Most described feeling less comfortable in their bodies and noticed a clinical shift—they engaged in fewer or shorter silences and talked more. She suggests there is a loss of data that is vital to the human connection, with a result that subtle online adjustments avoid or prevent the emergence of regressive states and thereby make it harder to access free-floating states of reverie, intuition, and fantasy. She notes that the screen makes it more difficult to introduce and unpack transferential dynamics, so much so that communications may be more easily ignored or disavowed. Note the enhancement of an overactive left and a deactivation of right hemispheric asymmetry in Zoom therapy.

Furthermore, in discussing "Zoom fatigue," Trub (2024) notes,

> Relating to people through a screen demands a higher cognitive load than doing it in-person. Because it is more difficult to send and receive signals through a screen the ease of natural communication becomes more effortful. People engage in compensatory behaviors, like exaggerated gestures that can be quite depleting. . . . *The neural circuitry in the brain that gets activated during face-to-face social interactions does not translate to the screen.* In contrast to in-person exchanges, remote interactions involve less pupil dilation—an indicator of increased arousal—and lower levels of synchronized neural activity. This led neuroscience

researchers at Yale University (Zhao et al., 2023) to refer to *Zoom* as *"an impoverished social communication system relative to in-person conditions* [emphasis added]."

Recall the work of Ünsalver et al. (2021) in Chapter 7 on face-to-face mutual eye contact, gaze synchronization, and involuntary autonomic pupil mimicry, as well as the research of Noah and his colleagues (2020) showing increased activity in the right temporoparietal junction in both partners viewing each other in a live and not video context (see Figure 8.2). Online as opposed to face-to-face work that diminishes interpersonal synchrony would thus reduce accessing right-brain-to-right-brain nonverbal communication, physiological synchrony, pupillary contagion, and levels of safety and trust within the therapeutic alliance.

With respect to individual psychoanalytic therapy, she states, "I am not suggesting that good therapeutic work cannot be achieved through a screen. It can and it does." This is especially so in patients who have a history of working face-to-face and synchronously cocreating a right-brain-to-right-brain alliance with a familiar therapist and then switching to Zoom or temporarily having an online session when direct contact is not possible. That said, therapists and patients alike should know that teletherapy, which prioritizes self-interest and convenience, has some important limitations compared to in-person work, as I have shown in the pages above. Trub concludes that technology limits our capacity for empathy, mutuality, recognition of self and other, and intimacy, and thereby shrinks the potentialities of the clinical situation. With all patients, particularly new patients, it stays on the surface of the conscious left mind, unable to directly access or change the deeper emotional attachment dynamics of the unconscious subjective right mind, the foundation of our human nature. Also, with an increased level of left brain dominance, the right brain therapeutic alliance does not strengthen over time in online therapy, as it does in the face-to-face context.

At the end of her article, Trub (2024) asks if remote work threatens the viability of deep psychoanalytic work. She boldly asserts that technology changes and limits our subjectivity and makes a clarion call for clinicians to return to in-person face-to-face treatment, especially in today's world where "concern for others has eroded and been replaced by low frustration tolerance and a greater absorption in concern for the self." Note this last observation directly relates to the earlier-mentioned increase of left hemispheric dominant narcissistic disorders in the United States.

In addition to limitations of teletherapy I would add my deep concerns about another highly controversial possible application of technology to psychotherapy, artificial intelligence (AI). Russell and Norvig (2021) contend AI mimics human behavior in that it thinks and acts rationally. Despite industry marketing and media hype (Firstpost, 2024) a continuing controversy exists about the limitations of AI, including current left brain large language models of AI-based chatbots. I suggest in the therapeutic context the use of AI simulation of the rational mind fosters an ersatz experience of connection and intimacy, but in actuality completely overlooks right brain social and emotional intelligence and the unconscious mind. Indeed authors are referring to an "algorithmic unconscious," whereby the unconscious mind of the coder is a source of projective identification that invisibly shapes and prejudices how he designs AI systems, thereby amplifying his own hidden unconscious biases (Messina, 2025). AI errors, "hallucinations," result from biases in the data used to train the model.

An AI model of treatment has no access to right brain emotions (Brookhouse, 2023) and bodily-based emotional empathy (Cocato, 2025), elements of therapeutic change common to all forms of psychotherapy. Authors assert, "People are increasingly willing, and even choosing, to settle for the illusion of being understood by a non-human entity that lacks the basic capacity for empathy" (Trub, 2024). AI cannot intersubjectively communicate and empathically share a subjective state nor spontaneously emotionally interact with a sentient human being. In essence, language-based AI amplifies the left brain false self involved in social compliance, at the expense of the right brain true self which acts as the source of emotional depth, creativity, autonomy, and moral decisions.

Without any direct access to right brain interpersonal neurobiology and emotional processes, AI emphasizes left brain explicit power functions over implicit affiliative functions, and thereby this hemispheric asymmetry is associated with an imbalanced relationship between the left and right cerebral hemispheres. In the treatment context, this is expressed in increased left-brain-to-left-brain verbal communications and decreased right-brain-to-right-brain nonverbal communications. Furthermore, the algorithmic procedures of AI large language models are specialized in creating persuasive and manipulative verbal narratives, including advertising narratives that attempt to create a compelling need for consumer products, as well as deceptive and untruthful political speech (Fede & Masia, 2025). Recall Damasio's (1999) observation, "The left cerebral hemisphere of humans is prone to fabricating verbal narratives that do not necessarily accord with the truth."

Twelve years after his first volume, McGilchrist (2021b) offered thoughts on our current left hemispheric world. Note the similarity to the description of the stressful changes in U.S. culture I described at the beginning of this book:

> Social cohesion is breaking down in the face of atomistic individualism; and we are experiencing an epidemic of depression, anxiety, and loneliness. . . . We neglect all that is implicit. . . . This is even affecting our ability to understand tone of voice and to read faces. There is a growth of machine-like inflexibility; loss of judgment and discretion, and a culture of petty rules that strangle initiative and affront our humanity. We are witnessing the triumph of black and white judgements, especially in the "culture wars," where there is no vestige of subtlety in our thinking, but rather anger and self-righteousness. We are newly beset by tyranny of literal-mindedness—affecting our capacity to understand metaphors, humour, and irony, which are increasingly being driven out of public conversation and out of our lives. . . . We have an insatiable need for control—approaching total control, not just of action but now of thought, through surveillance by both state and global capitalism. . . . Every aspect of this reflects, as the reader will recognize, a prepotency of the left hemisphere's *modus operandi*. (McGilchrist, 2021b, pp. 1312–1313)

Furthermore, he concludes, "The serious problem for humanity is that the left hemisphere is prone to . . . 'go it alone.' Not knowing what it is it doesn't know, it tends to be overconfident it is right" (p. 372). Indeed, he sees this overemphasis of left and underemphasis of right brain functions may be a sign that we are losing our humanity.

As the reader has seen, a large body of studies on the right brain's essential adaptive implicit unconscious functions in everyday life underscores the price we pay for the current ongoing left-right imbalance between the hemispheres—a significant loss of our right brain human nature. In light of my earlier Chapter 4 on the left over right hemispheric imbalance associated with repression, I suggest that this culture is generating increased numbers of left dominant highly repressed individuals. Recall that earlier I cited the general principle, "Efforts directed at reinforcing repression are usually associated with a constant failing of repressive barriers with a breakthrough and release of repressed material" (Wolberg, 1977). This would lead to increased acting out of repressed aggression in the culture in not only the individual but also in synchronously dysregulated groups of people, expressed in shared testosterone adrenaline-infused hyperaroused aggression and mob violence.

In order to reverse this current imbalance of the hemispheres, we need, *now*, to use recent scientific knowledge in order to reflect more broadly on what is required, at levels of the individual, family, and culture, to provide an optimal human context for both mental and physical health. In addition to culturally supporting the development of intellectual and cognitive abilities, we need to foster the individual's adaptive capacity to relate socially and emotionally to other human beings via the right brain functions of intersubjective communication, affective processing, empathy, stress regulation, love, and imagination. The large body of studies on the critical survival functions of the right brain can be applied not only to individuals but to cultures, including animal cultures, as I show in my work on elephants (Bradshaw et al., 2005; Bradshaw & Schore, 2007).

Throughout life, right brain dynamics, operating beneath levels of awareness, act as a fundamental psychobiological mechanism not only within individuals, dyads, or couples, but in all human group dynamics and in the organization of all cultures. Expanding this assertion, I apply my work on the role of unconscious right-brain-to-right-brain communications in a group psychotherapy session to an interpersonal neurobiological construct described by Carl Jung as a "collective unconscious" (Schore, 2020). Distinct from a personal unconscious, he used this term to represent a form of the unconscious mind, acting beneath awareness, which is common to humankind as a whole that originates in the inherited structure of the brain. He referred to the "psychic stratum which has been called the *collective unconscious*" (see Figure 2.3, and note it operates in the deep core of the right brain).

Jung's collective unconscious represents a construct of multiple psyches, which he says every individual is born with and is shared by all human beings due to ancestral experience (note the direct relevance to the origin of human nature, the central theme of this book). Jung asserted that the collective unconscious underpins and surrounds the personal unconscious and acts through instincts and archetypes, universal images that influence an individual's feelings and actions, shared ancestral memories that aren't obvious to the eye and therefore invisible. It embodies within itself the psychic life of our ancestors back to the earliest human beginnings.

Furthermore, the collective unconscious generates an "image of the world" and acts as the source of self-sufficiency, as it contains "all those elements that are necessary for the self-regulation of the psyche as a whole" (Jung, 1928/1943, p. 187). I suggest that the human collective unconscious encodes a right brain program of how one unconscious system can communicate with another unconscious, and thereby other members of the human species, beginning with the mother. The collective unconscious thus encodes developmental, communicational, and regulatory strategies associated with the evolution of the human species.

In line with Jung's ideas, my studies of right brain mechanisms in group psychotherapy focus on the central theoretical and clinical core construct of group psychotherapy, cohesion, defined as "the act of sticking together or cohering: a tendency to remain united," "indivisible," "holding together." Citing clinical material, I show that group cohesion is created at the intersection of multiple synchronized unconscious minds via a shared-group right-brain-to-right-brain communication system, a relational unconscious acting as a collective group unconscious mind (Schore, 2020). The construct of social synchrony that operates beneath awareness thus describes a collective human psyche. Applying this model to the groups within a culture, salient unconscious information about the social environment is communicated via a "sociological unconscious." Recall the *OED* defines psyche as "the collective, mental or psychological characteristics of a nation, people." Furthermore, in the larger cultural context of different groups this collective unconscious that is communicating between and shared by members of a culture is strongly impacted by the unconscious mind of a political leader, including those with a narcissistic personality disorder who display a motive for *retribution and revenge* (see Chapter 5). Extensive research documents narcissists are characterized by a sense of superiority over others, a desire for control, fantasies of grandeur, delusional thinking, paranoia, and conspiracy theories (Kay, 2021).

With respect to the elevated levels of stress in the U.S., I contend that the current rapid and seemingly unpredictable and uncontrollable changes we are now experiencing generate not only a loss of cohesion within the collective unconscious of American culture but also in the larger human collective unconscious across all human cultures. Earlier I cited McGilchrist's observation that social cohesion is breaking down. At levels beneath awareness, the daily bombardment of stressful evocative images of unpredictable changes mentioned at the beginning of this book creates a stressfully dysregulated emotional atmosphere shared by our society's unconscious minds and bodies. Recall that neuroscientists now refer to "brain interactions between individuals *transcending the boundary of the skull.*"

Due to the ongoing residual stressors of the recent pandemic, the current period of time represents a universal chronic stressor of the human collective unconscious, sensed by our right brain limbic and immune systems, each of which operates on an involuntary unconscious level. The COVID-19 respiratory virus transmitted face-to-face directly impacts the stress regulating orbitofrontal cortex and the emotion processing limbic system (Douaud et al., 2022; Thomasson et al., 2023), and thereby mental as well as physical health. Long COVID, a residue of the pandemic, is now understood as a pathogenesis of the vagus nerve (Zheng et al., 2024) and a hypothalamic-pituitary-adrenal-stress axis mitochondrial dysfunction (Camici et al., 2024). The social isolation of the pandemic and the masking of faces has generated a shared, stressed negatively charged collective unconscious that amplifies autoregulation over eye-to-eye interactive regulation and thereby diminishes survival skills for coping with the potential dysregulation of our right brains and bodies. This has defensively altered our ways of being with other humans, reduced positive right brain emotional interactions at close distance, and negatively impacted mental health. Research documents that climate change also negatively impacts mental health (Obradovich et al., 2018), inducing a risk for youth depression (Majeed & Lee, 2017), violence and aggression (Miles-Novelo & Anderson, 2019), and for "invisible injustice," inequities suffered by the most marginalized populations, groups, and individuals (Ingle & Mikulewicz, 2020).

Earlier I stated that neuroscientists are concluding that the amygdala is centrally involved in "invisible social force fields that regulate close physical proximity" (Todd & Anderson, 2009). According to these authors, the human amygdala acts as a fear center and threat detector of potentially harmful events. At levels beneath awareness, the current emotional atmosphere is impairing individual and communal levels of safety and trust, as well as generating more rigid forms of left hemispheric repression and thereby increasing our defensiveness and reducing our right brain empathy and creativity. Indeed, studies indicate that the number of insecure dismissive avoidant attachments and narcissistic personality disorders, both associated with a deficiency of right brain empathy, are increasing in the United States (see Schore, 2019a, 2019b). Twenge and Campbell (2009) have described a "narcissism epidemic" in America, and cite data showing that this rise in narcissism is occurring in both men and women (Twenge et al., 2008).

In the last section of this chapter, and indeed this book, I will share some other thoughts about how we can pragmatically apply what we've learned about the right brain and the depths of human nature to the current and future human condition. Recall that the social and empathic self and the continuous sense of self with depth of existence over time is more dependent on the right hemisphere, and that although the left hemisphere has a relatively limited capacity to understand human motivation and feeling, the right hemisphere is more able to understand the motivation of an action or behavior. In line with Sigmund Freud's fundamental discovery that the human unconscious mind is the primary driver of every human motivational and emotional state, I suggest that any adaptive or maladaptive human behavior can only be understood in terms of right brain unconscious systems operating beneath awareness within individuals and within a culture.

Throughout these chapters, I have offered neuroscience and clinical data that have dramatically expanded and scientifically validated Freud's model of the unconscious to include both its adaptive interpersonal functions between organisms as an omnipresent relational unconscious in everyday life that psychobiologically communicates with other right brains, as well as its essential intrapsychic functions that generate an unconscious self-image, a right brain cohesive, continuous, and unified sense of self that creates a capacity for reflective self-awareness.

The importance of self-awareness in the human condition traces back to the classical period of ancient Greece of Socrates and Plato. This essential aspect of human nature has been explored over the last 2,400 years by ensuing generations of philosophers and psychologists. According to Wikipedia, "Know thyself" (Greek: Γνῶθι σαυτόν, *gnōthi sauton*) is a philosophical maxim that was inscribed upon the Temple of Apollo in the ancient Greek precinct of Delphi. The inscription likely had its origin in a popular proverb. Furthermore,

> The late 19th and early 20th centuries saw the birth of psychoanalysis which would come to take "know thyself" as its watchword. The founder of the discipline, Sigmund Freud, quoted the maxim only once, in *The Psychopathology of Everyday Life* (1901), but in later decades it became a common assertion among practitioners in the field that to know oneself means to understand one's unconscious mind. Certain branches of psychoanalysis, based around object relation theory, focus on the role of interpersonal relationships in the development of the ego, allowing this application of the maxim to incorporate the idea that self-knowledge depends upon knowledge of others. (Gipps & Lacewing, 2019)

I suggest that the mind's ability to "know itself" is an ongoing continuous process that occurs across the changing stages of life. It is now well established that there are two human minds, two self-systems, a left hemispheric explicit mind of the conscious self as well as a right hemispheric implicit mind of the unconscious self. This knowing of self(s) involves more than knowing the conscious mind, but a familiarity with one's unconscious mind and its array of emotional states. In the parlance of Iain McGilchrist (2009), the left brain "emissary" comes more deeply to know the right brain "master."

As I have demonstrated in this volume, recent neuroscience can give us valuable new information about the operations of the right brain unconscious mind and emotion not only in early development and psychotherapy but in the various behaviors that define our humanity. I cited the neuroscientist Jill Bolte Taylor (2008) on how the right hemisphere generates a state of mind when "everything and everyone are connected together as one" in which "our right mind perceives each of us as equal members of the human family" and allows us to recognize "our relationship with this marvelous planet, which sustains our life."

Recall from the introduction that the right brain cortical and subcortical systems generate the highest levels of human abilities, including creativity, intuition, empathy, imagery, symbolic thought, imagination, humor, music, dance, poetry, art, morality, altruism, compassion, spirituality, and love. In pioneering neuropsychological split-brain research in Sperry's lab J. Bogen and G. Bogen (1969) concluded, "Creativity has not only made the human experience unique in Nature . . . it gives value and purpose to human experience." With regard to intuition, McGilchrist (2021a) suggests that "the product of intuition is insight," that "conscious executive processes play little role in insight," and that "we need to get conscious reason out of the way, if we are to make use of insight" (p. 762). Albert Einstein's words are still relevant: "The intuitive mind is a sacred gift and the rational mind is a faithful servant. We have created a society that honors the servant and has forgotten the gift" (Samples, 1976).

Indeed, a major finding of McGilchrist's massive overviews of brain laterality research indicates that "the rational workings of the left hemisphere should be subject to the intuitive wisdom of the right hemisphere" (2009, p. 203). He asserts that the adaptive capacity for imagination is supported by the expansions of the right frontal lobe:

> It is the faculty of imagination which comes into being between the two hemispheres, which enables us to take things back from the world of the left hemisphere and make them live again in the right. It is in this way . . . that things are made truly new once again. (p. 199)

More recently, he suggests, "*The right hemisphere has more of a grasp of moral values* [emphasis added], is apt to take responsibility rather than blame others, is more apt to inhibit our first impulse to what is simple and easy, is more intelligent, and complicates our simple mechanistic vision by its insight" (McGilchrist, 2021b, p. 1332).

This increased new knowledge generated by science of the emotional right brain, the deeper strata of our personalities, can be used both by the culture to collectively cope more effectively with ongoing social stressors and also by an individual to increase his or her own subjective self-awareness of the emotional core within each of us. The primary focus of the field of cultural neuroscience is the bidirectional relation between the culture and the brain, specifically the mechanisms by which culture influences how people experience, recognize, express, and regulate their emotions and how they infer the mental states of others (Chiao, 2009), as well as the neurobiological processes by which culture ascribes meaning and value to the self by emotion regulation and the way people feel in their interpersonal and intergroup interactions (Kim & Sasaki, 2014).

The neurobiological perspective of regulation theory also applies to current U.S. and world culture as described in the first paragraph of this book and to the shared unconscious fear and uncertainty that pervade the ambient human emotional atmosphere. Classic studies on emotional response without awareness demonstrate that even a rapid 30 millisecond, and thereby unconscious, presentation of stressful, frightening images can increase right brain autonomic physiological stress responses (Kimura et al., 2004), and that the right amygdala, the right anterior cingulate, and the right ventromedial prefrontal cortex detect fearful stimuli when they are presented unconsciously (Williams et al., 2009).

Indeed, research now establishes that the right amygdala is involved in fear conditioning (Baker & Kim, 2004) and in the processing of emotionally negative social information and its attendant stress states (Rifkin-Graboi et al., 2013). Furthermore, neurophysiological activity in the right amygdala correlates with negative mood (Abercrombie et al., 1998), suicide attempts (Spoletini et al., 2011), and depression severity (Drevets et al., 2002). The latter authors suggest that the elevated amygdala metabolism in major depressive disorder reflects increased transmission from "the caudal orbital cortex, the anterior insula and the ventral anterior cingulate, which are also hypermetabolic" (p. 440). Depression has recently increased in this country.

At levels beneath awareness, daily evocative images of nature-induced extreme weather, man-made destruction, and public violence between humans generate a stressfully dysregulated right amygdala, the deep unconscious that is shared by the culture's collective unconscious, and thereby its members' unconscious minds and bodies. The right amygdala, the deep unconscious that mediates "unseen" fear (Morris et al., 1999), functions as a gatekeeper that evaluates the social environment for threat cues and generates vigilance (Davis & Whalen, 2001), acting as "the border patrol of the self" (Kuhl et al., 2015) that "senses the invisible" and reacts to a traumatic context (Hendler et al., 2003). This ancient subcortical structure is fundamentally involved in emotional communications and autobiographical memory. It also plays an essential role in attachment security or insecurity (Lemche et al., 2006). My coauthor Ruth Lanius described early attachment trauma as "the hidden epidemic" (Lanius et al., 2010), and my colleague Clara Mucci (2013) has written on "collective trauma."

As stated earlier, we as individuals and as a culture are now experiencing rapid and unpredictable stressful changes in the physical environment, climate change in the natural world, in mass extinction of animals and plants, and in the external social environment and the unconscious internal world. To these I would add recent stressors by political figures that increase our anxiety about employment and economic insecurity, and that induce two-day six trillion dollar crashes in the U.S. stock market. These stressors are generating a shared subjective state of uncertainty that too commonly is accompanied by the troubling thought that the world we are living in and the people in it are coming apart at the seams, before our very eyes. Indeed, the cohesion of present culture in the United States has been fragmented and is leading to increased polarization, which the OED defines as a process that will "accentuate the *division* within (a group, system); *separate* into two (or more) *opposing groups, extremes of opinion.*" Sound familiar? Note how the description of these societal stressors applies to current U.S. politics and that it represents the opposite of a culture's cohesion, "a tendency to remain united."

It is now common knowledge that we are all connected. These chapters suggest that this is more than a metaphor, and that this connection is not cognitive but emotional. As the clinical material and neuroscience research in the previous chapters shows, this social connection occurs in everyday life in rapid right-brain-to-right-brain emotional communications that operate between us. We are unconsciously connected to each other by this early-forming ubiquitous evolutionary mechanism common to all humans.

That said, the extraordinary social *isolation* due to the pandemic continues to generate less face-to-face direct eye contact and thereby a significantly reduced intersubjective personal context for interpersonal brain synchrony and implicitly shared positive emotional states. These chapters suggest that the current epidemic of *loneliness, a basic painful longing for emotional reconnection with other humans*, is expressed in reduced levels of positively valenced intimate *right-brain-to-right-brain* nonverbal emotional communications within the collective unconscious of U.S. culture. This stressful ambient intersubjective context favors autoregulation and going at it alone over social connection, interactive regulation, and collaborating with trusted others as the primary emotional strategy.

Western cultures show a well-known bias toward left brain power, separateness, and independence over right brain connectedness and affiliation. Kuhl and Kazen (2008) state that power motivation "is contingent upon the control of means of influencing another person." In contrast, they state that a primary example of affiliation is "a sense [that] common humanity has united us." We urgently need respectful, two-way cultural conversations about a more optimal balance of these primary human needs. The challenge before us is whether the cultures we live in can *now* seriously address the current essential problems facing the human species, including those I have been discussing in this final chapter.

Observing that social cohesion is now breaking down, Iain McGilchrist convincingly argues that the left hemisphere is increasingly taking precedence in the modern world, with potentially disastrous consequences. I suggest we are at a conscious and indeed unconscious crossroad. The current stressful social context may increase even more the imbalance of the left hemisphere's role in individuality, power, and control, at the expense of the right hemisphere's being connected with others and seeking warm relationships, and thereby defensively alter our ways of being with other humans.

On the other hand, we may more creatively use our communal right brains to increase our resilient coping abilities and increase the joy of living in ourselves and in more members of our societies. During these trying times, we need to intimately come together for the common good, not only to truly listen to each other, but to raise our voices together and defend our institutions, and to openly share our hopes, dreams, joys, fears, vulnerability, and need for right-brain-to-right-brain deep emotional connections with the people closest to us, the people we love, like ourselves, human flaws and all.

References

Abel, K. M., Dalman, C., Svensson, A. C., Susser, E., Dal, H., Idring, S., et al. (2013). Deviance in fetal growth and risk of autism spectrum disorder. *American Journal of Psychiatry, 170*, 391–398.

Abelin, E. (1971). The role of the father in the separation-individuation process. In J. B. McDevitt & C. F. Settlage (Eds.), *Separation-individuation* (pp. 229–252). International Universities Press.

Abercrombie, H. C., Schaefer, S. M., Oakes, T. R., Lindgren, K. A., Holden, J. E., Krahn, D. D., et al. (1998). Metabolic rate in the right amygdala predicts negative affect in depressed patients. *NeuroReport, 9*, 3301–3307.

Abraham, E., Hendler, T., Shapira-Lechter, I., Kanat-Maymon, Y., Zagoory-Sharon, O., & Feldman, R. (2014). Father's brain is sensitive to childcare experiences. *Proceedings of the National Academy of Sciences USA, 111*, 9792–9797.

Adolphs, R. (2001). The neurobiology of social cognition. *Current Opinion in Neurobiology, 11*, 231–239.

Adolphs, R., Damasio, H., Tranel, D., Cooper, G., & Damasio, A. R. (2000). A role for somatosensory cortices in the visual recognition of emotion as revealed by three-dimensional lesion mapping. *Journal of Neuroscience, 20*, 2683–2690.

Aftanas, L. I., & Varlamov, A. A. (2007). Effects of alexithymia on the activity of the anterior and posterior areas of the cortex of the right hemisphere in positive and negative emotional activation. *Neuroscience and Behavioral Physiology, 37*, 67–73.

Ainsworth, M. D. S., Blehar, M. C., Waters, E., & Wall, S. (1978). *Patterns of attachment.* Lawrence Erlbaum.

Aitken, K. J., & Trevarthen, C. (1997). Self/other organization in human psychological development. *Development and Psychopathology, 9*, 653–677.

Allison, K. L., & Rossouw, P. J. (2013). The therapeutic alliance: Exploring the concept of "safety" from a neuropsychotherapeutic perspective. *International Journal of Neuropsychotherapy, 1*, 21–29.

Allman, J. M., Tetreault, N. A., Hakeem, A. Y., Manaye, K. F., Semendeferi, K., Erwin, J. M., et al. (2011). The von Economo neurons in fronto-insular and anterior cingulate cortex. *Annals of the New York Academy of Science, 1225*, 59–71.

Allman, J. M., Watson, K. K., Tetreault, N. A., & Hakeem, A. Y. (2005). Intuition and autism: A possible role for Von Economo neurons. *Trends in Cognitive Sciences, 9*, 367–373.

Ally, B. A., Hussey, E. P., & Donahue, M. J. (2013). A case of hyperthymesia: Rethinking the role of the amygdala in autobiographical memory. *NeuroCase, 19*, 166–181.

Altmann, U., Brummel, M., Meier, J., & Strauss, B. (2021). Movement synchrony and facial synchrony as facial features of depression: A pilot study. *Journal of Nervous and Mental Disease, 209*, 128–136.

Amid, B. (2024). At-one-ment and twoness are not opposites. *American Journal of Psychoanalysis, 84*, 16–41. doi: 10.1057/s11231-024-09434-0

Ammaniti, M., & Gallese, V. (2014). *The birth of intersubjectivity.* Norton.

Ammaniti, M., & Trentini, C. (2009). How new knowledge about parenting reveals the neurobiological implications of intersubjectivity: A conceptual synthesis of recent research. *Psychoanalytic Dialogues, 19*, 537–555.

Anderson, P. A., & Guerrero, L. K. (1998). Principles of communication and emotion in social interaction. In P. A. Anderson & L. K. Guerrero (Eds.), *Handbook of communication and emotion* (pp. 49–88). Academic Press.

Andrade, V. M. (2005). Affect and the therapeutic action in psychoanalysis. *International Journal of Psychoanalysis, 86*, 677–697.

Andrews, S. C., Hoy, K. E., Enticott, P. G., Daskalakis, Z. J., & Fitzgerald, P. B. (2011). Improving working memory: the effect of combining cognitive activity and anodal transcranial direct current stimulation to the left dorsolateral prefrontal cortex. *Brain Stimulation, 4*, 84–89.

Andrieux, P., Chevillard, C., Cunha-Neto, E., & Nunes, J. P. S. (2021). Mitochondria as a cellular hub in infection and inflammation. *International journal of Molecular Science, 22*, 11338. doi: 10.3390/ijms22211138

Annau, Z., & Kamin, L. J. (1961). The conditioned emotional response as a function of the intensity of the US. *Journal of Comparative and Physiological Psychology, 54*, 428–432.

Archer, J. (2006). Testosterone and human aggression: An evaluation of the challenge hypothesis. *Neuroscience and Biobehavioral Reviews, 30*, 319–345.

Aron, E. N., & Aron, A. (1996). Love and expansion of the self: The state of the model. *Personal Relationships, 3*, 45–58.

Aron, L., & Bushra, A. (1998). Mutual regression: Altered states in the psychoanalytic situation. *Journal of the American Psychoanalytic Association, 46*, 389–412.

Asamoah, M. K. (2014). Re-examination of the limitations associated with correlational research. *Journal of Educational Research and Reviews, 2*, 42–52.

Asari, T., Konishi, S., Jimura, K., Chikazoe, J., Nakamura, N., & Miyashita, Y. (2008). Right temporopolar activation associated with unique perception. *NeuroImage, 41*, 145–152.

Asperger. H. (1944). Die "Autistischen Psychoparhen" im Kindesalter. *Arch. Psychiatry Nervenkr, 117,* 76–136

Ayache, J., Connor, A., Marks, S., Kuss, D. J., Rhodes, D., Sumich, A., et al. (2021). Exploring the "dark matter" of social interaction: Systematic review of a decade of research in spontaneous interpersonal coordination. *Frontiers in Psychology, 12.* doi: 10.3389/fpsyg.2021.718237

Bach, S. (1985). *Narcissistic states and the therapeutic process.* Jason Aronson.

Back, M. D., Kufner, A. C. P., Dufner, M., Gerlach, T. M., Rauthmann, J. F., & Denissen, J. J. A. (2013). Narcissistic admiration and rivalry: Disentangling the bright and dark sides of narcissism. *Journal of Personality and Social Psychology, 105,* 1013–1037.

Back, M. D., Schmukle, S. C., & Egloff, B. (2010). Why are narcissists so charming at first sight? Decoding the narcissism-popularity link at zero acquaintance. *Journal of Personality and Social Psychology, 98,* 132–145.

Baier, A. L., Kline, A., & Feeny, N. C. (2020). Therapeutic alliance as a mediator of change: A systematic review and evaluation of research. *Clinical Psychology Review, 82.* doi: 10.1016/j.cpr.2020.101921

Baker, K. B., & Kim, J. J. (2004). Amygdala lateralization in fear conditioning: Evidence for greater involvement of the right amygdala. *Behavioral Neuroscience, 118,* 15–23.

Baker, S. C., Frith, C. D., & Dolan, R. J. (1997). The interaction between mood and cognitive function studied with PER. *Psychological Medicine, 27,* 565–578.

Bakermans-Kranenberg, M. J., & van IJzendoorn, M. H. (2009). The first 10,0000 Adult Attachment Interviews: Distributions of adult attachment representations in clinical and non-clinical groups. *Attachment and Human Relationship, 11,* 223–263.

Balint, M. (1968). *The basic fault: Therapeutic aspects of aggression.* Tavistock.

Balters, S., Miller, J. G., Li, R. H., Hawthorne, G., & Reiss, A. L. (2023). Virtual (Zoom) interactions alter conversational behavior and interbrain coherence. *Journal of Neuroscience, 43,* 2568–2578.

Bangen, K. J., Meeks, M. D., & Jeste, D. V. (2013). Defining and assessing wisdom: A review of the literature. *American Journal of Geriatric Psychiatry, 21,* 1254–1266.

Barbas, H. (1995). Anatomic basis of cognitive-emotional interactions in the primate prefrontal cortex. *Neuroscience and Biobehavioral Reviews, 19,* 499–510.

Bargh, J. A., & Morsella, E. (2008). The unconscious mind. *Perspectives on Psychological Science, 3,* 73–79.

Barish, K. (2020). The role of play in contemporary child psychotherapy. *Journal of Infant, Child, and Adolescent Psychotherapy, 19,* 148–158.

Bartels, A., & Zeki, S. (2004). The neural correlates of maternal and romantic love. *NeuroImage, 21,* 1155–1166.

Bartz, J. A., & Hollander, E. (2006). The neuroscience of affiliation: Forging links between basic and clinical research on neuropeptides and social behavior. *Hormones and Behavior, 50,* 518–528.

Basavaraju, R., France, J., Sigmon, H. C., Girgis, R. R., Brucato, G., Lieberman, J. A., et al. (2023). Increased parietal and occipital lobe gyrification predicts conversion to syndromal psychosis in a clinical high-risk cohort. *Schizophrenia Research, 255,* 246–255.

Basch, M. F. (1976). The concept of affect: A re-examination. *Journal of the American Psychoanalytic Association, 24,* 759–777.

Basch, M. F. (1983). The perception of reality and the disavowal of meaning. *Annual Review of Psychoanalysis, 11,* 125–154.

Baumeister, R. F., & Leary, M. R. (1995). The need to belong: Desire for interpersonal attachments as a fundamental human motivation. *Psychological Bulletin, 117,* 497–528.

Beebe, B., Jaffe, J., Markese, S., Buck, K., Chen, H., Cohen, P., et al. (2010). The origins of 12- month attachment: A microanalysis of 4-month mother-infant interaction. *Attachment and Human Development, 12,* 3–142.

Beebe, B., Lachmann, F. M., Maekese, S., Buck, K. A., Bahrick, L. E., & Chen, H. (2012). On the origins of disorganized attachment and internal working models: Paper II. An empirical microanalysis of 4-month mother-infant interaction. *Psychoanalytic Dialogues, 22,* 352–374.

Beebe, B., & Steele, M. (2013). How does microanalysis of mother-infant communication inform maternal sensitivity and infant attachment? *Attachment and Human Development, 15*(5–6), 583–602. doi: 10.1080/14616734.2013.841050

Bembich, S., Castelpietra, E., Cont, G., Travan, L., Cavasin, J., Dolliani, M., Traino, R., & Demarini, S. (2022). Cortical activation and oxygen perfusion in preterm newborns during kangaroo mother care: A pilot study. *Acta Paediatrica, 112,* 942–950. doi: 10.1111/apa.16695

Benedetti, F., Poletti, S., Radaelli, D., Ranieri, R., Genduso, V., Cavallotti, S., et al. (2015). Right hemisphere neural activations in the recall of waking fantasies and of dreams. *Journal of Sleep Research, 24,* 576–582.

Benedetti, G. (1987). Illuminations of the human condition in the encounter with the psychotic patient. In J. Sacksteder, D. P. Schwartz, & Y. Akabane (Ed.), *Attachment and the therapeutic process: Essays in honor of Otto Allen Will, Jr. M.D.* (pp. 185–196). International Universities Press.

Benjamin, J. (2017). *Beyond doer and done to: Recognition theory, intersubjectivity and the analytic third.* Routledge.

Benowitz, L. I., Bear, D. M., Rosenthal, R., Mesulam, M.-M., Zaidel, E., & Sperry, R. W. (1983). Hemispheric specialization in nonverbal communication. *Cortex, 19,* 5–11.

Berant, E., Mikulincer, M., Shaver, P. R., & Segal, Y. (2005). *Journal of Personality Assessment, 84,* 70–81.

Beren, P. (1992). Narcissistic disorders. *The Psychoanalytic Study of the Child, 47,* 265–278.

Bergman, A., & Fahey, M. F. (1999). *Ours, yours, and mine: Mutuality and the emergence of the separate self.* Jason Aronson.

Bergman, N. J., Linley, L. L., & Fawcus, S. R. (2004). Randomized controlled trial of skin-to-skin contact from birth versus conventional incubator for physiological stabilization in 1200- to 2199-gram newborns. *Acta Paediatrica, 93,* 779–785.

Berlucchi, G., & Marzi, C. A. (2024). Roger Sperry, the maverick brain scientist who was haunted by the psyche. *Front. Hum. Neurosci.* 18:1392660. doi:10.3389/fnhum.2024.1392660

Berrios, R., Totterdell, P., & Kellett, S. (2015). Eliciting mixed emotions: A meta-analysis comparing models, types, and measures. *Frontiers in Psychology, 6,* 428. doi: 10.3389/fpsyg.2015.00428

Berthier, M., Starkstein, S., & Leiguarda, R. (1987). Behavioral effects of damage to the right insula and surrounding regions. *Cortex, 23,* 673–678.

Bertini, M., Violani, C., Zoccolotti, P., Antonelli, A., & DiStefano, L. (1984). Right cerebral hemisphere activation in dreaming sleep: Evidence from a unilateral tactile recognition test. *Psychophysiology, 21,* 418–423.

Bilek, E., Ruf, M., Schafer, A., Akdentz, Calhoun, V. D., et al. (2015). Information flow between interacting brains: Identification, validation, and relationship to social expertise. *Proceedings of the National Academy of Sciences, USA, 112,* 5207–5212. https://doi.org/10.1073/pnas.1421831112

Bilek, E., Stoebel, G., Schafer, A., Clement, L., Ruf, M., et al. (2017). State-dependent cross-brain information flow in borderline personality disorder. *JAMA Psychiatry, 74,* 949–957.

Bion, W. R. (1957). Differentiation of the psychotic from the non-psychotic personalities. *International Journal of Psycho-Analysis, 38,* 266–275.

Bion, W. R. (1970). *Attention and interpretation.* Tavistock.

Bjorklund, D. F. (2020). *How children invented humanity: The role of development in human evolution.* Oxford University Press.

Black, R. S. A., Curran, D., & Dyer, K. F. W. (2013). The impact of shame on the therapeutic alliance and intimate relationships. *Journal of Clinical Psychology, 69,* 646–654.

Bleiberg, E. (1988). Developmental pathogenesis of narcissistic disorders in children. *Bulletin of the Menninger Clinic, 52,* 3–15.

Blickle, G., Schlegel, A., Fassbinder, P., & Klein, U. (2006). Some personality correlates of white collar crime. *Applied Psychology: An International Review, 55,* 220–223.

Blonder, L. X., Bowers, D., & Heilman, K. M. (1991). The role of the right hemisphere in emotional communication. *Brain, 114,* 1115–1127.

Blood, A. J., Zatorre, R. J., Bermudez, P., Evans, A. C. (1999). Emotional responses to pleasant and unpleasant music correlate with activity in paralimbic brain regions. *Nature Neuroscience, 2,* 382–387.

Bode, S., He, A. H., Soon, C. S., Trampel, R., Turner, R., & Haynes, J. D. (2011). Tracking the unconscious generation of free decisions using ultra-high field fMRI. *PLoS ONE* 6:e21612. doi: 10.1371/jour.pone.0021612

Boeck, C., Gumpp, A. M., Calzia, E., Radermacher, P., Waller, C., Karabatsiakis, A.,

& Kolassa, I.-T. (2018). The association between cortisol, oxytocin, and immune cell mitochondrial oxygen consumption in postpartum women with childhood maltreatment. *Psychoneuroendocrinology, 96*, 69–77.

Bogels, S., & Phares, V. (2008). Fathers' role in the etiology, prevention and treatment of child anxiety: A review and new model. *Childhood Psychology Review, 28*, 539–558.

Bogen, J. E., & Bogen, G. M. (1969). The other side of the brain III: The corpus callosum and creativity. *Bulletin of the Los Angeles Neurological Society, 34*, 175–195.

Bolger, N., & Amarel, D. (2007). Effects of social support visibility on adjustment to stress: Experimental evidence. *Journal of Personality and Social Psychology, 92*, 458–475.

Bond, M., & Perry, J. C. (2004). Long-term changes in defense styles with psychodynamic psychotherapy for depressive, anxiety, and personality disorders. *American Journal of Psychiatry, 161*, 1665–1671.

Booth, A., & Dabbs, J. M. (1993). Testosterone and men's marriages. *Social Forces, 72*, 463–477.

Bordin, E. S. (1979). The generalizability of the psychoanalytic concept of the working alliance. *Psychotherapy, 16*, 252–260.

Borgogno, F., & Vigna-Taglianti, M. (2008). Role-reversal: A somewhat neglected mirror of heritages of the past. *American Journal of Psychoanalysis, 68*, 313–328.

Bornstein, R. F. (1999). Source amnesia, misattributions, and the power of unconscious perceptions and memories. *Psychoanalytic Psychology, 166*, 155–178.

Bosch-Bayard, J., Biscay, R. J., Fernandez, T., Otero, G. A., Ricardo-Garcell, J., Aubert-Vazquez, E., et al. (2022). EEG effective connectivity during the first year of life mirrors brain synaptogenesis, myelination, and early right hemisphere predominance. *NeuroImage, 252*, 119035. doi: 10.1016/j.neuroimage.2022.119035

Bourne, V. J., & Todd, B. K. (2004). When left means right: An explanation of the left cradling bias in terms of right hemisphere specializations. *Developmental Science, 7*, 19–24.

Bowlby, J. (1953). *Child care and the growth of love*. Penguin.

Bowlby, J. (1969). *Attachment and loss: Vol. 1. Attachment*. Basic Books.

Bowlby, J. (1973). *Attachment and loss: Vol. 2. Separation: Anxiety and anger*. Basic Books.

Bowlby, J. (1988). *A secure base* (2nd ed). Basic Books.

Bradley, R. M., & Mistretta, C. M. (1975). Fetal sensory receptors. *Physiological Review, 55*, 352–382.

Bradley, R. T. (2010). Detecting the identity signature of secret social groups: Holographic processes and the communication of member affiliation. *World Futures, 66*, 124–162.

Bradley, R. T. (2024). Harnessing the force of all creation: Part one. The power of love to shape reality. *World Futures, 80*, 413–447.

Bradshaw, G. A., & Schore, A. N. (2007). How elephants are opening doors: Developmental neuroethology, attachment and social context. *Ethology, 113*, 426–436.

Bradshaw, G. A., Schore, A. N., Brown, J. L., Poole, J. H., & Moss, C. J. (2005). Elephant breakdown. Social trauma: Early disruption of attachment can affect the physiology, behaviour and culture of animals and humans over generations. *Nature, 443,* 807.

Bradshaw, J. L., & Nettleton, N. C. (1981). The nature of hemispheric specialization in man. *Behavioral and Brain Sciences, 4,* 51–91.

Brancucci, A., Lucci, G., Mazzatenta, A., & Tommasi, L. (2009). Asymmetries of the human social brain in the visual, auditory and chemical modalities. *Philosophical Transactions of the Royal Society of London. Series B, Biological Science, 364,* 895–914.

Brazelton, T. B., & Cramer, B. G. (1990). *The earliest relationship.* Addison-Wesley.

Brenner, C. (1957). The nature and development of the concept of repression in Freud's writings. *Psychoanalytic Study of the Child, 12,* 19–46.

Breuer, J., & Freud, S. (1955). Studies on hysteria. In J. Strachey (Ed. and Trans.), *The standard edition of the complete psychological works of Sigmund Freud.* Hogarth. (Original work published 1891)

Bromberg, P. M. (1979). Interpersonal psychoanalysis and regression. *Contemporary Psychoanalysis, 15,* 647–655.

Bromberg, P. M. (1986). The mirror and the mask: On narcissism and psychoanalytic growth. In A. P. Morrison (Ed.), *Essential papers on narcissism* (pp. 438–466). New York University Press.

Bromberg, P. M. (1991). On knowing one's patient inside out: The aesthetics of unconscious communication. *Psychoanalytic Dialogues, 1,* 399–422.

Bromberg, P. M. (1992). Some basic issues. *Contemporary Psychoanalysis, 28,* 495–402.

Bromberg, P. M. (2011). *The shadow of the tsunami and the growth of the relational mind.* Routledge.

Bromberg, P. M. (2017). Psychotherapy as the growth of wholeness: The negotiation of individuality and otherness. In M. Solomon & D. S. Siegel (Eds.), *How people change: relationships and neuroplasticity in psychotherapy* (pp. 1–36). Norton.

Bronowski, J. (1972). *Science and human values.* Harper and Row.

Brookhouse, O. (2023). Can artificial intelligence understand emotions? *Telefónica Tech.* https://telefonicatech.com/en/blog/can-artificial-intelligence-understand-emotions

Broucek, F. J. (1982). Shame and its relationship to early narcissistic developments. *International Journal of Psychoanalysis, 63,* 369–378.

Broucek, F. J. (1991). *Shame and the self.* Guilford.

Brunell, A. B., Staats, S., Barden, J., & Hupp, J. M. (2011). Narcissism and academic dishonesty: The exhibition dimension and the lack of guilt. *Personality and Individual Differences, 50,* 323–328.

Buchanan, M. (2009). Secret signals. *Nature, 457,* 528–530.

Buck, R. (1994). The neuropsychology of communication: Spontaneous and symbolic aspects. *Journal of Pragmatics, 22,* 265–278.

Bugental, J. F. (1987). *The art of the psychotherapist.* Norton.

Buklina, S. B. (2005). The corpus callosum, interhemispheric interactions, and the function of the right hemisphere of the brain. *Neuroscience and Behavioral Physiology, 35*, 473–480.

Burnham, T. C., Chapman, J. F., Gray, P. B., McIntyre, M. H., Lipson, S. F., & Ellison, P. T. (2003). Men in committed, romantic relationships have lower testosterone. *Hormones and Behavior, 44*, 119–122.

Bursten, B. (1973). Some narcissistic personality types. *International Journal of Psycho-Analysis, 54*, 287–300.

Cabrera, N., & Tamis-LeMonda, C. S. (2013). *Handbook of father involvement: Multidisciplinary perspectives.* Routledge.

Cain, N. M., Pincus, A. L., & Ansell, E. B. (2008). Narcissism at the crossroads: Phenotypic description of pathological narcissism across clinical theory, social/personality psychology, and psychiatric diagnosis. *Clinical Psychology Review, 28*, 638–656.

Camici, M., Del Duca, G., Brita, A. C., & Antinori, A. (2024). Connecting dots of long COVID-19 pathogenesis: a vagus nerve-hypothalamic-pituitary-adrenal-mitochondrial axis dysfunction. *Front.Cell. Infect. Microbiol.* 14:1501949. doi: 10.3389/fcimb.2024.1501949

Campbell, W. K., Bosson, J. K., Goheen, T. W., Chad, E., & Kernis, M. H. (2007). Do narcissists dislike themselves "deep down inside"? *Psychological Science, 18*, 227–229.

Capaldi, R. A. (2000). The changing role of mitochondrial research. *Trends in Biochemical Science, 25*, 212–214.

Carlson, K. S., & Gjerde, P. F. (2009). Preschool personality antecedents of narcissism in adolescence and young adulthood: A 20-year longitudinal study. *Journal of Research in Personality, 43*, 570–578.

Carlsson, J., Lagercrantz, H., Olson, L., Printz, G., & Baryocci, M. (2008). Activation of the right fronto-temporal cortex during maternal recognition in young infants. *Acta Paediatrica, 97*, 1221–1225.

Carr, L., Iacoboni, M., Dubeau, M. C., Mazziotta, J. C., & Lenzi, G. L. (2003). Neural mechanisms of empathy in humans: A relay from neural systems for imitation to limbic areas. *Proceedings of the National Academy of Sciences USA, 100*, 5497–5502.

Carretie, L., Hinojosa, J. A., Mercado, F., & Tapia, M. (2005). Cortical response to subjectively unconscious danger. *NeuroImage, 24*, 615–623.

Carson, R. (1962). *Silent spring.* Houghton Mifflin Harcourt.

Carter, R. M., & Huettel, S. A. (2013). A nexus model of the tempero-parietal junction. *Trends in Cognitive Science, 17*, 328–336.

Cartwright, C. (2011). Transference, countertransference, and reflective practice in cognitive therapy. *Clinical Psychologist, 15*, 112–120.

Casagrande, M., & Bertini, M. (2008). Night-time right hemisphere superiority and daytime left hemisphere superiority: A repatterning of laterality across wake-sleep-wake states. *Biological Psychology, 77*, 337–342.

Cassidy, J. (1994). Emotion regulation: Influences of attachment relationships. *Monographs of the Society of Child Development, 59*, 228–249.

Castenega, A., Iacobazzi, V., & Infantino, V. (2015). The mitochondrial side of epigenetics. *Physiological Genomics, 47*, 299–307.

Castonguay, L. G., & Hill, C. E. (2017). *How and why are some therapists better than others? Understanding therapist effects.* American Psychological Association.

Ceko, M., Kragel, P. A., Woo, C.-H., Lopez-Sola, M., & Wagner, T. D. (2022). Common and stimulus-type-specific brain representations of negative affect. *Nature Neuroscience, 25*, 760–770.

Cerqueira, J. J., Almeida, O. F. X., & Sousa, N. (2008). The stressed prefrontal cortex. Left? Right! *Brain, Behavior, and Immunity, 22*, 630–638.

Chan, A., Northoff, G., Karasik, R., Ouyang, J., & Williams, K. (2022). Flights and perchings of the brainmind: A temporospatial approach to psychotherapy. *Frontiers in Psychology, 13*. doi: 10.3389/tpsyg.2022.828035

Chapple, E. D. (1970). Experimental production of transients in human interaction. *Nature, 228*, 630–633.

Charpak, N., Tessier, R., Ruiz, J. G., Uriza, F., Hernandez, J. T., Cortes, D., & Montealegre-Pomar, A. (2022). Kangaroo mother care had a proactive effect on the volume of brain structures in young adults born preterm. *Acta Paediatrica, 111*, 1004–1014.

Chelazzi, L., Bisley, J. W., & Bartolomeo, P. (2018). The unconscious guidance of attention. *Cortex, 102*, 1–5.

Chen, L., & Hsiao, J. (2014). Right hemisphere dominance in nonconscious processing. *Journal of Vision, 14*, 1313. https://doi.org/10.1167/14.10.1313

Chiao, J. Y. (2009). Culture neuroscience: A once and future discipline. *Progress in Brain Research, 178*, 287–304.

Chiron, C., Jambaque, I., Nabbout, R., Lounes, R., Syrota, A., & Dulac, O. (1997). The right brain hemisphere is dominant in human infants. *Brain, 120*, 1057–1065.

Chodorow, J. (1991). *Dance therapy and depth psychology: The moving imagination.* Routledge.

Chugani, H. T., Phelps, M. E., & Mazziotta, J. C. (1987). Positron emission tomography study of human brain functional development. *Annals of Neurology, 22*, 487–497.

Cloninger, C. R., Cloninger, K. M., Zwir, I., & Keltikangas-Järvinen, L. (2019). The complex genetics and biology of human temperament: A review of traditional concepts in relation to new molecular findings. *Translational Psychiatry, 9*, 1–21.

Cocato, P. (2025). The limit of AI lies in its inability to understand complex contexts or show empathy. *Telefónica*. https://www.telefonica.com/en/communication-room/blog/limit-ai-lies-inability-understandcomplex-contexts-show-empathy/

Cole, J. (1998). *About face.* MIT Press.

Conde-Agudelo, A., Belizan, J. M., & Diaz-Rossello, J. (2011). Kangaroo mother care to reduce morbidity and mortality in low birthweight infants. *Cochrane Database of Systematic Reviews, 3*, CD002771.

Corballis, P. M. (2003). Visuospatial processing and the right-hemisphere interpreter. *Brain and Cognition, 53*, 171–176.

Corbetta, M., Patel, G., & Shulman, G. L. (2008). The reorienting system of the human brain: From environment to theory of mind. *Neuron, 58*, 306–324.

Corbetta, M., & Shulman, G. L. (2002). Control of goal-directed and stimulus-driven attention in the brain. *Nature Reviews Neuroscience, 3*, 201–215.

Corry, N., Merritt, R. D., Mrug, S., & Pomp, B. (2008). The factor structure of the Narcissistic Personality Inventory. *Journal of Personality Assessment, 90*, 593–600.

Cortina, M., & Liotti, G. (2007). New approaches to understanding unconscious processes: Implicit and explicit memory systems. *International Forum of Psychoanalysis, 16*, 204–212.

Costafreda, S. G., Brammer, M. J., David, A. S., & Fu, C. H. Y. (2008). Predictors of amygdala activation during the processing of emotional stimuli: A meta-analysis of 385 PET and fMRI studies. *Brain Research Reviews, 58*, 57–70.

Courtney, S. M., Petit, L., Haxby, J. V., & Ungerleider, L. G. (1998). The role of the prefrontal cortex in working memory: Examining the contents of consciousness. *Philosophical Transactions of the Royal Society of London Series B: Biological Sciences, 353*, 1819–1828.

Cozolino, L. (2010). *The neuroscience of psychotherapy: Healing the social brain.* Norton.

Cozolino, L. (2024). *The neuroscience of psychotherapy: Healing the social brain* (4th ed.). Norton.

Craig, A. D. (2003). Interoception: The sense of the physiological condition of the body. *Current Opinions in Neurobiology, 13*, 500–505.

Craig, A. D. (2010). The sentient self. *Brain Structure and Function, 214*, 563–577.

Craig, A. D. (2011). Significance of the insula for the evolution of human awareness of feelings from the body. *Annals of the New York Academy of Science, 1225*, 72–82.

Cramer, P. (2011). Young adult narcissism: A 20 year longitudinal study of the contribution of parenting styles, preschool precursors of narcissism and denial. *Journal of Research in Personality, 45*, 19–28.

Cramer, P. (2017). Childhood precursors of the narcissistic personality. *Journal of Nervous and Mental Health Disorders, 205*, 679–684.

Cramer, P. (2019). Narcissism and attachment: The importance of early parenting. *Journal of Mental Disease, 207*, 69–75.

Crouzet, S. M., Kirchner, H., & Thorpe, S. J. (2010). Fast saccades toward faces: Face detection in just 100 ms. *Journal of Vision, 10*, 16. doi: 10.1167/10.4.16

Dabbs, J. M., Jr., & Morris, R. (1990). Testosterone, social class, and antisocial behavior in a sample of 4,462 men. *Psychological Science, 1*, 209–211.

Dabbs, J. M., Jr., Ruback, R. B., Frady, R. L., Hopper, C. H., & Sgoudas, D. S. (1988). Saliva testosterone and criminal violence among women. *Personality and Individual Differences, 9*, 269–275.

Dagra, A., Barpujari, A., Bauer, A., Olowofela, B. O., Mohamed, S., McGrath, K., et al. (2022). Epigenetics of neurotrauma. *Neurology Current Research, 2*, 42–47.

Damasio, A. R. (1996). The somatic marker hypothesis and the possible functions of the prefrontal cortex. *Philosophical Transactions of the Royal Society, Series B 351*, 1413–1420.

Damasio, A. R. (1999). *The feeling of what happens: Body, emotion and the making of consciousness*. Heineman.

Damasio, A. R. (2012). *Self comes to mind: Constructing the conscious brain*. Pantheon/Random House.

Damasio, A. R. (2018). *The strange order of things: Life, feeling, and the making of cultures*. Pantheon.

Darwin, C. (1958). *The origin of species*. Signet Classics. (Original work published 1859)

Darwin, C. (1965). *The expression of emotion in man and animals*. University of Chicago Press. (Original work published 1872)

Davidson, R. J. (1985). Affect, cognition, and hemispheric specialization. In C. E. Izard, J. Kagan, & R. B. Zajonc (Eds.), *Emotions cognition, and behavior* (pp. 320–365). Cambridge University Press.

Davidson, R. J. (2008). Cerebral asymmetry and emotion: Conceptual and methodological conundrums. *Cognition and Emotion, 7*, 115–138.

Davis, M., & Whalen, P. J. (2001). The amygdala: Vigilance and emotion. *Molecular Psychiatry, 6*, 13–34.

Davis, P. J. (1987). Repression and the inaccessibility of affective memories. *Journal of Personality and Social Psychology, 53*, 585–593.

Dean, D. C., Planalp, E. M., Wooten, W., Schmidt, C. K., Kecskemeti, S. R., Frye, C., et al. (2018). Investigation of brain structure in one-month infant. *Brain Structure and Function, 223*, 1953–1970.

DeCasper, A. J., & Fifer, W. P. (1980). Of human bonding: Newborns prefer their mothers' voices. *Science, 208*, 1174–1176.

Decety, J., & Chaminade, T. (2003). When the self represents the other: A new cognitive neuroscience view on psychological identification. *Consciousness and Cognition, 12*, 577–596.

Decety, J., & Lamm, C. (2007). The role of the right temporoparietal junction in social interaction: How low-level computational processes contribute to metacognition. *Neuroscientist, 13*, 580–593.

de Gelder, B. (2005). Nonconscious emotions: New findings and perspectives on nonconscious facial expression recognition and its voice and whole-body contexts. In L. Feldman Barrett, P. M. Niedenthal, & P. Winkielman (Eds.), *Emotion and consciousness* (pp. 123–149). Guilford.

Dehaene, S., & Naccache, L. (2001). Towards a cognitive science of consciousness: Basic evidence and a workspace framework. *Cognition, 79*, 1–37.

de Heering, A., & Rossion, B. (2015). Rapid categorization of natural face images in the infant right hemisphere. *eLife, 4*, e06564.

Demaree, H. A., Everhat, D. E., Youngstrom, E. A., & Harrison, D. W. (2005). Brain lateralization of emotional processing: Historical roots and a future incorporating "dominance." *Behavioral and Cognitive Neuroscience Reviews, 4*, 3–20.

De Pisapia, N., Serra, M., Rigo, P., Jager, J., Papinutto, N., Esposito, G., Venuti, P., & Bornstein, M. H. (2014). Interpersonal competence in young adulthood and right laterality in white matter. *Journal of Cognitive Neuroscience, 26*, 1257–1265.

Derryberry, D., & Tucker, D. M. (1994). Motivating the focus of attention. In P. M. Niedentahl & S. Kiyayama (Eds.), *The heart's eye: Emotional influences in perception and attention* (pp. 167–196). Academic Press.

de Schonen, S., & Deruelle, C. (1991). Visual field asymmetries for pattern processing are present in infancy: A comment on T. Hatta's study on children's performances. *Neuropsychologia, 29*(4), 335–337.

Deutsch, G., Papanicolaou, A. C., Bourbon, T., & Eisenberg, H. M. (1988). Cerebral blood flow evidence of right cerebral activation in attention demanding tasks. *International Journal of Neuroscience, 36*, 23–28.

Devinsky, O. (2000). Right cerebral hemispheric dominance for a sense of corporeal and emotional self. *Epilepsy and Behavior, 1*, 60–73.

DeYoung, C. G., Grazioplene, R. G., & Peterson, J. B. (2012). From madness to genius: The Openness/Intellect trait domain as a paradoxical simplex. *Journal of Research in Personality, 46*, 63–78.

DeYoung, P. A. (2015). *Understanding and treating chronic shame: A relational/neurobiological approach.* Routledge.

Diamond, D., Levy, K. N., Clarkin, J. F., Fisher-Kern, M., Cain, N. M., Doering, S., Horz, S., & Buchheim, A. (2014). Attachment and mentalization in female patients with co-morbid narcissistic and borderline personality disorder. *Personality Disorders: Theory, Research, and Treatment, 5*, 428–433.

Diaz de Chumaceiro, C. L. (1995). Lullabies are "transferential transitional songs": Further considerations on resistance in music therapy. *The Arts in Psychotherapy, 22*, 553–557.

Dickinson, K. A., & Pincus, A. L. (2003). Interpersonal analysis of grandiose and vulnerable narcissism. *Journal of Personality Disorders, 17*, 188–207.

Dijksterhuis, A., & Meurs, T. (2006). Where creativity resides: The generative power of unconscious thought. *Consciousness and Cognition, 15*, 135–146.

Dikker, S., Michalareas, G., Oostrik, M., Serafimaki, A., Kahraman, H. M., Struiksma, M. E., et al. (2021). Crowdsourcing neuroscience: Inter-brain coupling during face-to-face interactions outside the laboratory. *NeuroImage, 227*, 117436. doi: 10.1016/j.neuroimage.2020.117436

Dimberg, U., & Ohman, A. (1996). Behold the wrath: Psychophysiological responses to facial stimuli. *Motivation and Emotion, 20*, 149–182.

Dimond, S. J., & Beaumont, J. G. (1974). *Hemisphere function in the human brain.* Elek Science.

Diseth, T. H. (2005). Dissociation in children and adolescents as reaction to trauma—an overview of conceptual issues and neurobiological factors. *Nordic Journal of Psychiatry, 59*, 79–91.

Dissanayake, E. (2001). Becoming *Homo aestheticus*: Sources of aesthetic imagination in mother-infant interactions. *SubStance, 94/95*, 85–103.

Dissanayake, E. (2017). Ethology and interpersonal neurobiology together with play provide insights into the evolutionary origin of the arts. *American Journal of Play, 9*, 143–168.

Dobbing, J., & Sands, J. (1973). Quantitative growth and development of human brain. *Archives of Diseases of Childhood, 48*, 757–767.

Dodge, N., Simon, B., Brauer, L., Grant, D. C., First, M., Brunshaw, J., et al. (2002). Psychoanalytic patients in the U.S., Canada, and Australia: I. DSM-III-R, previous treatment, medications and length of treatment. *Journal of American Psychoanalytic Association, 50*, 575–614.

Domash, L. (2010). Unconscious freedom and the insight of the analyst: Exploring neuropsychological processes underlying "Aha" moments. *Journal of the American Academy of Psychoanalysis and Dynamic Psychiatry, 38*, 315–339.

Donaldson, Z., & Young, L. J. (2016). The neurobiology and genetics of affiliation and social bonding in animal modes. In J. C. Gewirtz, & Y. K. Kim (Eds.), *Animal Models of Behavior Genetics* (pp. 101–134). Springer.

Donegan, N. H., Sanislow, C. A., & Blumberg, H. P. (2003). Amygdala hyperreactivity in borderline personality disorder: Implications for emotional dysregulation. *Biological Psychiatry, 54*, 1284–1293.

Doran, J. M. (2016). The working alliance: Where have we been, where are we going? *Psychotherapy Research, 26*, 146–163.

Dorpat, T. L. (2001). Primary process communication. *Psychoanalytic Inquiry, 3*, 448–463.

Dotta, B. T., & Persinger, M. A. (2011). Increased photon emission from the right but not the left hemisphere while imagining white light in the dark: The potential connection to consciousness and cerebral light. *Journal of Consciousness Exploration and Research, 2*, 1463–1473.

Douaud, G., Lee, S., Alfara-Almagro, F., Arthofer, C., Wang, C., McCarthy, P., et al. (2022). SARS-CoV-2 is associated with changes in brain structure in UK biobank. *Nature, 604*, 697–707. https://doi.org/10.1038/s41586-022-04569-5

Dowds, B. (2021). Going beyond sucking stones: Connections and emergent meaning in life and in therapy. In R. Tweedy (Ed.), *The divided therapist: Hemispheric difference and contemporary psychotherapy* (pp. 181–201). Routledge.

Downey, G., Freitas, A. L., Michaelis, B., & Khouri, H. (1998). The self-fulfilling prophecy in close relationships: Rejection sensitivity and rejection by romantic partners. *Journal of Personality and Social Psychology, 75*, 545–560.

Downey, T. W. (2001). Early object relations into new objects. *Psychoanalytic Study of the Child, 56*, 39–75.

Drevets, W. C., Price, J. L., Bardgett, M. E., Reich, T., Todd, R. D., & Raichle, M. E. (2002). Glucose metabolism in the amygdala in depression: Relationship to diagnostic subtype and plasma cortisol levels. *Pharmacology, Biochemistry, and Behavior, 71,* 431–447.

Dubois, D., Ameis, S. H., Lai, M. C., Casanova, M. F., & Desarkar, P. (2016). Interoception in autism spectrum disorder: A review. *International Journal of Developmental Neuroscience, 52,* 104–111.

Dufner, M., Rauthmann, J. F., Czarna, A. Z., & Denissen, J. A. (2013). Are narcissists sexy? Zeroing in on the effect of narcissism on short-term mate appeal. *Personality and Social Psychology Bulletin, 39,* 870–882.

Dumas, G. (2011). Towards a two-body neuroscience. *Communicative and Integrative Biology, 4,* 349–352. https://doi.org/10.4161/cib.4.3.15110

Dumas, G., Moreau, Q., Tognoli, E., & Kelso, J. A. S. (2020). The human dynamic clamp reveals the fronto-parietal network linking real-time social coordination and cognition. *Cerebral Cortex, 30,* 3271–3285.

Dumas, G., Nadel, J., Soussignan, R., Martinerie, J., & Garnero, L. (2010). Inter-brain synchronization during social interaction. *PLoS One, 5,* e12166. doi: 10.1371/journal.pone.0012166

Edelman, G. (1989). *The remembered present: A biological theory of consciousness.* Basic Books.

Edelstein, R. S., Newton, N. J., & Stewart, A. J. (2012). Narcissism in midlife: Longitudinal changes in and correlates of women's narcissistic personality traits. *Journal of Personality, 80,* 1179–1204.

Egan, J., & Kernberg, P. F. (1984). Pathological narcissism in childhood. *Journal of the American Psychoanalytic Association, 32,* 39-62.

Ehrenzweig, A. (1957). The creative surrender: A comment on Joanna Field's book on experiment in leisure. *American Imago, 14,* 193–210.

Ellis, R. J., & Thayer, J. F. (2010). Music and autonomic nervous system (dys)function. *Music Perception, 27,* 317–326.

Ellison, W. D., Levy, K. N., Cain, N. M., Ansell, E., & Pincus, A. J. (2013). The impact of pathological narcissism on psychotherapy utilization, initial symptom severity, and early-treatment symptom change: A naturalistic investigation. *Journal of Personality Assessment, 95,* 291–300.

Endevelt-Shapira, Y., Djalovski, A., Dumas, G., & Feldman, R. (2021). Maternal chemosignals enhace infant-adult brain-to-brain synchrony. *Scientific Advances, 7,* 1–11.

Engels, A. S., Heller, W., Mohanty, A., Herrington, J. D., Banich, M. T., Webb, A. G., & Miller, G. A. (2007). Specificity of brain activity in anxiety types during emotion processing. *Psychophysiology, 44,* 352–363.

Enriquez, P., & Bernabeu, E. (2008). Hemispheric laterality and dissociative tendencies: Differences in emotional processing in a dichotic listening task. *Consciousness and Cognition, 17,* 267–275.

Epstein, R. S. (1994). *Keeping boundaries: Maintaining safety and integrity in the psychotherapeutic process.* American Psychiatric Press.

Erikson, E. H. (1950). *Childhood and society.* Norton.

Esterling, B. A., Antoni, M. H., Kumar, M., & Schneiderman, N. (1993). Defensiveness, trait anxiety, and Epstein-Barr viral capsid antigen antibody titers in healthy college students. *Health Psychology, 12,* 132–139.

Eubanks, C. F., Muran, J. C., & Safran, J. D. (2018). Alliance rupture repair: A meta-analysis. *Psychotherapy, 55,* 508–519.

Euler, S., Nolte, T., Constantinou, M., Griem, J., Montague, P. R., & Fonagy, P. (2021). Interpersonal problems in borderline personality disorder: Associations with mentalizing, emotion regulation, and impulsiveness. *Journal of Personality Disorders, 35,* 177–193.

Exline, J. J., Baumeister, R. F., Bushman, B. J., Campbell, W. K., & Finkel, E. J. (2004). Too proud to let go: Narcissistic entitlement as a barrier to forgiveness. *Journal of Personality and Social Psychology, 87,* 894–912.

Farroni, T., Csibra, G., Simion, F., & Johnson, M. H. (2002). Eye contact detection in humans from birth. *Proceedings of the National Academy of Sciences USA, 99,* 9602–9605.

Fede, F., & Masia, V. (2025). The manipulative side of chatbots and AI. *American Scientist, 113,* 104–111.

Feinberg, T. E., & Keenan, J. P. (2005). Where in the brain is the self? *Consciousness and Cognition, 14,* 661–678.

Feldman, R. (2010). The relational basis of adolescent development: Trajectories of mother-child interactive behaviors from infancy through adolescence shapes adolescent's adaptation. *Attachment & Human Development, 12,* 173–192.

Feldman, R., Greenbaum, C. W., & Yirmiya, N. (1999). Mother-infant affect synchrony as an antecedent of the emergence of self-control. *Developmental Psychology, 35,* 223–231.

Feldman, R., Magori-Cohen, R., Galili, G., Singer, M., & Louzon, Y. (2011). Mother and infant coordinate heart rhythms through episodes of interaction synchrony. *Infant Behavior and Development, 34,* 569–577.

Feldman, R., Singer, M., & Zagoory, O. (2010). Touch attenuates infants' physiological reactivity to stress. *Brain and Behaviour, 13,* 271–278.

Ferber, S. G., Feldman, R., & Makhoul, I. R. (2008). The development of maternal touch across the first year of life. *Early Human Development, 84,* 363–370.

Ferenczi, S. (1980). *Further contributions to the theory and technique of psychoanalysis* (J. Rickman, Ed.; E. Mosbacher, Trans.). Brunner-Mazel. (Original work published 1926)

Ferenczi, S. (1988). *The clinical diary of Sandor Ferenczi* (E. Dupont, Ed.). Harvard University Press. (Original work published 1932)

Ferrario, R., Parisi, A., Tallarita, G., Parente, A., Pastori, C., & Giovagnoli, A. R. (2024). Sensitivity to moral and conventional rules in temporal lobe epilepsy. *Epilepsy and Behavior, 158,* 1–8.

Firstpost. (2024). How companies overhype the use of artificial intelligence | vantage on firstpost. YouTube. https://www.youtube.com/watch?v=2wp5Ksld5nQ

Fischer, K. W., & Pipp, S. L. (1984). Development of the structures of unconscious thought. In K. S. Bowers & D. Meichenbaum (Eds.), *The unconscious reconsidered* (pp. 88–148). Wiley.

Fiskum, C. (2019). Psychotherapy beyond all the words: Dyadic expansion, vagal regulation, and biofeedback in psychotherapy. *Journal of Psychotherapy Integration, 29*, 412–425.

Flanagan, L. M. (2022). Object relations theory. In J. Berzoff, L. M. Flanagan, & P. Hertz (Eds.), *Inside out and outside in: Psychodynamic clinical theory and psychopathology in contemporary multicultural contexts* (5th ed., pp. 92–124). Rowman & Littlefield.

Flanders, J. L., Herman, K. N., & Paquette, D. (2013). Rough-and-tumble play and the cooperation-competition dilemma: Evolutionary and developmental perspectives on the development of social competence. In D. Narvaez, J. Panksepp, A. Schore, & T. R. Gleason (Eds.), *Evolution, early experience and human development* (pp. 371–387). Oxford University Press.

Flanders, J. L., Simard, M., Paquette, D., Parent, S., Vitaro, F., Pihl, R. O., & Seguin, J. R. (2010). Rough-and-tumble play and the development of physical aggression and emotion regulation: A five-year follow-up study. *Journal of Family Violence, 25*, 357–367.

Flor-Henry, P., Shapiro, Y., & Sombrun, C. (2017). Brain changes during a shamanic trance: Altered modes of consciousness, hemispheric laterality, and systemic psychobiology. *Cogent Psychology, 4*, 1313522.

Fluckiger, C., Del Re, A., Wampold, B. E., & Horvath, A. O. (2018). The alliance in adult psychotherapy: A meta-analytic synthesis. *Psychotherapy, 55*, 316–340.

Forrester, G. S., Davis, R., Mareschal, D., Malatesta, G., & Todd, B. K. (2018). The left cradling bias: An evolutionary facilitator of social cognition? *Cortex, 118*, 116–131.

Fossati, A., Feeney, J., Pincus, A., Borroni, S., & Maffei, C. (2015). The structure of pathological narcissism and its relationships with adult attachment styles: A study of Italian and clinical adult participants. *Psychoanalytic Psychology, 32*, 403–431.

Foster, P. S., Drago, V., Ferguson, B. J., & Harrison, D. W. (2008). Cerebral moderation of cardiovascular functioning: A functional cerebral systems perspective. *Clinical Neurophysiology, 119*, 2846–2854.

Fox, K. C. R., Yih, J., Raccah, O., Pendekanti, S. L., Limbach, L. E., Maydan, D. D., & Parvizi, J. (2018). Changes in subjective experience elicited by direct stimulation of the human orbitofrontal cortex. *Neurology, 91*, e1519–e1527.

Fox, N. A., Calkins, S. D., & Bell, M. A. (1994). Neural plasticity and development in the first two years of life: Evidence from cognitive and socioemotional domains of research. *Developmental Psychopathology, 6*, 677–696.

Fraiberg, S. H., Adelson, E., & Shapiro, V. B. (1975). Ghosts in the nursery: A psychoanalytic approach to the problem of infant/mother relationships. *Journal of the American Academy of Child Psychiatry, 14*, 113–169.

Frankel, J. (1998). The play's the thing: How the essential processes of psychotherapy are seen most clearly in child therapy. *Psychoanalytic Dialogues, 8*, 149–182.

Frayn, D. (1990). Regressive transferences—a manifestation of primitive personality organization. *American Journal of Psychotherapy, 44*, 50–60.

Freud, S. (1953). A general introduction to psycho-analysis. In J. Strachey (Ed. &

Trans.), *The standard edition of the complete psychological works of Sigmund Freud* (Vol. 3). Hogarth. (Original work published 1920)

Freud, S. (1953). *A general introduction to psycho-analysis* (J. Riviere, Trans.). Edward L. Bernays. (Original work published 1935)

Freud, S. (1953). The interpretation of dreams. In J. Strachey (Ed. & Trans.), *The standard edition of the complete psychological works of Sigmund Freud* (Vols. 4 & 5, pp. 1–627). Hogarth. (Original work published 1900)

Freud, S. (1953). Three essays on the theory of sexuality. In J. Strachey (Ed. & Trans.), *The standard edition of the complete psychological works of Sigmund Freud* (Vol 7, pp. 135–243). Hogarth. (Original work published 1905)

Freud, S. (1957). On the history of the psycho-analytic movement. In J. Strachey (Ed. & Trans.), *The standard edition of the complete psychological works of Sigmund Freud* (Vol. 14, pp. 7–66). Hogarth. (Original work published 1914)

Freud, S. (1957). On narcissism: An introduction. In J. Strachey (Ed. & Trans.), *The standard edition of the complete psychological works of Sigmund Freud* (Vol 14, pp. 67–102). Hogarth. (Original work published 1914)

Freud, S. (1957). The unconscious. In J. Strachey (Ed. & Trans.), *The standard edition of the complete psychological works of Sigmund Freud* (Vol. 14, pp. 166–204). Hogarth. (Original work published 1915)

Freud, S. (1957). Thoughts for the times on war and death. In J. Strachey (Ed. & Trans.), *The standard edition of the complete psychological works of Sigmund Freud* (Vol 14, 275–288). Hogarth. (Original work published 1914–1916)

Freud, S. (1958). Recommendations to physicians practicing psycho-analysis. In J. Strachey (Ed. & Trans.), *The standard edition of the complete psychological works of Sigmund Freud* (Vol. 12, 111–120). Hogarth. (Original work published 1912)

Freud, S. (1958). On beginning the treatment. In J. Strachey (Ed. & Trans.). In *The standard edition of the complete psychological works of Sigmund Freud* (Vol. 12, pp. 23–144). Hogarth. (Original work published 1913)

Freud, S. (1958). The claims of psycho-analysis to scientific interest. In J. Strachey (Ed. & Trans.), *The standard edition of the complete psychological works of Sigmund Freud* (Vol. 20, pp. 87–174). Hogarth. (Original work published 1914)

Freud, S. (1961). Papers on techniques of psychotherapy. In J. Strachey (Ed. and Trans.), *The standard edition of the complete psychological works of Sigmund Freud* (Vol. 12). Hogarth. (Original work published 1915)

Freud, S. (1961). The ego and the id. In J. Strachey (Ed. & Trans.), *The standard edition of the complete psychological works of Sigmund Freud* (Vol. 19, pp. 3–68). Hogarth. (Original work published 1923)

Freud, S. (1961). The future of an illusion, civilization and its discontents, and other works. In J. Strachey (Ed. & Trans.), *The standard edition of the complete psychological works of Sigmund Freud* (Vol. 21, pp. 5–589). Hogarth. (Original work published 1927)

Freud, S. (1961). The question of lay analysis. In J. Strachey (Ed. & Trans.), *The standard edition of the complete psychological works of Sigmund Freud* (Vol. 20, 177–258). Hogarth. (Original work published 1926)

Freud, S. (1963). Introductory lectures on psycho-analysis. In J. Strachey (Ed. & Trans.), *The standard edition of the complete psychological works of Sigmund Freud* (Vols. 15 & 16). Hogarth. (Original work published 1916–1917)

Freud, S. (1964). An outline of psychoanalysis. In J. Strachey (Ed. & Trans.), *The standard edition of the complete psychological works of Sigmund Freud* (Vol 23, pp. 144–207). Hogarth. (Original work published 1940)

Freud, S. (1966). Project for a scientific psychology. In J. Strachey (Ed. & Trans.), *The standard edition of the complete psychological works of Sigmund Freud* (Vol. 1, pp. 295–397). Hogarth. (Original work published 1895)

Frewen, P., Brown, M., DePierro, J., D'Andrea, W., & Schore, A. (2015). Assessing the family dynamics of childhood maltreatment history with the Childhood Attachment and Relational Trauma Screen (CARTS). *European Journal of Psychotraumatology, 6*, 27792. https://dx.doi.org/10.3402/ejpt.v6.27792

Frewen, P. A., Evans, B., Goodman, J., Halliday, A., Boylan, J., Moran, G., Reiss, J., Schore, A., & Lanius, R. A. (2013). Development of a Childhood Attachment and Relational Trauma Screen (CARTS): A relational-socioecological framework for surveying attachment security and childhood trauma history. *European Journal of Psychotraumatology, 4*, 20232. https://dx.doi.org/10.3402/ejpt.v4i0.20232

Frijda, N. H. (1988). The laws of emotion. *American Psychologist, 43*, 349–358.

Fromm, E. (1956). *The art of loving.* Harper and Row.

Furedy, J. J., & Riley, D. (1987). Human Pavlovian autonomic conditioning and the cognitive paradigm. In G. Day (Ed.), *Cognitive processes and Pavlovian conditioning in humans.* Wiley.

Gabbard, G. O. (1989). Two subtypes of narcissistic personality disorder. *Bulletin of the Menninger Clinic, 53*, 527–532.

Gabbard, G. (2022). Narcissism and suicide risk. *Annals of General Psychiatry, 21*, 3.

Gabel, S. (1988). The right hemisphere in imagery, hypnosis, rapid eye movement sleep and dreaming: Empirical studies and tentative conclusions. *Journal of Nervous and Mental Disease, 176*, 323–331.

Gainotti, G. (1972). Emotional behavior and hemispheric side of the lesion. *Cortex 8*, 41–55.

Gainotti, G. (2005). Emotions, unconscious processes, and the right hemisphere. *Neuropsychoanalysis, 7*, 71– 81.

Gainotti, G. (2006). Unconscious emotional memories and the right hemisphere. In M. Mancia (Ed.), *Psychoanalysis and neuroscience* (pp. 151–173). Milan: Springer Milan.

Gainotti, G. (2012). Unconscious processing of emotions and the right hemisphere. *Neuropsychologia, 50*, 205–218.

Gainotti, G. (2019). A historical review of investigations on laterality of emotions in the human brain. *Journal of the History of the Neurosciences, 28*, 23–41.

Gainotti, G. (2020). *Emotions and the right side of the brain.* Springer.

Galbusera, L., Finn, M. T., & Fuchs, T. (2018). Interactional synchrony and negative symptoms: An outcome study of body-oriented psychotherapy for schizophrenia. *Psychotherapy Research, 28,* 457–469. doi: 10.1080/10503307.2016.1216624

Galin, D. (1974). Implications for psychiatry of left and right cerebral specializations: A neurophysiological context for unconscious processes. *Archives of General Psychiatry, 31,* 572–583.

Gallese, V. (2007). Dai neuroni, specchio alla consonanza intenzionale: Meccanismi neurofisiologici dell'intersoggettivita [From mirror neurons to intentional consonance: Neurophysiological mechanisms of intersubjectivity]. *Rivista di Psicoanalisi, 53,* 197–208.

Gallotti, M., & Frith, C. D. (2013). Social cognition in the we-mode. *Trends in Cognitive Sciences, 17,* 160–165.

Gebauer, L., Witek, M., Hansen, N. C., Thomas, J., Konvalinka, I., & Vuust, P. (2014). *The influence of oxytocin on interpersonal rhythmic synchronization and social bonding* [Poster presentation]. The Neurosciences and Music—V, Dijon.

Geller, S. M., & Porges, S. W. (2014). Therapeutic presence: Neurophysiological mechanisms mediating feeling safe in therapeutic relationships. *Journal of Psychotherapy Integration, 24,* 178–192.

Geng, J. J., & Vossel, S. (2013). Re-evaluating the role of TPJ in attentional control: Contextual updating? *Neuroscience and Biobehavioral Review, 37,* 2608–2620.

George, C., & Aikins, J. W. (2023). Developing a secure base in family intervention: Using the adult attachment projective system to assess attachment in family relationships. *Frontiers in Psychology, 14.* doi: 10.3389/fpsyg.2023.1291661

George, C., Kaplan, N., & Main, M. (1996). *Adult attachment interview* [Unpublished manuscript, 3rd ed.]. Department of psychology, University of California, Berkeley.

George, M. S., Parekh, P. I., Rosinsky, N., Ketter, T. A., Kimbrell, T. A., Heilman, K. M., Herscovitch, P., & Post, R. M. (1996). Understanding emotional prosody activates right hemispheric regions. *Archives of Neurology, 53,* 665–670.

Geschwind, N., & Galaburda, A. M. (1985). Cerebral lateralization: Biological mechanisms, associations, and pathology. I. A hypothesis and a program for research. *Archives of Neurology, 42,* 428–459.

Gettler, L. T., McDade, T. W., Feranil, A. B., & Kuzawaa, C. W. (2011). Longitudinal evidence that fatherhood decreases testosterone in human males. *Proceedings of the National Academy of Sciences USA, 108,* 16194–16199.

Ghashghaei, H. T., & Barbas, H. (2002). Pathways for emotion: Interactions of prefrontal and anterior temporal pathways in the amygdala of the rhesus monkey. *Neuroscience, 115,* 1261–1279.

Ghent, E. (1990). Masochism, submission, surrender: Masochism as a perversion of surrender. *Contemporary Psychoanalysis, 26,* 108–136.

Ghent, E. (1995). Interaction in the psychoanalytic situation. *Psychoanalytic Dialogues, 5,* 479–491.

Giesbrecht, G. F., Muller, U., & Miller, M. R. (2010). Psychological distancing in the development of executive functions and emotional regulation. In B. W. Sokel, U.

Muller, J. Carpendale, A. Young, & G. Iaroci (Eds.), *Self- and social-regulation: The development of social interaction, social understanding, and executive functions* (pp. 337–357). Oxford University Press.

Giljov, A., Karenina, K., & Malaschichev, Y. (2018). Facing each other: Mammal mothers and infants prefer the position favouring right hemisphere processing. *Biology Letters, 14*, 20170707. https://doi.org/10.1098/rsbl.2017.0707

Gill, M. M., & Brenman, M. (1959). *Hypnosis and related states*. International Universities Press.

Gilmore, J. H., Shi, F., Woolson, S. I., Knickmeyer, R. C., Short, S. J., Lin, S. J., et al. (2012). Longitudinal development of cortical and subcortical gray matter from birth to 2 years. *Cerebral Cortex, 22*, 2478–2485.

Giovacchini, P. L. (1990). Regression, reconstruction, and resolution: Containment and holding. In P. L. Giovacchini (Ed.), *Tactics and techniques in psychoanalytic therapy III: The implications of Winnicott's contributions* (pp. 226–264). Jason Aronson.

Giovacchini, P. L. (1991). The creative person as maverick. *Journal of the American Academy of Psychoanalysis, 19*, 174–188.

Gipps, R. G. T., & Lacewing, M. (2019). Introduction: Know thyself. In R. G. T. Gipps & M. Lacewing (Eds.), *The Oxford handbook of philosophy and psychoanalysis* (pp. 1–19). Oxford University Press.

Glasel, H., Leroy, F., Dubois, J., Hertz-Pannier, L., Mangin, J. F., & Dehaene-Lambertz, G. (2011). A robust cerebral asymmetry in the infant brain: The rightward superior temporal sulcus. *NeuroImage, 58*, 716–723.

Gnaulati, E. (2019). The ethics of neglecting clinical relationship and alliance building in trauma-focused treatments. *Ethical Human Psychology and Psychiatry, 21*, 104–116.

Gnaulati, E. (2021). Relational healing in psychotherapy: Reaching beyond the research. *Psychoanalytic Inquiry, 41*, 593–602.

Goldstein, P., Weissman-Fogel, I., Dumas, G., & Shamay-Tsoory, S. G. (2018). Brain-to-brain handholding is associated with pain reduction. *Proceedings of the National Academy of Sciences USA, 115*, E2528–E2537.

Goleman, D. (1995). *Emotional intelligence*. Bantam.

Gonzalez, C. L. R., van Rootselaar, N. A., & Gibb, R. L. (2018). Sensorimotor lateralization scaffolds cognitive specialization. *Progress in Brain Research, 238*, 405–433.

Goodkind, M. S., Solberger, M., Gyuark, A., Rosen, H. J., Rankin, K. B., Miller, B., et al. (2012). Tracking emotional valence: The role of the orbitofrontal cortex. *Human Brain Mapping, 33*, 753–762.

Gotti, M. (2024). From the gate to the gateway: Psychoanalytic navigations online. *The American Journal of Psychoanalysis, 84*, 229–249.

Goyal, M. S., Hawrylycz, M., Miller, J. A., Snyder, A. Z., & Raichle, M. E. (2014). Aerobic glycolysis in the human brain is associated with development and neotenous gene expression. *Cell Metabolism, 19*, 49–57.

Grabner, R. H., Fink, A., & Neubauer, A. C. (2007). Brain correlates of self-related originality of ideas: Evidence from event-related power and phase-locking changes in the EEG. *Behavioral Neuroscience, 121*, 224–230.

Grafanaki, S., Brennan, M., Holmes, S., Tang, K., & Alvarez, S. (2007). In search of flow in counseling and psychotherapy: Identifying the necessary ingredients of peak moments of therapy interaction. *Person-Centered and Experiential Psychotherapies, 6*, 240–255.

Gramzow, R., & Tangney, J. P. (1992). Proneness to shame and the narcissistic personality. *Personality and Social Psychology Bulletin, 18*, 369–376.

Granat, A., Gadassi, R., Gilboa-Schectman, E., & Feldman, R. (2017). Maternal depression and anxiety, social synchrony, and infant regulation of negative and positive emotions. *Emotion, 17*, 11–27. doi: 10.1037/emo0000204

Gray, P. B., Yang, C.-F. J., & Pope, H. G., Jr. (2006). Fathers have lower salivary testosterone levels than unmarried men and married non-fathers in Beijing, China. *Proceedings in Biological Science, 273*, 333–339.

Greenberg, D. L., Rice, H. J., Cooper, J. J., Cabeza, R., Rubin, D. C., & Labar, K. S. (2005). Co-activation of the amygdala, hippocampus, and inferior frontal gyrus during autobiographical memory retrieval. *Neuropsychologia, 43*, 659–674.

Greenberg, L. S. (2006). The clinical application of emotion in psychotherapy. In L. F. Barrett, M. Lewis, & J. M. Haviland-Jones (Eds.), *Handbook of emotions* (4th ed., pp. 670–684). Guilford.

Greenberg, L. S. (2014). The therapeutic relationship in emotion-focused therapy. *Psychotherapy, 51*, 350–357.

Greenson, R. (1978). *Explorations in psychoanalysis*. International Universities Press.

Grijalva, E., Harms, P. D., Newman, D. A., Gaddis, B. H., & Fraley, R. C. (2014). Narcissism and leadership: A meta-analytic review of linear and nonlinear relationships. *Personnel Psychology, 68*(1), 1–47. https://doi.org/10.1111/peps.12072

Grijalva, E., & Newman, D. A. (2014). Narcissism and counterproductive work behavior: Meta-analysis and consideration of collectivist culture, Big Five personality, and narcissism's facet structure. *Applied Psychology, 64*, 93–126.

Gromada, A., Rees, G., & Chzhen, Y. (2020). *Worlds of Influence: Understanding what shapes child well-being in rich countries*. Innocenti Report Card 16. UNICEF Office of Research.

Gross, J. J., & Thompson, R. A. (2007). Emotion regulation. Conceptual foundations. In J. J. Gross (Ed.), *Handbook of emotion regulation* (pp. 3–24). The Guilford Press.

Grossmann, T., Johnson, M. H., Lloyd-Fox, S., Blasi, A., Deligianni, F., Elwell, C., & Csibra, G. (2008). Early cortical specialization for face-to-face communication in human infants. *Proceedings of the Royal Society B: Biological Sciences, 275*, 2803–2811.

Grossmann, T., Oberecker, R., Koch, S. P., & Friederici, A. D. (2010). The developmental origins of voice processing in the human brain. *Neuron, 65*, 852–858.

Grossmark, R. (2012). The unobtrusive relational analyst. *Psychoanalytic Dialogues, 22*, 629–646.

Grupe, D. W., Oathes, D. J., & Nitschke, J. B. (2013). Dissecting the anticipation of aversion reveals dissociable neural networks. *Cerebral Cortex, 23*, 1874–1883.

Guedeney, A., Guedeney, N., Tereno, S., Dugravier, R., Greacen, T., Welniarz, B., & Saias, T. (2011). Infant rhythms versus parental time: Prompting parent-infant synchrony. *Journal of Physiology, Paris, 105*, 195–200.

Guile, J. M., Mbekou, V., & Lageix, P. (2004). Child and parent variables associated with treatment response in narcissistic youths: The role of self-blame and shame. *Canadian Child and Adolescent Psychiatry Review, 13*, 81–85.

Gumpp, A. M., Behnke, A., Ramo-Ferndez, L., Radermacher, P., Gundel, H., Ziegenhain, U., et al. (2022). Investigating mitochondrial bioenergetics in peripheral blood mononuclear cells of women with childhood maltreatment from post-partum period to one-year follow-up. *Psychological Medicine, 53*, 3793–3804.

Guntrip, H. (1969). *Schizoid phenomena, object relations and the self.* International Universities Press.

Guo, K., Meints, K., Hall, C., Hall, S., & Mills, D. (2009). Left gaze bias in humans, rhesus monkeys and domestic dogs. *Animal Cognition, 12*, 409–418.

Gupta, R. K., Hasan, K. M., Trivedi, R., Pradhan, M., Das, V., Parikh, N. A., & Narayana, P. A. (2005). Diffusion tensor imaging of the developing human cerebrum. *Journal of Neuroscience Research, 81*, 172–178.

Gur, R. C., Gunning-Dixon, F., Bilker, W. B., & Gur, R. E. (2002). Sex differences in temporo-limbic and frontal brain volumes in healthy adults. *Cerebral Cortex, 12*, 998–1003.

Hadamard, J. (1945). *The mathematician's mind: The psychology of invention in the mathematical field.* Princeton University Press.

Hakuno, Y., Pirazzoli, L., Biasi, A., Johnson, M. H., & Lloyd-Fox, S. (2018). Optical imaging during toddlerhood: Brain responses during naturalistic social interactions. *Neurophotonics, 5*(1), 011020.

Hall, J. J., Neal, T. J., & Dean, R. (2008). *Lateralization of cerebral functions* (3rd ed.). Springer.

Ham, J., & Tronick, E. (2006). Infant resilience to the stress of the still-face: Infant and maternal psychophysiology are related. *Annals of the New York Academy of Sciences, 1094*, 297–302.

Hamann, S. B., Ely, T. D., Grafton, S. T., & Kilts, C. D. (1999). Amygdala activity related to enhanced memory for pleasant and aversive stimuli. *Nature Neuroscience, 2*, 289–293.

Hammer, E. (1990). *Reaching the affect: Style in the psychodynamic therapies.* Jason Aronson.

Halonen, R., Kuula, L., Selin, M., Suutari, A., Antila, M., & Pesonen, A.-K. (2024). REM Sleep preserves affective response to social stress - Experimental study. *eNeuro, 11*(6). https://doi.org/10.1523/ENEURO.0453-23.2024

Hanson, J. L., Chung, M. K., Avants, B. B., Shirtcliff, E. A., Gee, J., Davidson, R. J., & Pollak, S. D. (2010). Early stress is associated with alterations in the orbitofrontal cortex: A tensor-based morphometry investigation of brain structure and behavioral risk. *Journal of Neuroscience, 30,* 7466–7472.

Happaney, K., Zelazo, P. D., & Stuss, D. T. (2004). Development of orbitofrontal function: Current themes and future directions. *Brain and Cognition, 55,* 1–10.

Harricharan, S., Rabellino, D., Frewen, P. A., Densmore, M., Theberge, J., McKinnon, M. C., Schore, A. N., & Lanius, R. A. (2016). fMRI functional connectivity of the periaqueductal gray in PTSD and its dissociative subtype. *Brain and Behavior, 6*(12), e00579. doi: 10.1002/brb3.579

Harris, J. J., Jolivet, R., & Atwell, D. (2012). Synaptic energy use and supply. *Neuron, 75,* 762–777.

Harrison, N. A., Singer, T., Rothstein, P., Dolan, R. J., & Critchley, H. D. (2006). Pupillary contagion: Central mechanisms engaged in sadness processing. *Social Cognitive and Affective Neuroscience, 1,* 5–17.

Hart, B. M., Taqvi, U., Gastrock, R. Q., Ruttle, J. E., Modchalingam, S., & Henriques, D. Y. P. (2024). Measures of implicit and explicit adaptation do not linearly add. *eNeuro, 11*(8). https://doi.org/10.1523/ENEURO.0021-23.2024

Hartikainen, K. M. (2021). Emotion-attention interaction in the right hemisphere. *Brain Science, 11,* 1006. https://doi.org/10.3390/brainsci11081006

Hassin, R. R. (2009). Implicit working memory. *Consciousness and Cognition, 18,* 665–678.

Hassin, R. R. (2013). Yes it can: On the functional abilities of the human unconscious. *Perspectives in Psychological Science, 8,* 195–207.

Hasson, H., Ghazanfar, A. A., Galantucci, B., Garrod, S., & Keysers, C. (2012). Brain-to-brain coupling: A mechanism for creating and sharing a social world. *Trends in Cognitive Science, 16,* 114–121.

Hatfield, E., Cacioppo, J. T., & Rapson, R. L. (1994). *Emotional contagion.* Cambridge University Press.

Håvås, E., Svartberg, M., & Ulvenes, P. (2015). Attuning to the unspoken: The relationship between therapist nonverbal attunement and attachment security in adult psychotherapy. *Psychoanalytic Psychology, 32,* 235–254.

Hazan, C., & Shaver, P. (1987). Romantic love conceptualized as an attachment process. *Journal of Personality and Social Psychology, 52,* 511–524.

Hecht, D. (2014). Cerebral lateralization of pro- and anti-social tendencies. *Experimental Neurobiology, 23,* 1–27.

Heilman, K. M., & van den Abell, T. (1979). Right hemispheric dominance for mediating cerebral activation. *Neuropsychologia, 17,* 315–321.

Heinrichs, M., Baumgartner, T., Kirschbaum, C., & Ehlert, U. (2003). Social support and oxytocin interact to suppress cortical and subjective responses to psychosocial stress. *Biological Psychiatry, 54,* 1389–1398.

Helmeke, C., Seidel, K., Poeggel, G., Bredy, T. W., Abraham, A., & Braun, K. (2009).

Paternal deprivation during infancy results in dendrite- and time-specific changes of dendritic development and spine formation in the orbitofrontal cortex of the biparental rodent *Octodon Degus*. *Neuroscience, 163,* 790–798.

Helton, W. S., Dorahy, M. J., & Russell, P. N. (2011). Dissociative tendencies and right-hemisphere processing load: Effects on vigilance performance. *Consciousness and Cognition, 20,* 696–702.

Hendler, T., Rotshtein, P., Yeshurun, Y., Weizmann, T., Kahn, I., Ben-Bashat, D., et al. (2003). Sensing the invisible: Differential sensitivity of visual cortex and amygdala to traumatic context. *NeuroImage, 19,* 587–600.

Hendriks, A. W., van Rijswijk, M., & Omtzigt, D. (2011). Holding-side influences on infant's view of mother's face. *Lateralty: Assymetries of Body, Brain and Cognition, 16,* 641–655.

Henry, J. P. (1993). Psychological and physiological responses to stress: The right hemisphere and the hypothalamo-pituitary-adrenal axis, an inquiry into problems of human bonding. *Integrative Physiological and Behavioral Science, 28,* 369–387.

Hermans, E. J., Putman, P., & van Honk, J. (2006). Testosterone administration reduces empathetic behavior: A facial mimicry study. *Psychoneuroendocrinology, 31,* 859–866.

Herpetz, E. A., Dietrich, T. M., Wenning, B., Krings, T., Erberich, S. G., Wilmes, K., et al. (2001). Evidence of abnormal amygdala functioning in borderline personality disorder: A functional MRI study. *Biological Psychiatry, 50,* 292–298.

Herzog, J. M. (2001). *Father hunger: Explorations with adults and children.* Analytic Press.

Hess, N. (2019). A neuroscientific perspective on the therapeutic alliance and how talking changes the brain: Supporting a common factors model of psychotherapy. *Psychotherapy and Counselling Journal of Australia, 7*(2). https://doi.org/10.59158/001c.71106

Hesse, E. (2010). The Adult Attachment Interview: Protocol, method of analysis, and empirical studies. In J. Cassidy & P. Shaver (Eds.), *Handbook of attachment: Theory, research and clinical applications* (pp. 552–598). Guilford.

Hilgard, E. R. (1984). The hidden observer and multiple personality. *International Journal of Clinical and Experimental Hypnosis, 32,* 248–253.

Hill, C. E., Hoffman, M. A., Kivlighan, D. M., Spiegel, S. B., & Gelso, C. J. (2017). Therapist expertise in psychotherapy revisited. *Counseling Psychologist, 45,* 7–53.

Hill, D. (2024). *Affect, consciousness, and self: A view from the bottom of the mind.* Routledge.

Hilsenroth, M. J., Holdwick, D. J., Castlebury, F. D., & Blais, M. A. (1998). The effects of *DSM-IV* cluster B personality disorder symptoms on the termination and continuation of psychotherapy. *Psychotherapy: Theory, Research, Practice, Training, 35,* 163–176.

Hoehl, S., Fairhurst, M., & Schirmer, A. (2021). Interactional synchrony: Signals, mechanisms and benefits. *Social Cognition and Affective Neuroscience, 16,* 5–18.

Hofer, M. A. (1984). Relationships as regulators: A psychobiological perspective on bereavement. *Psychosomatic Medicine, 46,* 183–197.

Hoffmann, M. (2021). The neurobiology of human super-communication: Insights for medicine and business. *World Journal of Neuroscience, 11*, 287–306.

Holland, D., Chang, L., Ernst, T. M., Curran, M., Buchtal, S. D., Alicata, D., et al. (2014). Structural growth trajectories and rates of change in the first 3 months of infant brain development. *JAMA Neurology, 71*(10), 1266–1274. doi: 10.1001/jamaneurol.2014.1638

Homae, F., Watanabe, H., Nakano, T., Asakawa, K., & Taga, G. (2006). The right hemisphere of sleeping infants perceives sentential prosody. *Neuroscience Research, 54*, 276–280.

Horney, K. (1937). *The neurotic personality of our time.* Norton.

Horowitz, M. J. (1992). Formulation of states of mind in psychotherapy. In N. G. Hamilton (Ed.), *From inner sources: New directions in object relations psychotherapy* (pp. 75–83). Jason Aronson.

Hosseini, E. (2021). Brain-to-brain communication: The possible role of brain electromagnetic fields (as a potential hypothesis). *Heliyon, 7*(3), e06363. https://doi.org/10.1016/j.heliyon.2021.e06363

Hove, M., & Risen, J. L. (2009). It's all in the timing: Interpersonal synchrony increases affiliation. *Social Cognition, 27*(6), 949–960. https://doi.org/10.1521/soco.2009.27.6.949

Howard, M. F., & Reggia, J. A. (2007). A theory of the visual system biology underlying development of spatial frequency lateralization. *Brain and Cognition, 64*, 111–123.

Howland, M. (2016). Reading minds and being invisible: The role of empathic accuracy in invisible support provision. *Social and Psychological and Personality Science, 7*, 149–156.

Howland, M., & Simpson, J. A. (2010). Getting in under the radar: A dyadic view of invisible support. *Psychological Science, 21*, 1878–1885.

Huang, P., Qui, L., Zhang, Y., Song, Z., Qi, Z., Gong, Q., & Xie, P. (2013). Evidence of a left-over-right inhibitory mechanism during figural creative thinking in healthy nonartists. *Human Brain Mapping, 34*, 2724–2732.

Hugdahl, K. (1995). Classical conditioning and implicit learning: The right hemisphere hypothesis. In R. J. Davidson & K. Hugdahl (Eds.), *Brain asymmetry.* MIT Press.

Hunter, R. G., Seligson, M., Rubin, T. G., Griffiths, B. B., Ozdemir, Y., Pfaff, D. W., et al. (2016). Stress and corticosteroids regulate rat hippocampal mitochondrial gene expression via the glucocorticoid receptor. *Proceedings of the National Academy of Sciences USA, 113*, 9099–9104.

Hurlemann, R., Patin, A., Onur, O. A., Cohen, M. X., Baumgartner, T., Metzler, S., et al. (2010). Oxytocin enhances amygdala-dependent, socially reinforced learning and emotional empathy in humans. *Journal of Neuroscience, 30*, 4999–5007.

Ingle, H. E., & Mikulewicz, M. (2020). Mental health and climate change: Tackling invisible injustice. *Lancet Planet Health, 4*, e435–436.

Izard, C. E. (1991). *The psychology of emotions.* Plenum.

Jackson, J. H. (1931). *Selected writings of John Hughlings Jackson* (Vols. 1 and 2). Hodder and Stoughton.

Jacobs, T. J. (1994). Nonverbal communications: Some reflections on their role in the psychoanalytic process and psychoanalytic education. *Journal of the American Psychoanalytic Association, 42*, 741–762.

Jacobson, E. (1964). *The self and the object world.* International Universities Press.

Jacques, C., & Rossion, B. (2009). The initial representation of individual faces in the right occipito-temporal cortex is holistic: Electrophysiological evidence from the composite face illusion. *Journal of Vision, 9*, 1–16.

Jaffe, J., Beebe, B., Feldstein, S., Crown, C. L., Jasnow, M. D., Rochat, P., & Stern, D. N. (2001). Rhythms of dialogue in infancy: Coordinated timing in development. *Monographs of the Society of Research in Child Development, 66*, 1–149.

Jamner, L. D., Schwartz, G. E., & Leigh, H. (1988). The relationship between repressive and defensive coping styles and monocyte, eosinophile, and serum glucose levels: Support for the opioid hypothesis of repression. *Psychosomatic Medicine, 50*, 567–575.

Jauk, E., Benedek, M., Koschutnig, K., Kedia, G., & Neubauer, A. C. (2017). Self-viewing is associated with negative affect rather than reward in highly narcissistic men: An fMRI study. *Scientific Reports, 7*, 5804. https://doi.org/10.1038/s41598-017-03935-y

Jauk, E., & Kanske, P. (2021). Can neuroscience help to understand narcissism? A systematic review of an emerging field. *Personality Neuroscience, 4*: e3. doi: 10.1017/pen.2021.1

Jiang, J., Chen, C., Dai, B., Shi, G., Ding, G., Liu, L., & Lu, C. (2015). Leader emergence through interpersonal neural synchronization. *Proceedings of the National Academy of Sciences USA, 112*, 4274–4279.

Johnsen, B. J., & Hugdahl, K. (1993). Right hemisphere representation of autonomic conditioning to facial emotional expressions. *Psychophysiology, 30*, 274–288.

Johnson Chacko, L., Pechriggl, E. J., Fritsch, H., Rask-Andersen, H., Blumer, M. J., Schrott-Fischer, A., et al. (2016). Neuroscience differentiation and innervation patterning in the human fetal vestibular end organs between the gestational weeks 8-12. *Frontiers in Neuroanatomy, 10*, 1–19.

Jones, B. P. (1993). Repression: The evolution of a psychoanalytic concept from the 1890's to the 1990's. *Journal of the American Psychoanalytic Association, 41*, 63–93.

Jones, E. (1953). *The life and work of Sigmund Freud: Vol. 2. The formative years and the great discoveries, 1856–1900.* Basic Books.

Jordan, J. V. (2000). The role of mutual empathy in relational/cultural therapy. *Journal of Clinical Psychology/In Session: Psychotherapy in Practice, 56*, 1005–1016.

Joseph, R. (1982). The neuropsychology of development: Hemispheric laterality, limbic language, and the origin of thought. *Journal of Clinical Psychology, 38*, 4–33.

Joseph, R. (1992). *The right brain and the unconscious: Discovering the stranger within.* Plenum.

Joseph, R. (1996). *Neuropsychiatry, neuropsychology, and clinical neuroscience* (2nd ed.). Williams & Wilkins.

Jostmann, N. B., Kuole, S. L., Vander Wulp, N. Y., & Fockenberg, D. A. (2005). Subliminal affect regulation: The moderating role of action- versus state-orientation. *European Psychologist, 10,* 209–217.

Jung, C. G. (1912). *The theory of psychoanalysis. Collected works 5.* Princeton University Press.

Jung, C. G. (1943). *Two essays on analytical psychology.* Meridian. (Original work published 1928)

Jung, C. G. (1946). *The psychology of the transference* (R. F. C. Hull, Trans.; Ark ed.). Routledge and Kegan Paul.

Jung, C. G. (1959). *Archetypes of the collective unconscious.* In G. Adler & R. F. C. Hull (Eds. & Trans.), *Collected works of C.G. Jung* (Vol. 9, pp. 3–41). Princeton University Press.

Kaffashi, F., Scher, M. S., Ludington-Hoe, S., & Loparo, K. A. (2013). An analysis of the kangaroo care intervention using neonatal EEG complexity: A preliminary study. *Clinical Neurophysiology, 124,* 238–246.

Kahneman, D. (2011). *Thinking fast and slow.* Farrar, Straus and Giroux.

Kaiser, N., & Butler, E. (2021). Introducing social breathing: A model of engaging in relational systems. *Frontiers in Psychology, 12,* 571298. doi: 10.3389/fpsyg.2021.571298

Kalin, N. H., Shelton, S. E., & Lynn, D. E. (1995). Opiate systems in mother and infant primates coordinate intimate contact during reunion. *Psychoneuroendocrinology, 20,* 735–742.

Kalsched, D. E. (2003). Daimonic elements in early trauma. *Journal of Analytic Psychology, 48,* 145–169.

Kandel, E. R. (1999). Biology and the future of psychoanalysis: A new intellectual framework for psychiatry revisited. *American Journal of Psychiatry, 156,* 505–524.

Kane, J. (2004). Poetry as right hemispheric language. *Journal of Consciousness Studies, 11,* 21–59.

Kanner, L. (1943). Autistic disturbances of affective contact. *Nervous Child, 2,* 217–250.

Kantrowitz, J. L., Katz, A. L., Greenman, D. A., Morris, H., Paolitto, F., Sashin, J., & Solomon, L. (1989). The patient-analyst match and the outcome of psychoanalysis: A pilot study. *Journal of the American Psychoanalytic Association, 37,* 893–919.

Kaplan-Solms, K., & Solms, M. (1996). Psychoanalytic observations on a case of frontal limbic disease. *Journal of Clinical Psychoanalysis, 5,* 405–438.

Karr-Morse, R., & Wiley, M. S. (1997). *Ghosts from the nursery: Tracing the roots of violence.* Atlantic Monthly Press.

Katyare, S. S., Balasubramanian, S., & Parmar, D. V. (2003). Effect of corticosterone treatment on mitochondrial oxidative energy metabolism in developing rat brain. *Experimental Neurology, 183,* 241–248.

Kaufman, G. (1992). *Shame: The power of caring.* Schenkman.

Keenan, J. P., Gallup, G. G., & Falk, D. (2003). *The face in the mirror: The search for the origins of consciousness.* HarperCollins.

Keenan, J. P., Nelson, A., O'Connor, M., & Pascual-Leone, A. (2001). Self-recognition and the right hemisphere. *Nature, 409,* 305.

Keenan, J. P., Rubio, J., Racioppi, C., Johnson, A., & Barnacz, A. (2005). The right hemisphere and the dark side of consciousness. *Cortex, 41,* 695–704.

Keenan, J. P., Wheeler, M. A., Gallup, G. G., Jr., Pascual-Leone, A. (2000). Self recognition and the right prefrontal cortex. *Trends in Cognitive Science, 4,* 338–344.

Kernberg, O. (1975). *Borderline conditions and pathological narcissism.* Aronson.

Kernberg, O. (1984). *Severe personality disorders: Psychotherapeutic strategies.* Yale University Press.

Kernberg, O. (1992). *Aggression in personality disorders and perversions.* Yale University Press.

Kernberg, O. F. (2010). Narcissistic personality disorders. In J. F. Clarkin, P. Fonagy, & G. P. Gabbard (Eds.), *Psychodynamic therapy for personality disorders.* University of Chicago Press.

Kernis, M. H., Lakey, C. L., & Heppner, W. L. (2008). Secure versus fragile self-esteem as a predictor of verbal defensiveness: Converging findings across three different markers. *Journal of Personality, 76,* 477–512.

Key, A. P. (2025). Treating patients with borderline personality disorders. *Monitor on Psychology, 56,* 37–41.

Killeen, L. A., & Teti, D. M. (2012). Mothers' frontal EEG asymmetry in response to infant emotion states and mother-infant emotional availability, emotional experience, and internalizing symptoms. *Development and Psychopathology, 24,* 9–21.

Kim, H. S., & Sasaki, J. Y. (2014). Cultural neuroscience: Biology of the mind in cultural contexts. *Annual Review of Psychology, 65,* 487–514.

Kim, P., Leckman, J. F., Mayes, L. C., Wang, X., & Swain, J. F. (2010). The plasticity of human maternal brain: Longitudinal changes in brain anatomy during the early postpartum period. *Behavioral Neuroscience, 124,* 695–700.

Kimura, Y., Yoshino, A., Takahashi, Y., & Nomura, S. (2004). Interhemispheric differences in emotional response without awareness. *Physiology and Behavior, 82,* 727–731.

King, A. C., Taylor, C. B., Albright, C. A., & Haskell, W. L. (1990). The relationship between repressive and defensive coping styles and blood pressure responses in healthy, middle-aged men and women. *Journal of Psychosomatic Research, 34,* 461–471.

Kinreich, S., Amir, D., Lior, K., Yoram, L., & Ruth, F. (2017). Brain-to-brain synchrony during naturalistic social interactions. *Science Reports, 7,* 1–12.

Kinsley, C. H., & Lambert, K. G. (2006). The maternal brain. *Scientific American, 294,* 72–79.

Kircher, T. T. J., Senior, C., Phillips, M. L., Rabe-Hesketh, S., Benson, P. J., Bullmore, E. T., Brammer, M., Simmons, A., Bartels, M., & David, A. S. (2001). Recognizing one's own face. *Cognition, 78,* B1–B5.

Kline, J. P., Allen, J. J. B., & Schwartz, G. E. (1998). Is left frontal brain activation in defensiveness gender specific? *Journal of Abnormal Psychology, 107,* 149–153.

Kobak, R. R., & Sceery, A. (1988). Attachment in late adolescence: Working models, affect regulation, and representations of self and others. *Child Development, 59*, 135–146.

Kohoutova, L., Atlas, L. Y., Buchel, C., Buhle, J. T., Geuter, S., Jepma, M., et al. (2022). Individual variability in brain representations of pain. *Nature Neuroscience, 25*, 749–759.

Kohut, H. (1971). *The analysis of the self.* International Universities Press.

Kohut, H. (1972). Thoughts on narcissism and narcissistic rage. *Psychoanalytic Study of the Child, 27*, 360–400.

Kohut, H. (1977). *The restoration of the self.* International Universities Press.

Kohut, H., & Wolf, E. S. (1978). The disorders of the self and their treatment: An outline. *International Journal of Psycho-analysis, 59*, 413–425.

Konrad, K., & Puetz, V. B. (2024). A context-dependent model of resilient functioning after childhood maltreatment—the case for flexible biobehavioral synchrony. *Translational Psychiatry, 14*, 388. https://doi.org/10.1038/s41398-024-03092-7

Konrath, S. H., Chopik, W. J., Hsing, C. K., & O'Brien, E. (2014). Changes in adult attachment styles in American college students over time: A meta-analysis. *Personality and Social Psychology Review, 18*, 326–348.

Koole, S. L., Atzil-Slonim, D., Butler, E., Dikker, S., Tschacher, W., & Wilderjans, T. (2020). In sync with your shrink. In J. P. Forgas, W. D. Crano, & K. Fiedler (Eds.), *Applications of social psychology: How social psychology can contribute to the solution of real-world problems* (pp. 161–184). Taylor and Francis AS. doi: 10.4324/9780367816407-9

Koole, S. L., & Jostmann, N. B. (2004). Getting a grip on your feelings: Effects of action orientation and external demands on intuitive affect regulation. *Journal of Personality and Social Psychology, 87*, 974–990.

Koole, S. L., & Tschacher, W. (2016). Synchrony in psychotherapy: A review and an integrative framework for the therapeutic alliance. *Frontiers of Psychology, 7*, 1–17.

Koole, S. L., Webb, T. L., & Sheeran, P. L. (2015). Implicit emotion regulation: feeling better without knowing why. *Current Opinion in Psychology, 3*, 6–10.

Kotikalapudi, R., Dricu, M., Andreas Moser, D., & Aue, T. (2022). Whole-brain white matter correlates of personality profiles predictive of subjective well-being. *Scientific Reports, 12*, 4558. https://doi.org/10.1038/s41598-022-08686-z

Krall, S. C., Rottschy, C., Oberwelland, E., Bzdok, D., Fox, P. T., Eickhoff, S. B., et al. (2015). The role of the right temporoparietal junction in attention and social interaction as revealed by ALE meta-analysis. *Brain Structure and Function, 220*, 587–604.

Kret, M. E., Fischer, A. H., & De Dreu, C. K. W. (2015). Pupil mimicry correlates with trust in in-group partners with dilating pupils. *Psychological Science, 26*, 1401–1410.

Kringelbach, M. (2005). The human orbitofrontal cortex: Linking reward to hedonic experience. *Nature Reviews Neuroscience, 6*, 691–702.

Kringelbach, M. L., Lehtonen, A., Squire, S., Harvey, A. G., Craske, M. G., Holliday,

I. E., et al. (2008). A specific and rapid neural signature for parental instinct. *PLoS One, 3*(2), e1664.

Kris, E. (1952). *Psychoanalytic explorations in art.* International Universities Press.

Kris, E. (1953). Psychoanalysis and the study of creative imagination. *Bulletin of the New York Academy of Medicine, 29,* 334–351.

Kuchinke, L., Jacobs, A. M., Vo, M. L. H., Conrad, M., Grubich, C., & Herrmann, M. (2006). Modulation of prefrontal cortex activation by emotional words in recognition memory. *NeuroReport, 17,* 1037–1041.

Kuhl, J., & Kazen, M. (2008). Motivation, affect, and hemispheric asymmetry: Power versus affiliation. *Journal of Personality and Social Psychology, 95,* 456–469.

Kuhl, J., Quirin, M., & Koole, S. L. (2015). Being someone: The integrated self as a neuropsychological system. *Social and Personality Psychology Compass, 9,* 115–132.

Kupper, Z., Ramseyer, F., Hoffmann, H., & Schacher, W. (2015). Nonverbal synchrony in social interactions of patients with schizophrenia indicates sociocommunicative deficits. *PLoS One, 10,* e0145882.

Kykyri, V.-L., Karvonen, A., Wahostrom, J., Kaartinen, M., & Seikkula, J. S. (2017). Soft prosody and embodied attunement in therapeutic interaction: A multimethod case study of a moment of change. *Journal of Constructivist Psychology, 30,* 211–234.

Ladavas, E., & Bertini, C. (2021). Right hemisphere dominance for unconscious emotionally salient stimuli. *Brain Science, 11,* 823. https://doi.org/10.3390/brainsci11070823

Lagercrantz, H., & Changeux, J.-P. (2009). The emergence of human consciousness: From fetal to neonatal life. *Pediatric Research, 65,* 255–259.

Lamb, M. E. (2004). *The role of the father in child development* (4th ed.). John Wiley.

Lambert, M. J. (2013). The efficacy and effectiveness in psychotherapy. In M. J. Lambert (Ed.), *Bergin and Garfield's handbook of psychotherapy and behavior change.* Wiley.

Lange, J., Crusius, J., & Hagemeyer, B. (2016). The evil queen's dilemma: Linking narcissistic admiration and rivalry to benign and malicious envy. *European Journal of Personality, 30,* 168–188.

Langer, R. (2024). The therapeutic relationship and retirement: A complex and challenging journey. *Practice Innovations, 9*(3), 215–222. https://doi.org/10.1037/pri0000245

Lanius, R. A., Vermetten, E., & Pain, C. (Eds.). (2010). *The impact of early life trauma on health and disease: The hidden epidemic.* Cambridge University Press.

Lapp, H. E., Bartlett, A. A., & Hunter, R. G. (2019). Stress and glucocorticoid receptor regulation of mitochondrial gene expression. *Journal of Molecular Endocrinology, 62,* R121–R128.

Lasch, C. (1979). *The culture of narcissism: American life in an age of diminishing expectations.* Norton.

Laurent, H. K., Stevens, A., & Ablow, J. C. (2011). Neural correlates of hypothalamic-pituitary-adrenal regulation of mothers with their infants. *Biological Psychiatry, 70,* 826–832.

Layard, R., Clark, A. E., Cornaglia, F., Powdthavee, N., & Vernoit, J. (2014). What predicts a successful life? A life-course model of well-being. *Economic Journal, 124*, F720–F738. doi: 10.1111/ecoj.12170

Lecanuet, J. P., & Schaal, B. (1996). Fetal sensory competencies. *European Journal of Obstetrics and Gynecology, 68*, 1–23.

Leckman, J. F., & March, J. S. (2011). Developmental neuroscience comes of age [Editorial]. *Journal of Child Psychology and Psychiatry, 52*, 333–338.

LeDoux, J. (2002). *Synaptic self: How our brains become who we are.* Viking.

Lee, J. H. N., Chong, E. S. K., Chui, H., Lee, T., Luk, S., Tao, D., & Lee, N. W. T. (2023). A curvilinear association between therapists' use of discourse particles and therapist empathy in psychotherapy. *Journal of Counseling Psychology, 70*, 562–570.

Lee, S. J., Ralston, H. J., Drey, E. A., Partridge, J. C., & Rosen, M. A. (2005). Fetal pain: A systematic multidisciplinary review of the evidence. *JAMA, 294*, 947–954.

Lee, S. M., & McCarthy, G. (2016). Functional heterogeneity and convergence in the right temporoparietal junction. *Cerebral Cortex, 26*, 1108–1116.

Le Grand, R., Mondloch, C., Maurer, D., & Brent, H. P. (2003). Expert face processing requires visual input to the right hemisphere during infancy. *Nature Neuroscience, 6*, 1108–1112.

Lehky, S. R. (2000). Fine discrimination of faces can be performed rapidly. *Journal of Cognitive Neuroscience, 12*, 848–855.

Leichsenring, F., Lyuten, P., Hilsenroth, M. J., Abass, A., Barber, J. P., Keefe, J. R., et al. (2015). Psychodynamic therapy meets evidence-based medicine: A systematic review using updated criteria. *Lancet Psychiatry, 2*, 648–660.

Leisman, G., Melillo, R., & Melillo, T. (2023). Prefrontal functional connectivities in autistic spectrum disorders: A connectopathic disorder affecting movement, interoception, and cognition. *Brain Research Bulletin, 198*, 65–76.

Lemaître, H., Augé, P., Saitovich, A., Vincon-Leite, A., Tacchella, J.-M., Fillon, J., et al. (2020). Rest functional brain maturation during the first year of life. *Cerebral Cortex, 31*, 1776–1785.

Lemche, E., Giampietro, V. P., Surguladze, S. A., Amaro, E. J., Andrew, C. M., Williams, S. C. R., et al. (2006). Human attachment security is mediated by the amygdala: Evidence from combined fMRI and psychophysiological measures. *Human Brain Mapping, 27*, 623–635.

Lemy, Z. C., Sousa, M. A., Matos, S. M., Garcia Marques, A. C., Lopez Pereira, M. U., Morsch, D. S., & Lamy-Filho, F. (2020). Kangaroo care in pre-term newborns: The perception of neonatal pain, its assessment and necessary approaches. *EC Paediatrics, 9*, 12–21.

Lenzi, D., Trentini, C., Pantano, P., Macaluso, E., Iacaboni, M., Lenzi, G. I., & Ammaniti, M. (2009). Neural basis of maternal communication and emotional expression processing during infant preverbal stage. *Cerebral Cortex, 19*, 1124–1133.

Lester, B. M., Hoffman, J., & Brazelton, T. B. (1985). The rhythmic structure of mother-infant interaction in term and preterm infants. *Child Development, 56*, 15–27.

Letourneau, N., Dewey, D., Kaplan, B. J., Ntanda, H., Novick, J., Thomas, J. C., et al. (2019). Intergenerational transmission of adverse childhood experiences via maternal depression and anxiety and moderation by child sex. *Journal of the Developmental Origin of Health and Disease, 10*, 88–99.

Levendosky, A. A., Turchan, J. E., Luo, X., & Good, E. (2022). A re-introduction of the psychodynamic approach to the standard clinical psychology curriculum. *Journal of Clinical Psychology, 79*(10), 2439–2451. https://doi.org/10.1002/jclp.23551

Levin, F. M. (1991). *Mapping the mind*. Analytic Press.

Levine, R. (2011). Progressing while regressing in relationships. *International Journal of Group Psychotherapy, 61*, 621–643.

Lev-Wiesel, R. (2007). Intergenerational transmission of trauma across three generations: A preliminary study. *Qualitative Social Work, 6*, 75–94.

Levy, J., Goldstein, A., & Feldman, R. (2017). Perception of social synchrony induces mother-child gamma coupling in the social brain. *Social Cognition and Affective Neuroscience, 157*, 1036–1046.

Levy, J., Heller, W., Banich, M. T., & Burton, L. A. (1983). Are variations among right-handed individuals in perceptual asymmetries caused by characteristic arousal differences between hemispheres? *Journal of Experimental Psychology: Human Perception and Performance, 9*, 329–359.

Lewis, H. B. (1971). *Shame and guilt in neurosis*. International Universities Press.

Lewis, M., Brooks-Gunn, J., & Jaskir, J. (1985). Individual differences in visual self-recognition as a function of mother-infant attachment relationship. *Developmental Psychology, 21*, 1181–1187.

Lichtenberg, J. D. (1989). *Psychoanalysis and motivation*. Analytic Press.

Lieberman, M. D. (2000). Intuition: A social neuroscience approach. *Psychological Bulletin, 126*, 109–137.

Lin, P.-Y., Roche-Labarbe, N., Dehaes, M., Fenoglio, A., Grant, P. E., & Franceschini, M. A. (2013). Regional and hemispheric asymmetries of cerebral hemodynamic and oxygen metabolism in newborns. *Cerebral Cortex, 23*, 339–348.

Livesley, W. J., Jang, K. I., Jackson, D. N., & Vernon, P. A. (1993). Genetic and environmental contributors to dimensions of personality disorder. *American Journal of Psychiatry, 150*, 1826–1831.

Lobbestael, J., Baumeister, R. F., Fiebig, T., & Eckel, L. A. (2014). The role of grandiose and vulnerable narcissism in self-reported and laboratory aggression and testosterone reactivity. *Personality and Individual Differences, 69*, 22–27.

Loewald, H. (1980). The ego and reality. In *Papers on psychoanalysis* (pp. 3–20). Yale University Press. (Original work published 1949)

Lu, J., Wu, J., Shu, Z., Zhang, X., Li, H., Liang, S., et al. (2024). Brain temporal-spectral functional variability reveals neural improvements of DBS treatment for disorders of consciousness. *IEEE Transactions on Neural Systems and Rehabilitation Engineering, 32*, 923–933.

Lueken, U., Leisse, M., Mattes, K., Naumann, D., Wittling, W., & Schweiger, E. (2009). Altered tonic and phasic cortisol secretion following unilateral stroke. *Psychoneuroendocrinology, 34,* 402–412.

Lundqvist, D., & Ohman, A. (2005). Caught by the evil eye: Nonconscious information processing, emotion, and attention to facial stimuli. In L. Feldman Barrett, P. M. Niedenthal, & P. Winkelman (Eds.), *Emotion and consciousness* (pp. 97–124). Guilford.

Luo, Y. L. L., Cai, H., Sedikides, C., & Song, H. (2014). Distinguishing communal narcissism from agentic narcissism: A behavior genetics analysis on the agency-communion model of narcissism. *Journal of Research in Personality, 49,* 52–58.

Luo, Y. L. L., Cai, H., & Song, H. (2014). A behavioral genetic study of intrapersonal and interpersonal dimensions of narcissism. *Plos One, 9*(4), e93403.

Luys, J. (1879). Etudes sur le dedoublement des operations et sur le role isole de chaque hemisphere dans les phenemenes de la pathologie mental. *Bulletin of the Academy of National Medicine, 8,* 547–565.

Luyten, P., Mayes, L. C., Blatt, S. J., Target, M., & Fonagy, P. (2015). *Theoretical and empirical foundations of contemporary psychodynamic approaches to psychopathology* (pp. 3–26). Guilford.

Lycke, C., Specht, K., Ersland, L., & Hugdahl, K. (2008). An fMRI study of phonological and spatial working memory using identical stimuli. *Scandinavian Journal of Psychology, 49,* 393–401.

Lynd, H. M. (1958). *On shame and the search for identity.* Harcourt Brace.

Lyons, D. M., Afarian, H., Schatzberg, A. F., Sawyer-Glover, A., & Moseley, M. E. (2002). Experience-dependent asymmetric variation in primate prefrontal morphology. *Behavioural Brain Research, 136,* 51–59.

Lyons-Ruth, K. (1999). The two-person unconscious: Intersubjective dialogue, enactive relational representation, and the emergence of new forms of relational organization. *Psychoanalytic Inquiry, 19,* 576–617.

Lyons-Ruth, K., & Block, D. (1996). The disturbed caregiving system: Relations among childhood trauma, maternal caregiving, an infant affect and attachment. *Infant Mental Health Journal, 17,* 257–275.

Machin, A. (2018). *The life of dad: The making of a modern father.* Simon and Schuster UK.

Maes, M., Ombelet, W., De Jongh, R., Kenis, G., & Bosmans, E. (2001). The inflammatory response following delivery is amplified in women who previously suffered from major depression, suggesting that major depression is accompanied by a sensitization of the inflammatory response system. *Journal of Affective Disorders, 63,* 85–92.

Mahler, M. S. (1967). Of human symbiosis and the vicissitudes of individuation. *Journal of the American Psychoanalytic Association, 15,* 740–763.

Mahler, M. S. (1980). Rapprochement subphase of the separation-individuation process. In R. Lax, S. Bach, & J. A. Burland (Eds.), *Rapprochement: The critical subphase of separation-individuation* (pp. 3–19). Jason Aronson.

Mahler, M., Pine, F., & Bergman, A. (1975). *The psychological birth of the human infant.* Basic Books.

Main, M., & Solomon, J. (1986). Discovery of an insecure-disorganized / disoriented attachment pattern. In T. B. Brazelton & M. W. Yogman (Eds.), *Affective development in infancy.* Ablex.

Main, M., & Stadtman, J. (1981). Infant response to rejection of physical contact by the mother: Aggression, avoidance and conflict. *Journal of the American Academy of Child Psychiatry, 20,* 292–307.

Main, M., & Weston, D. R. (1981). The quality of the toddler's relationship to mother and to father: Related to conflict behavior and the readiness to establish new relationships. *Child Development, 52,* 932–940.

Main, M., & Weston, D. R. (1982). Avoidance of the attachment figure in infancy: Descriptions and interpretations. In C. M. Parker & J. Stevenson-Hinde (Eds.), *The place of attachment in human behavior* (pp. 31–59). Basic Books.

Maisel, N. C., & Gable, S. L. (2009). The paradox of received social support: The importance of responsiveness. *Psychological Science, 20,* 928–932.

Majeed, H., & Lee, J. (2017). The impact of climate change on youth depression and mental health. *Lancet Planet Health, 1,* e94–e95.

Malatesta-Magai, C. (1991). Emotional socialization: Its role in personality and developmental psychopathology. In D. Cicchetti & S. L. Toth (Eds.), *Internalizing and externalizing expressions of dysfunction: Rochester symposium on developmental psychopatholgy* (Vol. 2, pp. 203–224). Lawrence Erlbaum.

Malatesta, G., Marzoli, D., Piccioni, C., & Tommasi, L. (2019). The relationship between the left-cradling bias and attachment to parents and partner. *Evolutionary Psychology,* 1–12.

Mancia, M. (Ed.) (2006). *Psychoanalysis and neuroscience* (pp. 151–173). Milan: Springer Milan.

Mandal, M. K., & Ambady, N. (2004). Laterality of facial expressions of emotions: Universal and culture-specific influences. *Behavioural Neurology, 15,* 23–34.

Manini, B., Cardone, D., Ebisch, S. J. H., Bafunno, D., Aureli, T., & Meria, A. (2013). Mom feels what her child feels: Thermal signatures of vicarious autonomic response while watching children in a stressful situation. *Frontiers in Human Neuroscience, 7,* 1–10. doi: 10.3389/fnhum.2013.00299

Manning, J. T., Trivers, R. L., Thornhill, R., Singh, D., Denman, J., Eklo, M. H., et al. (1997). Ear asymmetry and left-sided cradling. *Evolution and Human Behavior, 18,* 327–340.

Manoli, I., Alesci, S., Blackman, M. R., Su, Y. A., Rennert, O. M., & Chrousos, G. P. (2007). Mitochondria as key components of the stress response. *Trends in Endocrinology and Metabolism, 18,* 190–198.

Maquet, P., Ruby, P., Madoux, A., Albuoy, G., Stepenich, V., Dang-Vu, T., et al. (2005). Human cognition during REM sleep and the activity profile within frontal and parietal cortices: A reappraisal of functional neuroimaging data. *Progress in Brain Research, 150,* 219–227.

Marcus, D. M. (1997). On knowing what one knows. *Psychoanalytic Quarterly, 66*, 219–241.

Maret, S. M. (2009). *Introduction to prenatal psychology.* Church Gate.

Markin, R. (2014). Toward a common identity for relationally oriented clinicians: A place to hang one's hat. *Psychotherapy, 51*, 327–333.

Markowitsch, H. J., Reinkemeier, A., Kessler, J., Koyuncu, A., & Heiss, W. D. (2000). Right amygdalar and temporofrontal activation during autobiographical, but not fictitious memory retrieval. *Behavioral Neurology, 12*, 181–190.

Marks-Tarlow, T. (2012). *Clinical intuition in psychotherapy: The neurobiology of embodied response.* Norton.

Marks-Tarlow, T. (2021). Birds of a feather: The importance of interpersonal synchrony in psychotherapy. In D. J. Siegel, A. N. Schore, & L. Cozolino (Eds.) *Interpersonal neurobiology and clinical practice* (pp. 261–292). Norton.

Maroda, K. J. (2005). Show some emotion: Completing the cycle of affective communication. In L. Aron & A. Harris (Eds.), *Revolutionary connections: Relational psychoanalysis: Vol. 2. Innovation and expansion* (pp. 121–142). Analytic Press.

Marzoli, D., D'Anselmo, A., Malatesta, G., Lucato, C., Prete, G., & Tommasi, L. (2022). The intricate web of asymmetric processing of social stimuli in humans. *Symmetry, 14*, 1096.

Maslow, A. H. (1968). *Toward a psychology of being.* Van Nostrand.

Masterson, J. F. (1985). *The real self: A developmental, self, and object relations approach.* Bantam.

Matsuzawa, J., Matsui, M., Konishi, T., Noguchi, K., Gur, R. C., Bilker, W., & Miyawaki, T. (2001). Age-related volumetric changes of brain gray and white matter in healthy infants and children. *Cerebral Cortex, 11*, 335–342.

Maunder, R. G., & Hunter, J. J. (2009). Assessing patterns of adult attachment in medical patients. *General Hospital Psychiatry, 31*, 123–130.

Maurer, D. (1985). Infants' perception of facedness. In T. Field & N. Fox (Eds.), *Social perception in infants.* Ablex.

Mayseless, N., & Shamay-Tsoory, S. G. (2015). Enhancing verbal creativity: Modulating creativity by altering the balance between the right and left inferior frontal gyrus with tDCS. *Neuroscience, 291*, 167–176.

McCrae, R. R., & Costa, P. T., Jr. (1997). Conceptions and correlates of openness to experience. In R. Hogan, J. A. Johnson, & S. R. Briggs (Eds.), *Handbook of personality psychology* (pp. 825–847). Academic Press.

McCraty, R. (2004). The energetic heart: Bioelectromagnetic communication within and between people. In P. J. Rosch & M. S. Markov (Eds.), *Bioelectromagnetic medicine* (pp. 541–562). Marcel Dekker.

McEwen, B. S., & Wingfield, J. C. (2003). The concept of allostasis in biology and biomedicine. *Hormones and Behavior, 43*, 2–15.

McFadden, J. (2002). Synchronous firing and its influence on the brain's electromagnetic field. *Journal of Consciousness Studies, 9*, 23–50.

McGaugh, J. L. (2004). The amygdala modulates the consolidation of memories of emotionally arousing experience. *Annual Review of Neuroscience, 27*, 1–28.

McGilchrist, I. (2009). *The master and his emissary.* Yale University Press.

McGilchrist, I. (2015). Divine understanding and the divided brain. In J. Clausen & N. Levy (Eds.), *Handbook of neuroethics.* Springer Science.

McGilchrist, I. (2016). "Selving" and union. *Journal of Consciousness Studies, 23,* 196–213.

McGilchrist, I. (2021a). *The matter with things* (Vol. 1). Perspectiva Press.

McGilchrist, I. (2021b). *The matter with things* (Vol. 2). Perspectiva Press.

McNaughton, K. A., & Redcay, E. (2020). Interpersonal synchrony in autism. *Current Psychiatry Reports, 22*(3), 12. doi: 10.1007/s11920-020-1135-8

Meares, R. (1993). *The metaphor of play: Disruption and restoration in the borderline experience.* Aronson.

Meares, R. (2012). *A dissociation model of borderline personality disorder.* Norton.

Meares, R. (2016). *The poet's voice in the making of mind.* Routledge.

Meares, R. (2017). The disintegrative core of relational trauma and a way toward unity. In M. Solomon & D. J. Siegel (Eds.), *How people change: Relationships and neuroplasticity in psychotherapy* (pp. 135–150). Norton.

Meares, R., Schore, A., & Melkonian, D. (2011a). Is borderline personality a particularly right hemispheric disorder? A study of P3a using single trial analysis. *Australian and New Zealand Journal of Psychiatry, 45,* 131–139.

Medford, N., & Critchley, H. D. (2010). Conjoint activity of anterior insular and anterior cingulate cortex: Awareness and response. *Brain Structure and Function, 214,* 535–549.

Melges, F. T., & Swartz, M. S. (1989). Oscillations of attachment in borderline personality disorder. *American Journal of Psychiatry, 146,* 1115–1120.

Mento, G., Suppiej, A., Altoe, G., & Bisiacchi, P. S. (2010). Functional hemispheric asymmetries in humans: Electrophysiological evidence from infants. *European Journal of Neuroscience, 31,* 565–574.

Merced, M. (2015). Noticing indicators of emerging change in the psychotherapy of a borderline patient. *Clinical Social Work Journal, 44,* 293–308. doi: 10.1007/s10615-015-0547-0

Meuwissen, A. S., & Carlson, S. M. (2015). Fathers matter: The role of father parenting in preschoolers' executive function development. *Journal of Experimental Child Psychology, 140,* 1–15.

Messina, K. (2025). When AI amplifies gender bias. *TAP Magazine.*

Meyer-Lindenberg, A. (2008). Impact of prosocial neuropeptides on human brain function. *Progress in Brain Research, 170,* 463–470.

Meyers, B., & Pilkonis, P. A. (2011). Attachment theory and narcissistic personality disorder. In W. K. Campbell & J. D. Miller, *The handbook of narcissism and narcissistic personality disorder: Theoretical approaches, empirical findings, and treatment* (pp. 434–444). Wiley.

Miall, D., & Dissanayake, E. (2003). The poetics of baby talk. *Human Nature, 14,* 337–354.

Mihov, K. M., Denzler, M., & Forster, J. (2010). Hemispheric specialization and creative thinking: A meta-analytic review of lateralization of creativity. *Brain and Cognition, 72*, 442–448.

Mikulincer, M., & Shaver, P. R. (2003). The attachment behavioral system in adulthood: Activation, psychodynamics, and interpersonal processes. In M. P. Zanna (Ed.), *Advances in experimental social psychology* (Vol. 35, pp. 53–152). Academic.

Mikulincer, M., Shaver, P. R., & Pereg, D. (2003). Attachment theory and affect regulation: The dynamics, development, and cognitive consequences of attachment-related strategies. *Motivation and Emotion, 27*, 77–102.

Miles, L. K., Nind, L. K., & Macrae, C. N. (2009). The rhythm of rapport: Interpersonal synchrony and social perception. *Journal of Experimental Social Psychology, 45*(3), 585–589. https://doi.org/10.1016/j.jesp.2009.02.002

Miles-Novelo, A., & Anderson, C. A. (2019). Climate change and psychology: Effects of rapid global warming on violence and aggression. *Current Climate Change Reports, 5*, 36–46.

Miller, B. L., Seeley, W. W., Mychack, P., Rosen, H. J., Mena, I., & Boone, K. (2001). Neuroanatomy of the self: Evidence from patients with frontotemporal dementia. *Neurology, 57*, 817–821.

Miller, J. D., Hoffman, B. J., Gaughan, E. T., Gentile, B., Maples, J., & Cambpell, W. K. (2011). Grandiose and vulnerable narcissism: A nomological network analysis. *Journal of Personality, 79*, 5.

Miller, J. D., Lynam, D. R., Vize, C., Crowe, M., Sleep, C., Maples-Keller, J. L., et al. (2018). Vulnerable narcissism is (mostly) a disorder of neuroticism. *Journal of Personality, 86*, 186–199.

Miller, J. G., Xia, G., & Hastings, P. D. (2020). Right temporoparietal junction involvement in autonomic responses to the suffering of others: A preliminary transcranial magnetic stimulation study. *Frontiers in Human Neuroscience, 14*, 7. doi: 10.3389/fnhum.2020.00007

Miller, M., & Fry, W. F. (2009). The effect of mirthful laughter on the human cardiovascular system. *Medical Hypotheses, 73*, 636–639.

Miller, S. (1985). *The shame experience*. Analytic Press.

Miller, S. B. (1993). Cardiovascular reactivity in defensive individuals: The influence of task demands. *Psychosomatic Medicine, 55*, 79–85.

Mills, E. L., Kelly, B., & O'Neill, L. A. (2017). Mitochondria are the powerhouse of immunity. *Nature Immunology, 18*, 488–498.

Minagawa-Kawai, Y., Matsuoka, S., Dan, I., Naoi, N., Nakamura, K., & Kojima, S. (2009). Prefrontal activation associated with social attachment: Facial-emotion recognition in mothers and infants. *Cerebral Cortex, 19*, 284–292.

Mischel, W., Ayduk, O., Berman, M. G., Casey, B. J., Gotlib, I. H., Jonides, J., et al. (2011). "Willpower" over the lifespan: Decomposing self-regulation. *Social Cognitive and Affective Neuroscience, 6*, 252–256.

Mlot, C. (1998). Probing the biology of emotion. *Science, 280*, 1005–1007.

Mohaupt, H., Holgersen, H., Binder, P.-E., & Nielsen, G. H. (2006). Affect consciousness or mentalization? A comparison of two concepts with regard to affect development and affect regulation. *Scandinavian Journal of Psychology, 47*, 237–244.

Mohr, C., Rowe, A. C., & Crawford, M. T. (2007). Hemispheric differences in the processing of attachment words. *Journal of Clinical and Experimental Neuropsychology, 30*, 471–480.

Moll, H., Pueschel, E., Ni, Q., & Little, A. (2021) Sharing experiences in infancy: From primary intersubjectivity to shared intentionality. *Front. Psychol.* 12:667679. doi: 10.3389/fpsyg.2021.667679

Monk, C., Spicer, J., & Champagne, F. A. (2012). Linking prenatal maternal adversity to developmental outcomes in infants: The role of epigenetic pathways. *Developmental Psychopathology, 24*, 1361–1376.

Montirosso, R., Cozzi, P., Tronick, E., & Borgatti, R. (2012). Differential distribution and lateralization of infant gestures and their relation to maternal gestures in the face-to-face still-face paradigm. *Infant Behavior and Development, 35*, 819–828.

Moore, G. A., & Calkins, S. D. (2004). Infants' regulation in the still-face paradigm is related to dyadic coordination of mother-infant interaction. *Developmental Psychology, 40*, 1068–1080.

Moore, G. A., Hill-Soderlund, A. L., Propper, C. B., Calkins, S. D., Mills-Koonce, W. R., & Cox, M. J. (2009). Mother-infant vagal regulation in the face-to-face still-face paradigm is moderated by maternal sensitivity. *Child Development, 80*, 209–223.

Morf, C. C., & Rhodewalt, F. (2001). Expanding the dynamic self-regulatory processing model of narcissism: Research directions for the future. *Psychological Inquiry, 12*, 243–251.

Mori, K., & Iwanaga, M. (2014). Pleasure generated by sadness: Effects of sad music on the emotions induced by happy music. *Psychology of Music, 42*, 643–652.

Morishima, Y., Schunk, D., Bruhn, A., Ruff, C. C., & Fehr, E. (2012). Linking brain structure and activation in temporoparietal junction to explain the neurobiology of human altruism. *Neuron, 75*, 73–79.

Morita, T., Itakura, S., Saito, D. N., Nakashita, S., Harada, T., Kochiyama, T., & Sadato, N. (2008). The role of the right prefrontal cortex in self-evaluation of the face: A functional magnetic resonance imaging study. *Journal of Cognitive Neuroscience, 20*, 342–355.

Morita, T., Tanabe, H. C., Sasaki, A. T., Shimada, K., Kakigi, R., & Sadato, N. (2014). The anterior insular and anterior cingulate cortices in emotional processing for self-face recognition. *Social Cognitive and Affective Neuroscience, 9*(5), 570–579. doi: 10.1093/scan/nst011

Morris, J. S., Ohman, A., & Dolan, R. J. (1998). Conscious and unconscious emotional learning in the human amygdala. *Nature, 393*, 467–470.

Morris, J. S., Ohman, A., & Dolan, R. J. (1999). A subcortical pathway to the right amygdala mediating "unseen" fear. *Proceedings of the National Academy of Sciences USA, 96*, 1680–1685.

Morrison, A. P. (1984). Working with shame in psychoanalytic treatment. *Journal of the American Psychoanalytic Association, 32,* 479–505.

Mu, Y., Guo, C., & Han, S. (2016). Oxytocin enhances inter-brain synchrony during social coordination in male adults. *Social Cognitive and Affective Neuroscience, 11,* 1882–1893.

Mucci, C. (2013). *Beyond individual and collective trauma: Intergenerational transmission, psychoanalytic treatment and the dynamics of forgiveness.* Karnac.

Mucci, C. (2018). *Borderline bodies: Affect regulation theory for personality disorders.* Norton.

Mucci, C. (2021). Dissociation vs repression: A new neuropsychoanalytic model for psychopathology. *American Journal of Psychoanalysis, 81,* 82–111. https://doi.org/10.1057/s11231-021-09279-x

Mucci, C. (2022). *Resilience and survival: Understanding and healing intergenerational trauma.* Confer Books.

Mucci, C. (2023). Therapy for trauma of human agency: "What has been damaged in a relationship needs to be healed in a relationship." In A. Rachman & C. Mucci, *Ferenczi's confusion of tongues theory of trauma* (pp. 170–189). Routledge.

Mucci, C., & Scalabrini, A. (2021). Traumatic effects beyond diagnosis: The impact of dissociation on the mind-body-brain system. *Psychoanalytic Psychology, 38,* 279–289.

Muran, J. C., & Barber, J. P. (2010). *The therapeutic alliance.* Guilford.

Muratori, F., Apicella, F., Muratori, P., & Maestro, S. (2011). Intersubjective disruptions and caregiver-infant interactions in early autistic disorder. *Research in Autism Spectrum Disorders, 5,* 408–417.

Murray, L., & Trevarthen, C. (1985). Emotional regulation of interaction between two-month-olds and their mothers. In T. Field & N. Fox (Eds.), *Social perception in infants* (pp. 177–197). Ablex.

Music, G. (2023). Brainy kids skating on thin ice: New thoughts on psych-soma and how minds over-develop to cope with trauma. *Psychoanalytic Study of the Child, 77,* 41–59. doi: 10.1080/00797308.2023.2229716

Nagy, E. (2006). From imitation to conversation: The first dialogues with human neonates. *Infant and Child Development, 15,* 223–232.

Nakato, E., Otsuka, Y., Kanazawa, S., Yamaguchi, M. K., Watanabe, S., & Kakigi, R. (2009). When do infants differentiate profile face from frontal face? A near infrared spectroscopic study. *Human Brain Mapping, 30,* 462–472.

Naoi, N., Minagawa-Kawai, Y., Kobayashi, A., Takeuchi, R., Nakamura, K., Yamamoto, J., & Kojima, S. (2011). Cerebral responses to infant-directed speech and the effect of talker familiarity. *NeuroImage, 59,* 1735–1744.

Narvaez, D. (2014). *Neurobiology and the development of human morality: Evolution, culture, and wisdom.* Norton.

Nathanson, D. L. (1987). A timetable for shame. In D. L. Nathanson (Ed.), *The many faces of shame* (pp. 1–63). Guilford.

Naviaux, R. K. (2008). Mitochondrial control of epigenetics. *Cancer Biology and Therapy, 7*, 1191–1193.

Naviaux, R. K. (2019). Metabolic features and regulation of the healing cycle—a new model for chronic disease pathogenesis and treatment. *Mitochondrion, 46*, 278–297.

Naviaux, R. K. (2020). Perspective: Cell danger response biology—the new science that connects environmental health with mitochondria and the rising tide of chronic illness. *Mitochondrion, 51*, 40–45.

Nemeroff, C. B. (2016). Paradise lost: The neurobiological and clinical consequences of child abuse and neglect. *Neuron, 89*, 892–909.

Nemiah, J. C. (1989). Janet redivivus: The centenary of l'automatisme psychologique. *American Journal of Psychiatry, 146*, 1527–1529.

Neumann, D., Spezio, M. L., Priven, J., & Adolphs, R. (2006). Looking you in the mouth: Abnormal gaze in autism resulting from impaired top-down modulation of visual attention. *Social Cognition and Affective Neuroscience, 1*, 194–202.

New, A. S., Hazlett, E. A., Buchsbaum, M. S., Goodman, M., Mitelmaan, S. A., Newmark, R., et al. (2007). Amygdala-prefrontal disconnection in borderline personality disorder. *Neuropsychopharmacology, 32*, 1629–1640.

Newman, L. S., & Hedberg, D. A. (1999). Repressive coping and the inaccessibility of negative autobiographical memories: Converging evidence. *Personality and Individual Differences, 27*, 45–53.

Newmeyer, D. D., & Ferguson-Miller, S. (2003). Mitochondria: Releasing power for life and unleashing the machineries of death. *Cell, 112*, 481–490.

Nichelli, P., Grafman, J., Pietrini, P., Clark, K., Lee, K. Y., & Miletich, R. (1995). Where the brain appreciates the moral of a story. *NeuroReport, 6*, 2309–2313.

Nicholson, K. G., Baum, S., Kilgour, A., Koh, C. K., Munhall, K. G., & Cuddy, L. L. (2003). Impaired processing of prosodic and musical patterns after right hemisphere damage. *Brain and Cognition, 52*, 382–389.

Nijhuis, J. G. (2003). Fetal behavior: The brain and behavior in different stages of human life. *Neurobiology of Aging, 24*, S41–S46.

Nishida, M., Pearsall, J., Buckner, R. L., & Walker, M. P. (2008). REM sleep, prefrontal theta, and the consolidation of human emotional memory. *Cerebral Cortex, 19*, 1158–1166.

Nishitani, S., Doi, H., Koyama, A., & Shinohara, K. (2011). Differential response to infant facial emotions in mothers compared to non-mothers. *Neuroscience Research, 70*, 183–188.

Nitschke, J. B., Nelson, E. E., Rusch, B. D., Fox, A. S., Oales, T. R., & Davidson, R. J. (2004). Orbitofrontal cortex tracks positive mood in mothers viewing pictures of their newborn infants. *NeuroImage, 21*, 583–592.

Noah, J. A., Zhang, X., Dravida, S., Ono, Y., Naples, A., McPartland, J. C., & Hirsch, J. (2020). Real-time eye-to-eye contact is associated with cross-brain neural coupling in angular gyrus. *Frontiers in Human Neuroscience, 14.* https://doi.org/10.3389/fnhum.2020.00019

Nolte, T., Hudac, C., Mayes, L. C., Fonagy, P., Blatt, S. J., & Pelphrey, K. (2010). The effect of attachment-related stress on the capacity to mentalize: An fMRI investigation of the biobehavioral switch model. *Journal of the American Psychoanalytic Association, 58,* 566–573.

Norcross, J. C. (Ed.). (2011). *Psychotherapy relationships that work* (2nd ed.). Oxford University Press.

Norcross, J. C., & Lambert, M. J. (2018). Psychotherapy relationships that work III. *Psychotherapy, 55,* 303–315.

Norhayati, M. N., Hazlina, N., Asrenee, A. R., & Wan Emilin, W. M. A. (2014). Magnitude and risk factors for postpartum symptoms: A literature review. *Journal of Affective Disorders, 175,* 34–52.

Noriuchi, M., Kikuchi, Y., Mori, K., & Yoko, K. (2019). The orbitofrontal cortex modulates parenting stress in the maternal brain. *Scientific Reports, 9,* 1658.

Noriuchi, M., Kikuchi, Y., & Senoo, A. (2008). The functional neuroanatomy of maternal love: Mother's response to infant's attachment behaviors. *Biological Psychiatry, 2008,* 63, 415–423.

Northoff, G., Bermpohl, F., Scheneich, F., & Boeker, H. (2007). How does our brain constitute defense mechanisms? First-person neuroscience and psychoanalysis. *Psychotherapy and Psychosomatics, 76,* 141–153.

Novakovic, B., Wong, N. C., Sibson, M., Ng, H. K., Morley, R., Manuelpillai, U., et al. (2010). DNA methylation-mediated down-regulation of DNA methyltransferase-1 (DNMT1) is coincident with, but not essential for, global hypomethylation in human placenta. *Journal of Biological Chemistry, 285,* 9583–9593.

Obradovich, N., Migliorini, R., Paulus, M. P., & Rahwan, I. (2018). Empirical evidence of mental health risks posed by climate change. *Proceedings of the National Academy of Sciences USA, 115,* 10953–10958.

Ochsner, K., & Gross, J. J. (2007). The neural architecture of emotion regulation. In J. Gross (Ed.), *Handbook of emotion regulation* (pp. 131–157). Guilford.

Ogden, T. H. (1994a). The analytical third: Working with intersubjective clinical facts. *International Journal of Psychoanalysis, 75,* 3–20.

Ogden, T. H. (1994b). The concept of internal object relations. In J. S. Grotstein & D. B. Rinsley, *Fairbairn and the origins of object relations* (pp. 88–111). Guilford.

Olson, I. R., Plotsker, A., & Ezzyat, Y. (2007). The enigmatic temporal pole: A review of findings on social and emotional processing. *Brain, 130,* 1718–1731.

Ongur, D., & Price, J. L. (2000). The organization of networks within the orbital and medial prefrontal cortex of rats, monkeys, and humans. *Cerebral Cortex, 10,* 206–219.

Opie, J. E., McIntosh, J. E., Esler, T. B., Duschinsky, R., George, C., Schore, A. N. et al. (2020). Early childhood attachment stability and change: a meta-analysis. *Attachment & Human Development,* https://doi.org/10.1080/14616734.2020.1800769

Orlinsky, D. E., & Howard, K. I. (1986). Process and outcome in psychotherapy. In

S. L. Garfield & A. E. Bergin (Eds.), *Handbook of psychotherapy and behavior change* (3rd ed.). Wiley.

Ornstein, P. H. (1999). Conceptualization and treatment of rage in self psychology. *Journal of Clinical Psychology, 55,* 283–293.

Ornstein, R. O. (1997). *The right mind: Making sense of the hemispheres.* Harcourt Brace.

Ota, C., & Nakano, T. (2021). Self-face activates the dopamine reward pathway without awareness. *Cerebral Cortex, 31,* 4420–4426.

Othmer, S., & Othmer, S. (2020). Toward a theory of infra-low frequency neurofeedback. In H. Kirk (Ed.), *Restoring the brain* (2nd ed.). Taylor and Francis.

Otsuka, Y., Nakato, E., Kanazawa, S., Yamaguchi, M. K., Watanabe, S., & Kakigi, R. (2007). Neural activation to upright and inverted faces in infants measured by near infrared spectroscopy. *NeuroImage, 34,* 399–406.

Ovenstad, K. S., Orrmhaug, S. M., Shirk, S. R., & Jensen, T. K. (2020). Therapists' behaviors and youths' therapeutic alliance during trauma-focused cognitive behavioral therapy. *Journal of Consulting and Clinical Psychology, 88,* 350–361.

Ovtscharoff, W., Jr., & Braun, K. (2001). Maternal separation and social isolation modulate the postnatal development of synaptic composition in the infralimbic cortex of *Octodon degus. Neuroscience, 104,* 33–40.

Ovtscharoff, W., Jr., Helmeke, C., & Braun, K. (2006). Lack of paternal care affects synaptic development in the anterior cingulate cortex. *Brain Research, 1116,* 58–63.

Pagani, L. S., Harandian, K., Necsa, B., & Harbec, M.-J. (2023). Prospective associations between maternal depressive symptoms during early infancy and growth deficiency from childhood to adolescence. *International Journal of Environmental Research and Public Health, 20,* 7117. https://doi.org/10.3390/ijerph20237117

Paladino, M. P., Mazzurega, M., Pavani, F., & Schubert, T. W. (2010). Synchronous multisensory stimulation blurs self-other boundaries. *Psychological Science, 21,* 1202–1207. http://doi.org/10.1177/0956797610379234

Panksepp, J. (1998). *Affective neuroscience: The foundations of human and animal emotions.* Oxford University Press.

Papeo, L., Longo, M. R., Feurra, M., & Haggard, P. (2010). The role of the right temporoparietal junction in intersensory conflict: Detection or resolution? *Experimental Brain Research, 206,* 129–139.

Papousek, H., & Papousek, M. (1987). Intuitive parenting: A dialectic to the infant's integrative competence. In J. D. Osofsky (Ed.), *Handbook of infant development* (pp. 669–720). Wiley.

Papousek, H., Papousek, M., Suomi, S. J., & Rahn, C. W. (1991). Preverbal communication and attachment: Comparative views. In J. L. Gewirtz & W. M. Kurtines (Eds.), *Intersection with attachment* (pp. 97–122). Erlbaum.

Parise, E., & Csibra, G. (2013). Neural responses to multimodal ostensive signals in 5-month-old infants. *PLoS One, 8,* 72360.

Parkin, A. (1985). Narcissism: Its structures, systems and affects. *International Journal of Psycho-analysis, 66,* 143–156.

Pellis, S. M., & Pellis, V. C. (2007). Rough-and-tumble play and the development of the social brain. *Current Directions in Psychological Science, 16*, 95–98.

Perani, D., Saccuman, M. C., Scifo, P., Spada, D., Andreolli, G., Rovelli, R., et al. (2010). Functional specializations for music processing in the human newborn brain. *Proceedings of the National Academy of Sciences USA, 107*, 4758–4763.

Peretz, I., & Zatorre, R. J. (2005). Brain organization for music processing. *Annual Review of Psychology, 56*, 89–114.

Perez-Cruz, C., Simon, M., Czeh, B., Flugge, G., & Fuchs, E. (2009). Hemispheric differences in basilar dendrites and spines of pyramidal neurons in the rat prelimbic cortex: Activity- and stress-induced changes. *European Journal of Neuroscience, 29*, 738–747.

Perini, T., Ditzen, B., Hengartner, M., & Ehlert, U. (2012). Sensation seeking in fathers: The impact of testosterone and paternal investment. *Hormones and Behavior, 61*, 191–195.

Phelkos, J. L., Belsky, J., & Crnic, K. (1998). Earned security, daily stress, and parenting: A comparison of five alternative models. *Development and Psychopathology, 10*, 21–38.

Philips, R. (2013). The sacred hour: Uninterrupted skin-to-skin contact immediately after birth. *Newborn and Infant Nursing Reviews, 13*, 67–72.

Picard, M., Juster, R., & McEwen, B. S. (2014). Mitochondrial allostatic load put the "gluc" back in glucocorticoids. *Nature Reviews Endocrinology, 10*, 303–310.

Picard, M., McManus, M. J., Gray, J. D., Nasca, C., Moffat, C., Kopinski, P. K., et al. (2015). Mitochondrial functions modulate neuroendocrine, metabolic, inflammatory, and transcriptional responses to acute psychological stress. *Proceedings of the National Academy of Sciences USA, 112*, E6614–E6623.

Pileggi, L.-A., Storey, S., & Malcolm-Smith, S. (2020). Depressive symptoms disrupt leftward cradling. *Journal of Adolescent Mental Health, 32*, 35–43.

Pincus, D., Freeman, W., & Modell, A. (2007). A neurobiological model of perception: Consideration for transference. *Psychoanalytic Psychology, 24*, 623–640.

Pincus, A. L., & Lukowitsky, M. R. (2010). Pathological narcissism and narcissistic personality disorder. *Annual Review of Clinical Psychology, 6*, 421–446.

Pine, F. (1980). On the expansion of the affect array: A developmental description. In R. Lax, S. Bach, & J. A. Burland (Eds.), *Rapprochement: The critical subphase of separation-individuation* (pp. 217–233). Jason Aronson.

Pine, F. (1992). Some refinements of the separation-individuation concept in light of research on infants. *Psychoanalytic Study of the Child, 47*, 103–116.

Pistole, M. C. (1995). Attachment style and narcissistic vulnerability. *Psychoanalytic Psychology, 12*, 115–126.

Platek, S. M., Loughead, J. W., Gur, R. C., Busch, S., Ruparel, K., Phend, N., Panyavin, I. S., & Langleben, D. D. (2006). Neural substrates for functionally discriminating self-face from personally familiar faces. *Human Brain Mapping, 27*, 91–98.

Podolan, M., & Gelo, O. C. G. (2024). The role of safety in change-promoting therapeutic relationships: An integrative relational approach. *Clinical Neuropsychiatry, 21*, 403–417.

Porges, S. W. (2011). *The polyvagal theory: Neurophysiological foundations of emotions, attachment, communication, self-regulation.* Norton.

Porges, S. (2020). *How polyvagal theory helps us manage our reactions to Covid-19.* Master Class on psychology and psychotherapy, Liquid Plan srl, Webinar, November 3, 2020.

Porges, S. W., & Carter, S. (2010). Neurobiological basis of social behavior across the lifespan. In M. E. Lamb, A. M. Freund, & R. M. Lerner (Eds.), *The handbook of life-span development: Vol. 2. Social and emotional development* (pp. 9–50). John Wiley.

Posner, M. (1994). Attention: The mechanisms of consciousness. *Proceedings of the National Academy of Sciences, 91*, 7398–7404.

Potter-Effron, R. T. (1989). *Shame, guilt and alcoholism: Treatment issues in clinical practice.* Haworth.

Prechtl, H. F. (1985). Ultrasound studies of human fetal behaviour. *Early Human Development, 12*, 91–98.

Premkumar, P. (2012). Are you being rejected or excluded? Insights from neuroimaging studies using different rejection paradigms. *Clinical Psychopharmacology and Neuroscience, 10*, 144–154.

Pribram, K. H., Lennox, M. A., & Dunsmore, R. H. (1950). Some connections of the orbito-frontal-temporal, limbic and hippocampal areas of *Macaca mulatta. Journal of Neurophysiology, 13*, 127–135.

Priebe, S., Conneely, M., McCabe, R., & Bird, V. (2019). What can clinicians do to improve outcomes across psychiatric treatments: A conceptual review of non-specific components. *Epidemiology and Psychiatric Sciences, 29*, 1–8.

Priel, A., Djalovski, A., Zagoory-Sharon, O., & Feldman, R. (2019). Maternal depression impacts child psychopathology across the first decade of life: Oxytocin and synchrony as markers of resilience. *Journal of Child Psychiatry and Psychiatry, 60*, 30–42.

Prochazkova, E., & Kret, M. E. (2017). Connecting minds and sharing emotions through mimicry: A neurocognitive model of emotional contagion. *Neuroscience and Biobehavioral Reviews, 80*, 99–114.

Prodan, C. I., Orbelo, D. M., Testa, J. A., & Ross, E. D. (2001). Hemispheric differences in recognizing upper and lower facial displays of emotion. *Neuropsychiatry, Neuropsychology and Behavioral Neurology, 14*, 206–212.

Prokasy, W. F. (1965). Classical eyelid conditioning: Experimenter operations, task demands, and response shaping. In W. F. Prokasy (Ed.), *Classical conditioning.* Appleton-Century-Crofts.

Proust, M. (1923/1981). *Remembrance of things past.* Translated by C. K. Moncrief. Random House.

Psarra, A. M., & Sekeris, C. E. (2011). Glucocorticoids induce mitochondrial gene transcription in HepG2 cells: Role of the mitochondrial glucocorticoid receptor. *Biochimica Biophysica Acta, 1813*, 1814–1821.

Purves-Tyson, T. D., Owens, S. J., Double, K. L., Desai, R., Handelsman, D. J., &

Weickert, C. S. (2014). Testosterone induces molecular changes in dopamine signaling pathway molecules in the adolescent rat nigrostriatal pathway. *PLoS One, 9*(3), e91151. doi: 10.1371/journal.pone.0091151

Quinones-Camacho, L. E., Fishburn, F. A., Belardi, K., Williams, D. L., Huppert, E. J., & Perlman, S. B. (2021). Dysfunction in interpersonal neural synchronization as a mechanism for social impairment in autism spectrum disorder. *Autism Research, 14*, 1585–1596. doi: 10.1002/aur.2513

Quirin, M., Dusing, R., & Kuhl, J. (2013). Implicit affiliation motive predicts correct intuitive judgment. *Journal of Individual Differences, 34*, 24–31.

Quirin, M., Frohlich, S., & Kuhl, J. (2018). Implicit self and the right hemisphere: Increasing implicit self-esteem and implicit positive affect by left hand contractions. *European Journal of Social Psychology, 48*, 4–16.

Quirin, M., Gruber, T., Kuhl, J., & Dusing, R. (2013). Is love right? Prefrontal resting brain asymmetry is related to the affiliation motive. *Frontiers in Human Neuroscience, 7*, 902.

Quirin, M., Jais, M., Di Domenico, S. I., Kuhl, J., & Ryan, R. M. (2021). Effortless willpower? The integrative self and self-determined goal pursuit. *Frontiers in Psychology, 12*, 653458. doi: 10.3389/fpsyg.2021.653458

Quirin, M., Meyer, F., Heise, N., Kuhl, J., Kustermann, E., Struber, D., & Cacioppo, J. T. (2013). Neural correlates of social motivation: An FMRI study on power versus affiliation. *International Journal of Psychophysiology, 88*, 289–295.

Rabellino, D., Densmore, M., Theberge, J., McKinnon, M. C., & Lanius, R. A. (2018). The cerebellum after trauma: Resting-state functional connectivity of the cerebellum in posttraumatic stress disorder and its dissociative subtype. *Human Brain Mapping, 39*, 3354–3374.

Rabeyron, T. (2022). Psychoanalytic psychotherapies and the free energy principle. *Front. Hum. Neuroscience, 16*, 929940. doi: 10.3389/fnhum.2022.929940.

Racker, H. (1968). *Transference and countertransference*. International Universities Press.

Rangaraju, V., Calloway, N., & Annau, T. A. (2014). Activity-driven local ATP synthesis is required for synaptic function. *Cell, 156*, 825–835.

Rank, O. (2010). *The trauma of birth*. Routledge. (Original work published 1924)

Ranotte, S., Elliot, R., Abel, K. M., Mitchell, R., Deakin, F. W., & Appleby, L. (2004). The neural basis of maternal responsiveness to infants: An fMRI function. *NeuroReport, 15*, 1825–1829.

Ratnarajah, N., Rifkin-Graboi, A., Fortier, M. V., Chong, Y. S., Kwek, K., Saw, S.-M., et al. (2013). Structural connectivity in the neonatal brain. *NeuroImage, 75*, 187–194.

Rausch, J., Gabel, A., Nagy, K., Kleindienst, N., Herpetz, S. C., & Bertsch, K. (2015). Increased testosterone and cortisol awakening responses in patients with borderline personality disorder: Gender and trait aggressiveness matter. *Psychoneuroendocrinology, 55*, 116–127.

Rauthmann, J. F., & Kolar, G. P. (2013). Positioning the Dark Triad in the interpersonal complex: The friendly-dominant narcissist, hostile-submissive Machiavellian, and hostile-dominant psychopath? *Personality and Individual Differences, 54,* 622–627.

Ray, D., Roy, D., Sindhu, B., Sharan, P., & Banerjee, A. (2017). Neural substrate of group mental health: Insights from multi-brain reference frame in functional neuroimaging. *Frontiers in Psychology, 8,* 1627. doi: 10.3389/fpsyg.2017.01627

Redcay, E., Dodell-Feder, D., Pearrow, M. J., Mavros, P. L., Kleiner, M., Gabrieli, J. D. E., et al. (2010). Live face-to-face interaction during fMRI: A new tool for social cognitive neuroscience. *NeuroImage, 50,* 1639–1647.

Reed, S. F., Ohel, G., David, R., & Porges, S. W. (1999). A neural explanation of fetal heart rate patterns: A test of the polyvagal theory. *Developmental Psychobiology, 35,* 108–118.

Reich, A. (1960). Pathologic forms of self-esteem regulation. *Psychoanalytic Study of the Child, 15,* 215–234.

Reik, T. (1956). Adventures in psychoanalytic discovery. In M. Sherman (Ed.), *The search within* (pp. 473–626). Aronson.

Reinhard, D. A., Konrath, S. H., Lopez, W. D., & Cameron, H. G. (2012). Expensive egos: Narcissistic males have higher cortisol. *PLoS One, 7*(7). https://doi.org/10.1371/annotation/1c60eca3-794f-4a09-8a82-e43ed3cc2009

Reis, B. (2018). Being-with: From infancy through philosophy in psychoanalysis. *Psychoanalytic Inquiry, 38,* 130–137.

Reitav, J., & Thirlwell, C. (2025). *Putting trauma to sleep: Attachment-based neuromodulatory interventions for stabilizing the brains stem.* Norton.

Rentoul, R. W. (2010). *Ferenczi's language of tenderness: Working with disturbances from the earliest years.* Jason Aronson.

Rich, E. L., & Wallis, J. D. (2016). Decoding subjective decisions from orbitofrontal cortex. *Nature Neuroscience, 19,* 973–980.

Rifkin-Graboi, A., Bai, J., Chen, H., Hameed, W. B., Sim, L. W., et al. (2013). Prenatal maternal depression associates with microstructure of right amygdala in neonates at birth. *Biological Psychiatry, 74,* 837–844.

Rigas, D. (2008). Silent dialogues in the analytic relationship. *International Forum of Psychoanalysis, 17,* 37–43.

Rilke, R. M. (1929/2012). *Letters to a young poet.* Penguin Books.

Rinsley, D. B. (1989). *Developmental pathogenesis and the treatment of borderline and narcissistic personalities.* Jason Aronson.

Risse, G. L., & Gazzaniga, M. S. (1978). Well-kept secrets of the right hemisphere: A carotid amytal study of restricted memory transfer. *Neurology, 28,* 950–953.

Robbins, M. (2018). The primary process: Freud's profound yet neglected contribution to the psychology of consciousness. *Psychoanalytic Inquiry, 38,* 186–197.

Rodman, F. R. (2003). *Winnicott: Life and work.* Perseus.

Rogers, C. T. (1954). Toward a theory of creativity. *A Review of General Semantics, 11,* 249–260.

Rogers, C. T. (1957). The necessary and sufficient conditions of therapeutic personality change. *Journal of Consulting Psychology, 21,* 95–103.

Rogers, C. T. (1958). The characteristic of a helping relationship. In C.T. Rogers, *On becoming a person* (pp. 39–58). Houghton Mifflin.

Rogers, C. R. (1975). Empathic: An unappreciated way of being. *Counseling Psychologist, 5,* 2–10.

Rogers, C. T. (1989). A client-centered/person-centered approach to therapy. In H. Kirschenbaum & V. Land Henderson (Eds.), *The Carl Rogers reader* (pp. 135–152).Houghton Mifflin.

Rolls, E. T., & Grabenhorst, F. (2008). The orbitofrontal cortex and beyond: from affect to decision-making. *Progress in Neurobiology, 86,* 216–244.

Rolls, E. T., Hornak, J., Wade, D., & McGrath, J. (1994). Emotion-related learning in patients with social and emotional changes associated with frontal lobe damage. *Journal of Neurology, Neurosurgery, and Psychiatry, 57,* 1518–1524.

Ronningstam, E. (2009). Narcissistic personality disorder: Facing DSM-V. *Psychiatric Annals, 39,* 111–121.

Ronningstam, E., Weinberg, I., Goldblatt, M., Schechter, M., & Herbstman, B. (2018). Suicide and self-regulation in narcissistic personality disorder. *Psychodynamic Psychiatry, 46,* 491–510.

Rosa, C., Lassonde, M., Pinard, C., Keenan, J. P., & Belin, P. (2008). Investigations of hemispheric specialization of self-voice recognition. *Brain and Cognition, 68,* 204–214.

Rosenbaum, R. (2011). Exploring the other dark continent: Parallels between psi phenomena and the psychotherapeutic process. *Psychoanalytic Review, 98,* 57–90.

Ross, E. D. (1983). Right-hemisphere lesions in disorders of affective language. In A. Kertesz (Ed.), *Localization in neuropsychology* (pp. 493–508). Academic Press.

Ross, E. D., & Monnot, M. (2008). Neurology of affective prosody and its functional-anatomic organization in right hemisphere. *Brain and Language, 104,* 51–74.

Rotenberg, V. S. (1993). Richness against freedom: Two hemisphere functions and the problem of creativity. *European Journal of High Creativity, 4,* 11–19.

Rotenberg, V. S. (1995). Right hemisphere insufficiency and illness in the context of search activity concept. *Dynamic Psychiatry, 150/151,* 54–63.

Rotenberg, V. S. (2004). The peculiarity of the right-hemisphere function in depression: Solving the paradoxes. *Progress in Neuro-psychopharmacology and Biological Psychiatry, 28,* 1–13.

Rotenberg, V. S. (2021). The formation of two types of context by the brain hemispheres as a basis for a new approach to the mechanisms of psychotherapy. In R. Tweedy (Ed.), *The divided therapist: Hemispheric difference and contemporary psychotherapy* (pp. 258–278). Routledge.

Rotenberg, V. S., & Weinberg, I. (1999). Human memory, cerebral hemispheres, and limbic system: A new approach. *Genetic, Social and General Psychology Monographs, 125,* 45–70.

Roth, T. L., & Sweatt, J. D. (2011). Annual research review: Epigenetic mechanism and environmental shaping of the brain during sensitive periods of development. *Journal of Child Psychology and Psychiatry, 52*, 398–408.

Roy, M., Shohamy, D., & Wager, T. D. (2012). Ventromedial prefrontal subcortical systems and the generation of affective meaning. *Trends in Cognitive Science, 16*, 147–156.

Rubik, B., Muehsam, D., Hammerschlag, R., & Jain, S. (2015). Biofield science and healing: History, terminology, and concepts. *Global Advances in Health Medicine, 4*, 8–14.

Rudebeck, P. H., & Murray, E. A. (2014). The orbitofrontal oracle: Cortical mechanisms for the prediction and evaluation of specific behavioral outcomes. *Neuron, 84*, 1143–1156.

Rusch, N., Lieb, K., Gottler, M. D., Hermann, C., Schramm, E., Richter, H., et al. (2007). Shame and implicit self-concept in women with borderline personality disorder. *American Journal of Psychiatry, 164*, 500–508.

Rusch, N., Schultz, D., Valerius, G., Steil, R., Bohus, M., & Schmahl, C. (2010). Disgust and implicit self-concept in women with borderline personality disorder and posttraumatic stress disorder. *European Archives of Psychiatry and Clinical Neuroscience, 261*, 369–376. doi: 10.1007/s00406-010-0174-2

Russell, G. I. (2015). *Screen relations: The limits of computer-mediated psychoanalysis and psychotherapy.* Karnac.

Russell, P. (1998). The role of paradox in the repetition compulsion. In J. G. Teicholz & D. Kriegman (Eds.), *Trauma, repetition, and affect regulation: The work of Paul Russell* (pp. 1–22). Other Press.

Russel, S., & Norvig, P. (2021). *Artificial intelligence: A modern approach.* (4th ed.). Prentice Hall.

Ryan, R. (2007). Motivation and emotion: A new look and approach to two reemerging fields. *Motivation and Emotion, 31*, 1–3.

Sachs, M. E., Damasio, A., & Habibi, A. (2015). The pleasures of sad music: A systematic review. *Frontiers in Human Neuroscience, 9*, 404. doi: 10.3389/fnhum.2015.00404

Salavert, J., Gasol, M., Vieta, E., Cervantes, A., Trampal, C., & Gispert, J. D. (2011). Fronto-limbic dysfunction in borderline personality disorder: A 18F-Fdg positron emission tomography study. *Journal of Affective Disorders, 131*, 260–267.

Salmi, J., Roine, U., Glerean, E., Lahnakoski, J., Nieminen-von Wendt, T., Tani, P., et al. (2013). The brains of high functioning autistic individuals do not synchronize with those of others. *NeuroImage: Clinical, 3*, 489–497.

Salva, O. R., Regolin, L., Mascalzoni, E., & Vallortigara, G. (2012). Cerebral and behavioural asymmetries in animal social cognition. *Comprehensive Cognition and Behavioral Review, 7*, 110–138.

Samples, B. (1976). *The metaphoric mind: A celebration of creative consciousness.* Addison-Wesley.

Samson, D., Apperly, I. A., Chiavarino, C., & Humphreys, G. W. (2004). Left temporoparietal junction is necessary for representing someone else's belief. *Nature Neuroscience, 7,* 499–500.

Sander, K., Roth, P., & Scheich, H. (2003). Left-lateralized fMRI activation in the temporal lobe of high repressive women during the identification of sad prosodies. *Cognitive Brain Research, 16,* 441–456.

Sands, S. (1997). Self psychology and projective identification—whither shall they meet? A reply to the editors. *Psychoanalytic Dialogue, 7,* 651–668.

Santiestaban, I., Banissy, M. J., Catmur, C., & Bird, G. (2012). Enhancing social ability by stimulating right temporoparietal junction. *Current Biology, 22,* 2274–2277.

Saroka, K. S., Dotta, B. T., & Persinger, M. A. (2013). Concurrent photon emission, changes in quantitative brain activity over the right hemisphere, and alterations in the proximal geomagnetic field while imagining white light. *International Journal of Life Science and Medical Research, 3,* 30–34.

Sartre, J.-P. (1957). *Being and nothingness.* Methuen.

Sato, W., & Aoki, S. (2006). Right hemisphere dominance in processing unconscious emotion. *Brain and Cognition, 62,* 261–266.

Satoh, M., Nakase, T., Nagata, K., & Tomimoto, H. (2011). Musical anhedonia: Selective loss of emotional experience in listening to music. *Neurocase, 17,* 410–417.

Saugstad, L. F. (1998). Cerebral lateralisation and rate of maturation. *International Journal of Psychophysiology, 28,* 37–62.

Saxe, R., & Wexler, A. (2005). Making sense of another mind: The role of the right temporo-parietal junction. *Neuropsychologia, 43,* 1391–1399.

Scalabrini, A., Wolman, A., & Northof, G. (2021). The self and its right insula—differential topography and dynamic of right vs. left insula. *Brain Science, 11,* 1312. https://doi.org/10.3390/brainsci11101312

Scatliffe, N., Casavant, S., Vitner, D., & Cong, X. (2019). Oxytocin and early parent-infant interactions: A systematic review. *International Journal of Nursing Science, 6,* 445–453.

Schafer, R. (1958). Regression in the service of the ego: The relevance of a psychoanalytic concept for personality assessment. In G. Lindzey (Ed.), *Assessment of human motives.* Grove.

Schaffer, H. R., & Emerson, P. E. (1964). The development of social attachments in infancy. *Monograms for the Society of Research in Child Development, 29,* 1–77.

Scheller, K., Sekeris, C. E., Krohne, G., Hock, R., Hansen, I. A., & Scheer, U. (2000). Localization of glucocorticoid hormone receptors in mitochondria of human cells. *European Journal of Cell Biology, 79,* 299–307.

Schepman, A., Rodway, P., & Pritchard, H. (2016). Right-lateralized unconscious, but not conscious, processing of affective environmental sounds. *Laterality: Asymmetry. Body, Brain, Cognition, 21,* 606–632.

Schiepek, G. K., Tominschek, I., & Heinzel, S. (2014). Self-organization in psychotherapy: Testing synergetic model in change processes. *Frontiers in Psychology, 5,* 1089. doi: 10.3389/fpsyg.2014.01089

Schoenherr, D., Paulick, J., Strauss, B. M., Deisenhofer, A. K., Schwartz, B., Lutz, W., et al. (2019). Nonverbal synchrony predicts premature termination of psychotherapy for social anxiety disorder. *Psychotherapy, 56,* 503–513.

Schore, A. N. (1991). Early superego development: The emergence of shame and narcissistic affect regulation in the practicing period. *Psychoanalysis and Contemporary Thought, 14,* 187–250.

Schore, A. N. (1996). The experience-dependent maturation of a regulatory system in the orbital prefrontal cortex and the origin of developmental psychopathology. *Development and Psychopathology, 8,* 59–87.

Schore, A. N. (1997a). A century after Freud's Project: Is a rapprochement between psychoanalysis and neurobiology at hand? *Journal of the American Psychoanalytic Association, 45,* 841–867.

Schore, A. N. (1997b). Early organization of the nonlinear right brain and development of a predisposition to psychiatric disorders. *Development and Psychopathology, 9,* 595–631.

Schore, A. N. (2000a). Attachment and the regulation of the right brain. *Attachment and Human Development, 2,* 23–47.

Schore, A. N. (2000b). Foreword. In J. Bowlby, *Attachment and loss: Vol. I. Attachment.* Basic Books.

Schore, A. N. (2000c). The seventh Annual John Bowlby memorial lecture. Minds in the making: Attachment, the self-organizing brain, and developmentally oriented psychoanalytic psychotherapy. *British Journal of Psychotherapy, 17,* 199–328.

Schore, A. N. (2001a). The effects of a secure attachment relationship on right brain development, affect regulation, and infant mental health. *Infant Mental Health Journal, 22,* 7–66.

Schore, A. N. (2001b). The effects of relational trauma on right brain development, affect regulation, and infant mental health. *Infant Mental Health Journal, 22,* 201–269.

Schore, A. N. (2002a). Dysregulation of the right brain: A fundamental mechanism of traumatic attachment and the psychopathogenesis of posttraumatic stress disorder. *Australian and New Zealand Journal of Psychiatry, 36,* 9–30.

Schore, A. N. (2002b). The right brain as the neurobiological substratum of Freud's dynamic unconscious. In D. Scharff (Ed.), *The psychoanalytic century: Freud's legacy for the future* (pp. 61–88). Other Press.

Schore, A. N. (2003a). *Affect dysregulation and disorders of the self.* Norton.

Schore, A. N. (2003b). *Affect regulation and the repair of the self.* Norton.

Schore, A. N. (2005). A neuropsychoanalytic viewpoint: Commentary on paper by Steven H. Knoblauch. *Psychoanalytic Dialogues, 15,* 829–854.

Schore, A. N. (2009a, August 8). The paradigm shift: The right brain and the relational unconscious. Invited plenary address to the American Psychological Association 2009 Convention, Toronto, Canada. https://www.allanschore.com/pdf/SchoreAPAPlenaryFinal09.pdf

Schore, A. N. (2009b). Relational trauma and the developing right brain: An interface of psychoanalytic self psychology and neuroscience. *Annals of the New York Academy of Sciences, 1159,* 189–203.

Schore, A. N. (2011). The right brain implicit self lies at the core of psychoanalysis. *Psychoanalytic Dialogues, 21,* 75–100.

Schore, A. N. (2012). *The science of the art of psychotherapy.* Norton.

Schore, A. N. (2013). Regulation theory and the early assessment of attachment and autistic spectrum disorders: A response to Voran's clinical case. *Journal of Infant, Child, and Adolescent Psychotherapy, 12,* 164–189.

Schore, A. N. (2014a). Early interpersonal neurobiological assessment of attachment and autistic spectrum disorders. *Frontiers in Psychology, 5,* article 1049. doi: 10.3389/fpsyg.2014.01049

Schore, A. N. (2014b). The right brain is dominant in psychotherapy. *Psychotherapy, 51,* 388–397.

Schore, A. N. (2016). *Affect regulation and the origin of the self: The neurobiology of emotional development* (Classic ed.). Routledge. (Original work published 1994)

Schore, A. N. (2017a). All our sons: The developmental neurobiology and neuroendocrinology of boys at risk. *Infant Mental Health Journal, 38*(1). doi: 10.1002/imhj.21616

Schore, A. N. (2017b). Playing on the right side of the brain: An interview with Allan N. Schore. *American Journal of Play, 9,* 105–142.

Schore, A. N. (2019a). *The development of the unconscious mind.* Norton.

Schore, A. N. (2019b). *Right brain psychotherapy.* Norton.

Schore, A. N. (2020). Forging connections in group psychotherapy through right brain-to-right brain emotional communications: Part I. Theoretical models of right brain therapeutic action. Part II: Clinical case analyses of group right brain regressive enactments. *International Journal of Group Psychotherapy, 70,* 29–88.

Schore, A. N. (2021a). The interpersonal neurobiology of intersubjectivity. *Frontiers in Psychology, 12,* 648616. https://doi.org/10.3389/fpsyg.2021.648616

Schore, A. N. (2021b). The interpersonal neurobiology of therapeutic mutual regressions in reenactments of early attachment trauma. In D. J. Siegel, A. N. Schore, & L. Cozolino (Eds.), *Interpersonal neurobiology and clinical practice* (pp. 27–58). Norton.

Schore, A. N. (2022). Right brain-to-right brain psychotherapy: Recent scientific and clinical advances. *Annals of General Psychiatry, 21,* 46. https://doi.org/10.1186/s12991-022-00420-3

Schore, A. N., & Marks-Tarlow, T. (2018). How love opens creativity, play, and the arts through early right brain development. In T. Marks-Tarlow, M. Solomon, & D. J. Siegel (Eds.), *Play and creativity in psychotherapy* (pp. 64–91). Norton.

Schore, A. N., & Newton, R. P. (2012). Using modern attachment theory to guide clinical assessments of early attachment relationships. In J. E. Bettmann & D. Freedman (Eds.), *Attachment-based clinical work with children and adolescents* (pp. 61–96). Norton.

Schore, J. R., & Schore, A. N. (2008). Modern attachment theory: The central role of affect regulation in development and treatment. *Clinical Social Work Journal, 36*, 9–20.

Schultz, S. M. (2016). Neural correlates of heart-focused interoception: A functional magnetic resonance imaging meta-analysis. *Philosophical Transactions of the Royal Society of London: Series B, Biological Science, 371*, 1708.

Schultz, W. (2002). Getting formal with dopamine and reward. *Neuron, 36*, 241–263.

Schumann, C. M., Bauman, M. D., & Amaral, D. G. (2011). Abnormal structure or function of the amygdala is a common component of neurodevelopmental disorders. *Neuropsychologia, 49*, 745–759.

Schwartz, C. E., Kunwar, P. S., Greve, D. N., Kagan, J., Snidman, N. C., & Bloch, R. B. (2012). A phenotype of early infancy predicts reactivity of the amygdala in male adults. *Molecular Psychiatry, 17*, 1042–1050.

Schwartz, L., Levy, J., Endevelt-Shapira, Y., Djalovski, A., Hayut, O., Dumas, G., & Feldman, R. (2022). Technologically-assisted communication attenuates interbrain synchrony. *NeuroImage, 264*, 119677.

Sehgal, A., Nitzan, I., Jayawickreme, N., & Menaham, S. (2020). Impact of skin-to-skin parent-infant care on preterm circulatory physiology. *Journal of Pediatrics, 222*, 91–97.e2.

Semrud-Clikeman, M., Fine, J. G., & Zhu, D. C. (2011). The role of the right hemisphere for processing of social interactions in normal adults using functional magnetic resonance imaging. *Neuropsychobiology, 64*, 47–51.

Sened, H., Zilcha-Mano, S., & Shamay-Tsoory, S. (2022). Inter-brain plasticity as a biological mechanism of change in psychotherapy: A review and integrative model. *Frontiers in Human Neuroscience, 16*. 955238. doi: 10.3389//fnhum.2022 .955238

Settlage, C. F. (1977). The psychoanalytic understanding of narcissistic and borderline personality disorders: Advances in developmental theory. *Journal of the American Psychoanalytic Association, 25*, 805–833.

Shamay-Tsoory, S.G. (2022). Brains that fire together wire together: Interbrain plasticity underlies learning in social interactions. *The Neuroscientist, 28*, 543–551.

Shamay-Tsoory, S. G., Aharon-Peretz, J., & Perry, D. (2009). Two systems for empathy: A double dissociation between emotional and cognitive empathy in inferior frontal gyrus versus ventromedial prefrontal lesions. *Brain, 132*, 617–627.

Shamay-Tsoory, S. G., Tomer, R., Berger, B. D., & Aharon-Peretz, J. (2003). Characterization of empathy deficits following prefrontal brain damage: The role of the right ventromedial prefrontal cortex. *Journal of Cognitive Neuroscience, 15*, 324–337.

Shammi, P., & Stuss, D. T. (1999). Humor appreciation: A role of the right frontal lobe. *Brain, 122*, 657–666.

Shankle, W. R., Rafii, M. S., Landing, B. H., & Fallon, J. H. (1999). Approximate doubling of numbers of neurons in postnatal human cerebral cortex and in 35 specific cytoarchitectural areas from birth to 72 months. *Pediatric Developmental Pathology, 2*, 244–259.

Shedler, J. (2010). The efficacy of psychodynamic psychotherapy. *American Psychologist, 65*, 98–109.

Shedler, J. (2011). Getting to know me. *Scientific American Mind, 21*, 52–57.

Shirtcliff, E. A., Granger, D. A., & Likos, A. (2002). Gender differences in the validity of testosterone measured in saliva by immunoassay. *Hormones and Behavior, 42*, 62–69.

Shirvalkar, P., Prosky, J., Chin, G., Ahmadipour, P., Sani, O. G., Desai, M., et al. (2023). First-in-human prediction of chronic pain state using intracranial neural biomarkers. *Nature Neuroscience, 26*, 1090–1099. doi: 10.1038/s41593-023-01338-z

Shuren, J. E., & Grafman, J. (2002). The neurology of reasoning. *Archives of Neurology, 59*, 916–919.

Siegel, D. J. (1999). *The developing mind: Toward a neurobiology of interpersonal experience.* Norton.

Siegel, D. J. (2012). *The developing mind: How relationships and the brain interact to shape who we are* (2nd ed.). Guilford.

Sieratzki, J. S., & Woll, B. (1996). Why do mothers cradle their babies on the left? *Lancet, 347*, 1746–1748.

Silbereis, J. C., Pochareddy, S., Zhu, Y., Li, M., & Sestan, N. (2016). The cellular and metabolic landscapes of the developing human central nervous system. *Neuron, 89*, 248–268.

Silver, K. L., & Singer, P. A. (2014). A focus on child development [Editorial]. *Science, 345*, 120.

Slomian, J., Honvo, G., Emonts, P., Reginster, J.-Y., & Bruyère, O. (2019). Consequences of maternal postpartum depression: A systematic review of maternal and infant outcomes. *Women's Health, 15*, 1–55.

Smiraglia, D. J., Kulawiec, M., Bistulfi, G. I., Gupta, S. G., & Singh, K. K. (2008). A novel role for mitochondria for regulating epigenetic modification in the nucleus. *Cancer Biology and Therapy, 7*, 1182–1190.

Solms, M. (2021). *The hidden spring: A journey to the source of consciousness.* Norton.

Solms, M., & Turnbull, O. (2002). *The brain and inner world.* Other Press.

Sonnby-Borgström, M., & Jönsson, P. (2004). Dismissing-avoidant pattern of attachment and mimicry reactions at different levels of information processing. *Scandinavian Journal of Psychology, 45*, 103–113.

Sopp, M. R., Michael, T., Weeb, H. G., & Mecklinger, A. (2017). Remembering specific features of emotional events across time: the role of REM sleep and prefrontal theta oscillations. *Cognitive Affective and Behavioral Neuroscience, 17*, 1186–1209.

Spalding, L. R., & Hardin, C. D. (1999). Unconscious unease and self-handicapping: Behavioral consequences of individual differences in implicit and explicit self-esteem. *Psychological Science, 10*, 535–539.

Sparks, J. A., Duncan, B. L., & Miller, S. D. (2008). Common factors in psychotherapy. In J. L. Lebow (Ed.). *Twenty-first century psychotherapies: Contemporary approaches to theory and practice* (pp. 453–497). John Wiley & Sons.

Spence, J. T., & Helmreich, R. L. (1978). *Masculinity and femininity: Their psychological dimensions, correlates, and antecedents.* University of Texas Press.

Spencer, J., Goode, J., Penix, E., Trusty, W., & Swift, J. K. (2019). Developing a collaborative relationship with clients during the initial sessions of psychotherapy. *Psychotherapy, 56,* 7–10.

Spengler, F. B., Scheele, D., March, N., Kofferath, C., Flach, A., Schwartz, S., et al. (2017). Oxytocin facilitates reciprocity in social communication. *Social Cognitive and Affective Neuroscience, 12,* 1325–1333.

Spiegel, D., & Cardena, E. (1991). Disintegrated experience: The dissociative disorders revisited. *Journal of Abnormal Psychology, 100,* 366–378.

Spitzer, C., Wilert, C., Grabe, H.-J., Rizos, T., & Freyberger, H. J. (2004). Dissociation, hemispheric asymmetry, and dysfunction of hemispheric interaction: A transcranial magnetic approach. *Journal of Neuropsychiatry and Clinical Neurosciences, 16,* 163–169.

Spoletini., I., Piras, F., Fagioli, S., Rubino, I. A., Martinotti, G., Siracusano, A., et al. (2011). Suicidal attempts and increased right amygdala volume in schizophrenia. *Schizophrenia Research, 125,* 30–40.

Stenberg, G., Wiking, S., & Dahl, M. (1998). Judging words at face value: Interference in word processing task reveals automatic processing of affective facial stimuli. *Cognition and Emotion, 12,* 755–782.

Sterling, P., & Eyer, J. (1988). Allostasis: A new paradigm to explain arousal pathology. In S. Fisher & J. Reason (Eds.), *Handbook of life stress, cognition, and health* (pp. 629–649). John Wiley.

Stern, D. B. (1997). *Unformulated experience: From dissociation to imagination in psychoanalysis.* Analytic Press.

Stern, D. B. (2009). Dissociation and unformulated experience: A psychoanalytic model of mind. In P. F. Dell & J. A. O'Neil (Eds.), *Dissociation and the dissociative disorders: DSM-V and beyond* (pp. 653–663). Routledge.

Stern, D. N. (1977). *The first relationship.* Harvard University Press.

Stern, D. N. (1985). *The interpersonal world of the infant.* Basic Books.

Stern, D. N. (1990). Joy and satisfaction in infancy. In R. A. Glick & S. Bone (Eds.), *Pleasure beyond the pleasure principle* (pp. 13–25). Yale University Press.

Stern, D. N. (2004). *The present moment in psychotherapy and everyday life.* Norton.

Stern, D. N., Morgan, A. C.., Nahum, J. P., Sander, L., & Tronick, E. Z. (1998). The process of therapeutic change involving implicit knowledge: Some implications of developmental observations for adult psychotherapy. *Infant Mental Health Journal, 19,* 300–308.

Stevenson, C. W., Halliday, D. M., Marsden, C. A., & Mason, R. (2008). Early life programming of hemispheric lateralization and synchronization in the adult medial prefrontal cortex. *Neuroscience, 155,* 852–863.

Stiglmayr, C. E., Shapiro, D. A., Stiglitz, R. D., Limberger, M. F., & Bohus, M. (2001). Experience of aversive tension and dissociation in female patients with borderline personality disorder—a controlled study. *Journal of Psychiatric Research, 35*, 111–118.

Stolk, A., Noordzij, M. L., Verhagen, L., Volman, L., Schoffen, J.-M., Oostenveld, R., et al. (2014). Cerebral coherence between communicators marks the emergence of meaning. *Proceedings of the National Academy of Sciences USA, 111*, 18183–18188.

Stolorow, R. D., Brandshaft, B., & Atwood, G. E. (1987). *Psychoanalytic treatment: An intersubjective approach.* Routledge.

Storey, A. E., Walsh, C. J., Quinton, R. L., & Wynne-Edwards, K. E. (2000). Hormonal correlates of paternal responsiveness in new and expectant fathers. *Evolution and Human Behavior, 21*, 79–95.

Strogatz, S. (2008). *Sync: How order emerges from chaos in the universe, nature and daily life.* Paw Prints.

Stromsted, T. (2025). *Soul's body. Active imagination, authentic movement, and embodiment in psychotherapy.* Routledge.

Stumpfogger, N., & Panagiotopoulou, E. (2021). Blurred body boundaries of first-time mothers: An interpretative phenomenological analysis. *Neuropsychoanalysis, 23*, 97–109.

Sturm, W., de Simone, A., Krause, B., Specht, K., Hesselman, V., Redernacher, I., et al. (1999). Functional anatomy of intrinsic alertness: Evidence for a fronto-parietal-thalamic-brainstem network in the right hemisphere. *Neuropsychologia, 37*, 797–805.

Sullivan, H. S. (1953). *The interpersonal theory of psychiatry.* Norton.

Sullivan, R. M., & Gratton, A. (2002). Prefrontal cortical regulation of hypothalamic-pituitary-adrenal function in the rat and implications for psychopathology: Side matters. *Psychoneuroendocrinology, 27*, 99–114.

Sulloway, F. S. (1979). *Freud, biologist of the mind: Beyond the psychoanalytic legend.* Basic Books.

Sun, T., Patoine, C., Abu-Khalil, A., Visader, J., Sum, E., Cherry, T. J., et al. (2005). Early asymmetry of gene transcription in embryonic human left and right cerebral cortex. *Science, 308*, 1794–1798.

Suter, S. E., Huggenberger, H. J., & Schachinger, H. (2007). Cold pressor stress reduces left cradling preference in nulliparous human females. *International Journal of the Biology of Stress, 10*, 45–51.

Symeonides, C., Vacy, K., Thomson, S., et al. (2024). Male autism spectrum disorder is linked to brain aromatase disruption by prenatal BPA in multimodal investigations and 10HDA ameliorates the related mouse phenotype. *Nat Commun 15*, 6367. https://doi.org/10.1038/s41467-024-48897-8

Szymanska, M., Schneider, M., Chateau-Smith, C., Nezelof, S., & Vulliez-Coady, L. (2017). Psychophysiological effects of oxytocin on parent-child interactions: A literature review on oxytocin on parent-child interactions. *Psychiatry and Clinical Neuroscience, 71*, 690–705.

Takahashi, Y. K., Chang, C. Y., Lucantonio, F., Haney, R. Z., Berg, B. A., Yau, H.-J., et al. (2013). Neural estimates of imagined outcomes in the orbitofrontal cortex drive behavior and learning. *Neuron, 80,* 507–518.

Takatani, T., Takahashi, Y., Yoshida, R., Imai, R., Uchiike, T., Yamazaki, M., et al. (2018). Relationship between frequency spectrum of heart rate variability and autonomic nervous activities during sleep in newborns. *Brain and Development, 40,* 165–171.

Talia, A., Muzi, L., Lingiari, V., & Taubner, S. (2020). How to be a secure base: therapists' attachment representations and their link to attunement in psychotherapy. *Attachment and Human Development, 22,* 189–206.

Tamietto, M., & de Gelder, B. (2010). Neural basis of the non-conscious perception of emotional signals. *Nature Reviews Neuroscience, 11,* 97–709.

Tanaka, C., Matsui, M., Uematsu, A., Noguchi, K., & Miyawaki, T. (2012). Developmental trajectories of the fronto-temporal lobes from infant to early adulthood in healthy individuals. *Developmental Neuroscience, 34,* 477–487.

Tang, H., Mai, X., Wang, S., Zhu, C., Krueger, F., & Liu, C. (2016). Interpersonal brain synchronization in the right temporoparietal junction during face-to-face economic exchange. *Social Cognitive Affective Neuroscience, 157,* 314–330.

Tangney, J. P., Wagner, P., Fletcher, C., & Gramzow, R. (1992). Shamed into anger? The relation of shame and guilt to anger and self-reported aggression. *Journal of Personality and Social Psychology, 62,* 669–675.

Tanzilli, A., Muzi, L., Ronningstam, E., & Lingardi, V. (2017). Countertransference when working with narcissistic personality disorder: An empirical investigation. *Psychotherapy, 54,* 184–194.

Tarullo, A. R., & Gunnar, M. R. (2006). Child maltreatment and the developing HPA axis. *Hormones and Behavior, 50,* 632–639.

Tau, G. Z., & Peterson, B. S. (2010). Normal development of brain circuits. *Neuropsychopharmacology, 35,* 147–168.

Taylor, J. B. (2008). *My stroke of insight: A brain scientist's personal journey.* Viking Penguin.

Teasdale, J. D., Howard, R. J., Cox, S. G., Ha, Y., Bramner, M. J., Williams, S. C. R., & Checkley, S. A. (1999). Functional MRI study of the cognitive generation of affect. *American Journal of Psychiatry, 156,* 209–215.

Terburg, D., Morgan, B., & van Honk, J. (2009). The testosterone-cortisol ratio: A hormonal marker for proneness to social aggression. *International Journal of Law and Psychiatry, 32,* 216–223.

Thatcher, R. W. (1994). Cyclical cortical reorganization: Origins of human cognitive development. In G. Dawson & K.W. Fischer (Eds.), *Human behavior and the developing brain* (pp. 232–266). Guilford.

Thatcher, R. W. (1996). Neuroimaging of cyclical cortical reorganization during human development. In R.W. Thatcher, C. Reid Lyon, J. Rumsey, & N. Krasnegor (Eds.), *Developmental neuroimaging. Mapping the development of brain and behavior* (pp. 91–106). Academic Press.

Thatcher, R. W., Walker, R. A., & Giudice, S. (1987). Human cerebral hemispheres develop at different rates and ages. *Science, 236,* 1110–1113.

Thoma, M. V., La Marca, R., Bronnimann, R., Finkel, L., Ehlert, U., & Nater, U. M. (2013). The effect of music on the human stress response. *PLOS ONE, 8,* 1–11.

Thomasson, M., Voruz, P., Cionca, A., de Alantara, I.J., Nuber-Champier, A., Allali, G., et al. (2023). Markers of limbic system damage following SARS-CoV-2 infection. *Brain Communications,* https//doi.org/10.1093/braincomms/fcad177

Thurow, R. (2016). *The first 1,000 days: A crucial time for mothers and children and the world.* Public Affairs.

Todd, R. M., & Anderson, A. K. (2009). Six degrees of separation: The amygdala regulates social behavior and perception. *Nature Neuroscience, 12,* 1217–1218.

Tomer, R., Goldstein, R. Z., Wang, G. J., Wong, C., & Volkow, N. D. (2008). Incentive motivation is associated with striatal dopamine asymmetry. *Biological Psychology, 77,* 98–101.

Tomkins, S. (1963). *Affect / imagery / consciousness: Vol. 2. The negative affects.* Springer.

Tomkins, S. (1987). Shame. In D. L. Nathanson (Ed.), *The many faces of shame* (pp. 133–161). Guilford.

Tong, F., Nakayama, K., Moscovictch, M., Weinrib, O., & Kanwisher, N. (2000). Response properties of the human fusiform face area. *Cognitive Neuropsychology, 17,* 2572–2580.

Tracy, J. L., Cheng, J. T., Robins, R. W., & Trzesniewski, K. H. (2009). Authentic and hubristic pride: The affective core of self-esteem and narcissism. *Self and Identity, 8,* 196–213.

Tranel, D., Bechara, A., & Denburg, N. L. (2002). Asymmetric functional roles of right and left ventromedial, prefrontal cortices in social conduct, decision-making, and emotional processing. *Cortex, 38,* 589–612.

Trevarthen, C. (1990). Growth and education of the hemispheres. In C. Trevarthen (Ed.), *Brain circuits and functions of the mind* (pp. 334–363). Cambridge University Press.

Trevarthen, C. (1993). The self born in intersubjectivity: The psychology of an infant communicating. In U. Neisser (Ed.), *The perceived self: Ecological and interpersonal sources of self-knowledge* (pp. 121–173). Cambridge University Press.

Trevarthen, C. (1994). Roger W. Sperry (1913-1994). *Trends in Neuroscience, 17,* 402–404.

Trevarthen, C. (1996). Lateral asymmetries in infancy: Implications for the development of the hemispheres. *Neuroscience and Biobehavioral Review, 20,* 571–586.

Trevarthen, C., & Aitken, K. J. (2001). Infant intersubjectivity: Research, theory, and practice. *Journal of Child Psychology and Psychiatry, 42,* 3–48.

Tronick, E. (2004). Why is connection with others so critical? The formation of dyadic states of consciousness and the expansion of individuals' states of consciousness: Coherence governed selection and the co-creation of meaning out of messy meaning making. In J. Nadel & D. Muir (Eds.), *Emotional development* (pp. 293–315). Oxford University Press.

Tronick, E. (2007). *The neurobehavioral and social-emotional development of infants and children.* Norton.

Tronick, E. D., Als, H., & Brazelton, T. B. (1977). Mutuality in mother-infant inter-action. *Journal of Communication, 27*, 74–79.

Tronick, E. Z., Bruschweiler-Stern, N., Harrison, A. M., Lyons Ruth, K., Morgan, A. C., Nahum, J. P., et al. (1998). Dyadically expanded states of consciousness and the process of therapeutic change. *Infant Mental Health Journal, 19*, 290–299.

Trub, L. R. (2024). The elephant in the Zoom: Will psychoanalysis survive the screen? *American Journal of Psychoanalysis, 84*, 203–228.

Tsakiris, M., Constantini, M., & Haggard, P. (2008). The role of the right temporoparietal junction in maintaining a coherent sense of one's body. *Neuropsychologia, 46*, 3014–3018.

Tschacher, W., Greenwood, S., Ramakrishnan, S., Trondle, M., Wald-Fuhrmann, M., Seibert, C., et al. (2023). Audience synchronies in live concerts illustrate the embodiment of music experience. *Scientific Reports, 13*, 14843. https://doi.org/10.1038/s41598-023-41960-2

Tschacher, W., & Meier, D. (2019). Physiological synchrony in psychotherapy sessions. *Psychotherapy Research, 30*, 558–573.

Tschacher, W., Ramseyer, F., & Koole, S. L. (2018). Sharing the now: Duration of nonverbal synchrony is linked with personality. *Journal of Personality, 86*, 129–138.

Tschacher, W., Schildt, M., & Sander, K. (2010). Brain connectivity in listening to affective stimuli: A functional magnetic resonance imaging (fMRI) study and implications for psychotherapy. *Psychotherapy Research, 20*, 576–588.

Tschanz, B. T., Morf, C. C., & Turner, C. W. (1998). Gender differences in the structure of narcissism: A multi-sample analysis of the narcissistic personality inventory. *Sex Roles, 38*, 863–870.

Tschopp, J. (2011). Mitochondria: Sovereign of inflammation? *European Journal of Immunology, 41*, 1196–1202.

Tucker, D. M., Liu, P., & Pribram, K. H. (1995). Social and emotional self-regulation. *Annals of the New York Academy of Science, 769*, 213–239.

Tucker, D. M., & Moller, L. (2007). The metamorphosis: Individuation of the adolescent brain. In D. Romer & E. F. Walker (Eds.), *Adolescent psychopathology and the developing brain: Integrating brain and prevention science* (pp. 85–102). Oxford University Press.

Tucker, D. M., & Williamson, P. A. (1984). Asymmetric neural control systems in human self-regulation. *Psychological Review, 91*, 185–215.

Tummula-Narra, P., Li, Z., Chang, J., Yang, E. J., Jiang, J., Sagherian, M., et al. (2018). Developmental and contextual correlates of mental health and help-seeking among Asian American college students. *American Journal of Orthopsychiatry, 88*, 636–649.

Tweedy, R. (2021). *The divided therapist: Hemispheric difference and contemporary psychotherapy*. Routledge.

Twenge, J. M., & Campbell, W. K. (2009). *The narcissism epidemic: Living in the age of entitlement*. Free Press.

Twenge, J. M., Gentile, B., DeWall, C. N., Ma, D., Lacefield, K., & Schurtz, D. R.

(2010). Birth cohort increases in psychopathology among young Americans, 1938–2007: A cross-temporal meta-analysis of the MMPI. *Clinical Psychology Review, 30*, 145–154.

Twenge, J. M., Konrath, S., Foster, J. D., Campbell, W. K., & Bushman, B. J. (2008). Egos inflating over time: A cross-temporal meta-analysis of the narcissistic personality inventory. *Journal of Personality, 76*, 875–902.

Tzourio-Mazoyer, N., De Schonen, S., Crivello, F., Reutter, B., Aujard, Y., & Mazoyer, B. (2002). Neural correlates of woman face processing by 2-month infants. *NeuroImage, 15*, 454–461.

Uddin, L. Q., Kaplan, J. T., Molnar-Szakacs, I., Zaidel, E., & Iacoboni, M. (2005). Self face recognition activates a frontoparietal "mirror" network in the right hemisphere: An event-related fMRI study. *Neuroimage, 25*, 926–935.

Ulanov, A. B. (2001). *Finding space: Winnicott, God, and psychic reality*. Westminster John Knox Press.

Unconscious. (n.d.). In *Oxford English Dictionary*. https://www.oed.com/dictionary/unconscious_adj?tl=true

Ünsalver, B. Ö., Evrensel, A., Yertutanol, F. D. K., Dönmez, A., & Ceylan, M. E. (2021). The changeable positioning of the couch and repositioning to face-to-face arrangement in psychoanalysis to facilitate the experience of being seen. *Frontiers in Psychology, 12*, 718319. doi: 10.3389/fpsyg.2021.718319

Urakawa, S., Takamoto, K., Ishikawa, A., One, T., & Nishijo, H. (2015). Selective medial prefrontal cortex responses during live mutual gaze interactions in human infants: An fNIRS study. *Brain Topography, 28*, 691–701.

Uvnas-Moberg, K. (1996). Neuroendocrinology of the mother-child interaction. *Trends in Endocrinology and Metabolism, 7*, 126–131.

Vaillant, G. E. (1994). Ego mechanisms of defense and personality psychopathology. *Journal of Abnormal Psychology, 103*, 44–50.

Valdesolo, P., & Desteno, D. (2011). Synchrony and the social tuning of compassion. *Emotion, 11*, 262–266. https://doi.org/10.1037/a0021302

Valent, P. (2018). Paradigm shift in psychiatry: What may it involve? *Australasian Psychiatry, 26*, 73–75.

Valentine, L., & Gabbard, G. O. (2014). Can the use of humor in psychotherapy be taught? *Academic Psychiatry, 38*, 75–81.

Vallortigara, G., & Rogers, L. J. (2005). Survival with an asymmetrical brain: Advantage and disadvantages of brain lateralization. *Behavioral and Brain Sciences, 28*, 575–633.

van Lancker Sidtis, D. (2006). The right hemisphere processes a holistic mode for nonliteral expressions and a compositional mode for novel language. *Metaphor and Symbol, 21*, 213–244.

Varendi, H., Porter, R. H., & Winberg, J. (2002). The effect of labor on olfactory exposure learning within the first postnatal hour. *Behavioral Neuroscience, 116*, 206–211.

Vauclair, J., & Donnot, J. (2005). Infant holding biases and their relations to hemispheric specializations for processing facial emotions. *Neuropsychologia, 43, 564–571.* doi: 10.1016/j.neuropsychologia.2004.07.005

Vecera, S. P. (2006). Gaze direction and the cortical processing of faces: Evidence from infants and adults. *Visual Cognition, 2, 59–87.*

Vervloed, M. P. J., Hendriks, A. W., & Van der Eijnde, E. (2011). The effects of mothers' past infant-holding preferences on their adult children's face processing lateralization. *Brain and Cognition, 75, 248–254.*

Vignal, J. P., Maillard, L., McGonical, A., & Chauvet, P. (2007). The dreamy state: Hallucinations of autobiographic memory evoked by temporal lobe stimulations and seizures. *Brain, 130, 88–99.*

Wagner, A. D., Poldrack, R. A., Eldridge, L. L., Desmond, J. E., Glover, G. H., & Gabrieli, J. D. D. (1998). Material-specific lateralization of prefrontal activation during episodic encoding and retrieval. *Neuroreport, 9, 3711–3717.*

Wagner, U., Gais, S., & Born, J. (2001). Emotional memory formation is enhanced across sleep intervals with high amounts of rapid eye movement sleep. *Biological Psychiatry, 60, 788–790.*

Walker, M. P. (2009). The role of sleep in cognition and emotion. *Annals of the New York Academy of Science, 1156, 168–197.*

Walker-Andrews, A. S., & Bahrick, L. E. (2001). Perceiving the real world: Infants' detection of and memory for social information. *Infancy, 2, 469–481.*

Wampold, B. E. (2015). How important are the common factors in psychotherapy? An update. *World Psychiatry, 14, 270–277.*

Wampold, B. E., Baldwin, S. A., Holtforth, M. G., & Imsel, Z. E. (2017). What characterizes effective therapists? In L. G. Castonguay & C. E. Hill (Eds.), *How and why are some therapists better than others? Understanding therapist effects.* American Psychological Association.

Wampold, B. E., & Fluckiger, C. (2023). The alliance in mental health care: Conceptualizations, evidence and clinical applications. *World Psychiatry, 22, 25–41.*

Wampold, B. E., & Imel, Z. (2015). *The great psychotherapy debate.* Routledge.

Wang, J., Rao, H., Wetmore, G. S., Furlan, P. M., Korczykowski, M., Dinges, D. F., & Detre, J. A. (2005). Perfusion functional MRI reveals cerebral blood flow pattern under psychological stress. *Proceedings of the National Academy of Sciences USA, 102, 17804–17809.*

Wang, Y., Ramsey, R., & Hamilton, A. F. (2011). The control of mimicry by eye contact is mediated by medial prefrontal cortex. *Journal of Neuroscience, 31, 12001–12010.*

Ward, H. P. (1972). Shame: A necessity for growth in therapy. *American Journal of Psychotherapy, 26, 232–243.*

Wass, S. V., Smith, C. G., Clackson, K., Gibb, C., Eitzenberger, J., & Mirza, F. U. (2019). Parents mimic and influence their infant's autonomic state through dynamic affective state matching. *Current Biology, 29, 2415–2422.*

Watson, K. K., Jones, T. K., & Allman, J. M. (2006). Dendritic architecture of the Von Economo neurons. *Neuroscience, 141*, 1107–1112.

Watt, D. F. (1986). Transference: A right hemispheric event? An inquiry into the boundary between behavioral neurobiology, neuropsychology, and psychoanalysis. *Psychoanalysis and Contemporary Thought, 9*, 43–77.

Watt, D. F. (2003). Psychotherapy in an age of neuroscience: Bridges to affective neuroscience. In J. Corrigall & H. Wilkinson (Eds.), *Revolutionary connections: Psychotherapy and neuroscience* (pp. 79–115). Karnac.

Weaver, I. C. G., Cervoni, N., Champagne, F. A., D'Alessio, A. C., Sharma, S., Seckl, J. R., Dymov, S., Szyf, M., & Meaney, M. J. (2004). Epigenetic programming by maternal behavior. *Nature Neuroscience, 7*, 847–854.

Weber, A. M., Harrison, T., & Steward, D. K. (2012). Schore's regulation theory: Maternal-infant interaction in the NICU as a mechanism for reducing the effects of allostatic load on neurodevelopment in premature infants. *Biological Research for Nursing, 14*, 375–386.

Weinberg, I. (2000). The prisoners of despair: Right hemisphere deficiency and suicide. *Neuroscience and Biobehavioral Reviews, 24*, 799–815.

Weinberg, I. (2024). Building hope for treatment of narcissistic personality disorder. *Journal of Clinical Psychology, 80*, 721–732.

Weise, K. L., & Tuber, S. (2004). The self and object representations of narcissistically disturbed children: An empirical investigation. *Psychoanalytic Psychology, 21*, 244–258.

Weiss, S. J. (2005). Haptic perception and the psychosocial functioning of preterm, low birth weight infants. *Infant Behavior and Development, 28*, 329–359.

Welch, M. G. (2016). Calming cycle theory: The role of visceral/autonomic learning in early mother and infant/child behaviour and development. *Acta Paediatrica, 105*, 1266–1274.

Welling, H. (2005). The intuitive process: The case of psychotherapy. *Journal of Psychotherapy Integration, 15*, 19–47.

Westen, D., & Arkowitz-Westen, L. (1998). Limitations of Axis ll in diagnosing personality pathology in clinical practice. *American Journal of Psychiatry, 155*, 1767–1771.

Wexler, B. E., Warrenburg, S., Schwartz, G. E., & Janer, L. D. (1992). EEG and EMG responses to emotion-evoking stimuli processed without conscious awareness. *Neuropsychologia, 30*, 1065–1079.

Whitehead, C. C. (2006). Neo-psychoanalysis: A paradigm for the 21st century. *Journal of the Academy of Psychoanalysis and Dynamic Psychiatry, 34*, 603–627.

Whitehead, R. (1991). Right hemisphere processing superiority during sustained visual attention. *Journal of Cognitive Neuroscience, 3*, 329–334.

Wicker, B., Michel, F., Henaff, M. A., & Decety, J. (1998). Brain regions involved in the perception of gaze: A PET study. *Neuroimage, 8*, 221–227.

Widiger, T., & Frances, A. (1989). Epidemiology, diagnosis, and comorbidity of borderline personality disorder. *American Psychiatric Press Review of Psychiatry, 8*, 8–24.

Wilkinson, A. R., & Jiang, Z. D. (2006). Brainstem auditory evoked response in neonatal neurology. *Seminars in Fetal & Neonatal Medicine, 11*, 444–451.

Williams, L. M., Gatt, J. M., Schofield, P. R., Olivieri, G., Peduto, A., & Gordon, E. (2009). Negativity bias in risk for depression and anxiety: Brain-body fear circuitry correlates, 5-HTT-LPR and early life stress. *NeuroImage, 47*, 804–814.

Williams, R. B., Haney, T. L., Lee, K. L., Blumenthal, J. A., & Whalen, R. E. (1980). Type A behavior, hostility, and atherosclosis. *Psychosomatic Medicine, 42*, 539–549.

Wilson, D. F. (2017). Oxidative phosphorylation: Regulation and role in cellular and tissue metabolism. *Journal of Physiology, 595*, 7023–7038.

Wink, P. (1991). Two faces of narcissism. *Journal of Personality and Social Psychology, 61*, 590–597.

Winnicott, D. W. (1955). Metapsychological and clinical aspects of regression within the psycho-analytical set-up. *International Journal of Psychoanalysis, 36*, 16–26.

Winnicott, D. W. (1958a). The capacity to be alone. *International Journal of Psychoanalysis, 39*, 416–420.

Winnicott, D. W. (1958b). *Through pediatrics to psychoanalysis*. Tavistock.

Winnicott, D. W. (1960a). Ego distortion in terms of true and false self. In *The maturational processes and the facilitating environment* (pp. 140–152). International Universities Press.

Winnicott, D. W. (1960b). The theory of the parent-infant relationship. In *The maturational processes and the facilitating environment*. International Universities Press.

Winnicott, D. W. (1974). Fear of breakdown. *International Review of Psychoanalysis, 1*, 103–107.

Wittling, W. (1997). The right hemisphere and the human stress response. *Acta Physiologica Scandinavica, 640* (Suppl.), 55–59.

Wittling, W., & Roschmann, R. (1993). Emotion-related hemisphere asymmetry: Subjective emotional responses to laterally presented films. *Cortex, 29*, 431–448.

Wolberg, L. R. (1977). *The technique of psychotherapy*. Grune and Stratton.

Wolitzky, D. L., & Eagle, M. N. (1999). Psychoanalytic theories of psychotherapy. In P. L. Wachtel & S. B. Messer (Eds.), *Theories of psychotherapy: Origins and evolution* (pp. 39–96). American Psychoanalytic Association.

Wong-Riley, M. T. T. (1989). Cytochrome oxidase: An endogenous metabolic marker for neuronal activity. *Trends in Neuroscience, 12*, 94–101.

Woodhead, J. (2004). Shifting triangles: Images of father in sequences from parent-infant psychotherapy. *International Journal of Infant Observation and Its Applications, 7*, 76–90.

Woody, M. L., Feurer, C., Sosoo, E. E., & Gibb, B. F. (2016). Synchrony of physiological activity during mother-child interaction: Moderation by maternal history of major depressive disorder. *Journal of Child Psychology and Psychiatry, 57*, 843–850. doi: 10.1111/jcpp.12562

Wright, K. (1991). *Vision and separation: Between mother and baby*. Jason Aronson.

Wurmser, L. (1981). *The mask of shame*. Johns Hopkins University Press.

Wurst, S. N., Gerlach, T. M., Dufner, M., Rauthmann, J. F., Grosz, M. P., Kufner, A. C. P., et al. (2017). Narcissism and romantic relationships: The differential impact of narcissistic admiration and rivalry. *Journal of Personality and Social Psychology, 112*, 280–306.

Yamada, H., Sadato, N., Konishi, Y., Kimura, K., Tanaka, M., Yonekura, Y., et al. (1997). A rapid brain metabolic change in infants by fMRI. *NeuroReport, 8*, 3775–3778.

Yang, Z., Zhao, J., Jiang, Y., Li, C., Wang, J., Weng, X., & Northoff, G. (2011). Altered negative unconscious processing in major depressive disorder: An exploratory neuropsychological study. *PLoS One, 6*, e21881.

Yoshida, M., Yokoo, H., Tanaka, T., Mizoguchi, K., Emoto, H., Ishii, H., & Tanaka, M. (1993). Faciliatory modulation of mesolimbic dopamine neuronal activity by mu-opioid agonist and nicotine as examined with in vivo microdyalysis. *Brain Research, 624*, 277–280.

Yoshimura, S., Ueda, K., Suzuki, S., Onoda, K., Okamato, Y., & Yamawki, S. (2009). Self-referential processing of negative stimuli within the ventral anterior cingulate gyrus and right amygdala. *Brain and Cognition, 69*, 218–225.

Yovel, G. (2016). Neural and cognitive face-selective markers: An integrative review. *Neuropsychologia, 83*, 5–13.

Zak, P. J., Kurzban, R., & Matzner, W. T. (2005). Oxytocin is associated with human trustworthiness. *Hormones and Behavior, 48*, 522–527.

Zeigler-Hill, V. (2021). A homeostatic perspective on narcissistic personality dynamics. *Psychological Inquiry, 32*, 263–266.

Zelazo, P. D. (2004). The development of conscious control in childhood. *Trends in Cognitive Sciences, 8*, 12–17.

Zhang, Y., Meng, T., Hou, Y., Pan, Y., & Hu, Y. (2018). Interpersonal brain synchronization associated with working alliance during psychological counseling. *Psychiatry Research Neuroimaging, 282*, 103–109. doi: 10.1016/j.pscychresns.2018.09.007

Zhang, Y., Meng, T., Yang, Y., & Hu, Y. (2020). Experience-dependent counselor-client brain synchronization during psychological counseling. *eNeuro, 7*(5). doi: 10.1523/ENEURO.0236-20.2020

Zhao, N., Zhang, X., Noah, J. A., Tiede, M., & Hirsch, J. (2023). Separable processes for live "in-person" and live "Zoom-like" faces. *Imaging Neuroscience, 1*, 1–17. https://doi.org/10.1162/imag_a_00027

Zheng, J., & Meister, M. (2024). The unbearable slowness of being: Why do we live at 10 bits/s? *Neuron, 113*, 1–13.

Zheng, Z. S., Simonian, N., Wang, J., & Rosario, E. R. (2024). Transcutaneous vagus nerve stimulation improves long COVID symptoms in a female cohort: a pilot study. *Front. Neurol.* 15:1393371. doi: 10.3389/fneur.2024.1393371

Ziegler-Hill, V., Clark, C. B., & Pickard, J. D. (2008). Narcissistic subtypes and contingent self-esteem: Do all narcissists base their self esteem on the same domains? *Journal of Personality, 76*, 753–774.

Zilcha-Mano, S. (2021). Toward personalized psychotherapy: The importance of the trait-like/state-like distinction for understanding therapeutic change. *American Psychologist, 76*, 516–528.

Zilcha-Mano, S., & Errazuriz, P. (2017). Early development of mechanisms of change as predictor of subsequent change and treatment outcome: The case of working alliance. *Journal of Consulting and Clinical Psychology, 85*, 508–520.

Zilcha-Mano, S., Shamay-Tsoory, S., Dolev-Amit, T., Zagoory-Sharon, O., & Feldman, R. (2020). Oxytocin as a biomarker of the foundation of therapeutic alliance in psychotherapy and counseling psychology. *Journal of Counseling Psychology, 67*, 523–535.

Index

agentic characteristics
  defined, 122
aggression
  grandiose narcissistic, 121–22, 134
  internalized, 126–27
  toxic, 129
  vulnerable narcissism and, 134
aggressive behaviors
  testosterone levels related to, 312
"Aha!" moments, 160–61
"Aha!" self-recognition, 160
AI. *see* artificial intelligence (AI)
Aikins, J. W., xix–xx, 108
Ainsworth, M. D. S., xix, 120
Aitken, K. J., 183, 197
"alert inactivity," 190
alertness
  "quiet," 190
"algorithmic unconscious," 324
"alliance rupture repair"
  oxytocin synchrony and, 269
Allman, J. M., 56, 193
allostasis
  fundamental principle of, 77
Ambady, N., 53, 261
American Psychological Association, 227
  Distinguished Practice Award from
    Division of Trauma Psychology of,
    92
  Division of Psychotherapy of, 295–96
Amid, B., 188, 271–74
Ammaniti, M., 209, 216
amygdala
  central. *see* central amygdala
  communication with orbitofrontal cortex,
    312
  in earliest stage of postnatal develop-
    ment, 190
  early rearing experiences impact on,
    192
  function of, 328–29
  right. *see* right amygdala
  role in autobiographical memory,
    46
"analog amplifier"
  emotion as, 159
"an arrogant face," 115
Anderson, A. K., 192–93, 270
Anderson, P. A., 27, 125–26

Andrade, V. M., 55
anger
  shame and, 148
"animated mutual play," 210
anterior insula
  in emotional processing of self-face rec-
    ognition, 27
anxiety
  vulnerable narcissism and, 126
anxious attachment
  insecure. *see* insecure anxious
    attachment
  vulnerable narcissism and, 127
anxious-preoccupied attachments
  vulnerable narcissism and, 125–26
apoptosis
  mitochondrial activation in, 77–78
apprehension
  verbal anxious, 96
archaic
  defined, 53
"a relationship of care," 296
Aron, A., 220
Aron, E. N., 220
Aron, L., 72
arousal
  described, 76
  of emotion, 76
  "mutual regulatory system of," 196
  regulation of, 17
artificial intelligence (AI)
  in psychotherapy, 324–25
Asperger's syndrome
  autistic spectrum disorders overlap
    with, 280–81
asymmetry
  hemispheric. *see* hemispheric
    asymmetry
"at-one-ment," 271–74
ATP. *see* adenosine triphosphate (ATP)
attachment(s)
  anxious-preoccupied. *see* anxious-
    preoccupied attachments
  avoidant. *see* avoidant attachment
  control system of, 15
  described, 10–11
  dismissive, 121, 138
  disorganized. *see* disorganized
    attachment

communal characteristics
  defined, 122
communication(s)
  attachment. *see* attachment
    communications
  emotional. *see* emotional
    communication(s)
  eye-to-eye, 189
  face-to-face. *see* face-to-face
    communication
  "human super-," 316
  implicit-procedural body-to-body, 189
  intersubjective, 233–44
  mother–infant attachment, 21, 75,
    180–81
  mutual gaze in, 19
  "new forms of," 273
  nonverbal. *see* nonverbal
    communication(s)
  between orbitofrontal cortex and amyg-
    dala, 312
  primary-process, 261
  prosodic, 54–55
  rapid nonverbal, 85
  right-brain–right-brain, 226–74.
    see also right-brain–right-brain
    communications
  "technologically-assisted," 315–23
competence
  "interpersonal," 172
"compulsive self-reliance," 121
"conceptual self," 166
conditioning
  Pavlovian classical, 6–7
conflict(s)
  "bearable intrapsychic," 174
  "superego," 174
conscious awareness
  unconscious shame into, 151
consciousness
  "dyadic expansion of," 158
  "dyadic state of," 197
  "primary," 197
  "stepping into the light" and, 151
conscious self-image
  left brain, 111–12
conscious shame, 142, 143
"constructive creativity," 163

contact
  "psychological," 159
  skin-to-skin, 189
contagion
  emotional, 261
control
  "omnipotent," 121
control system of attachment
  Bowlby's, 15
conversation(s)
  proto-. *see* protoconversation(s)
  "spontaneous emotion-laden," 224
"conversational play," 218
core self, 207–9, 216
  subjective, xvi
cortex
  orbitofrontal. *see* orbitofrontal cortex
  right anterior cingulate, 193
  right orbitofrontal, 26–27
  right temporoparietal, 202–8
  ventromedial, 16
Cortina, M., 48
countertransference
  defined, 47
  described, 47–48
COVID
  long, 327
COVID-19 pandemic
  online Zoom sessions during, 314–15
  social isolation related to, 333–34
Cozolino, L., 45–46, 246
"crack in my universe"
  shame-triggered, 148
cradling
  left-sided, 182, 191–92
Craig, A. D., 256
Cramer, P., 37, 117, 130
creative mutual regressions. *see also* syn-
    chronized mutual regressions
  in rebalancing of hemispheres,
    162–69
creative storytelling
  intersubjective play of, 218
"creative unconscious," 163
creativity
  "constructive," 163
  defined, 137, 152, 155–56
  right brain, 137

violence
  defined, 311
  described, 311–13
  interpersonal aspect of, 311
visual-facial attachment communications, 24
visual-facial nonverbal communications, 181–82
vital
  defined, 200
"vitality affects," 195
voice
  spontaneous bidirectional nonverbal communication of, 275–77, 277*f*
von Economo neurons (VENs), 193
vulnerability
  in regulating stress/resilience, xiv
vulnerable narcissism, 116–34
  aggression/behavioral tendencies associated with, 134
  anxiety/depression with, 126
  anxious attachment in, 127
  anxious-preoccupied attachment and, 125–26
  attachment deactivation strategy in, 120
  attachment neurobiology of, 120–34, 125*f*
  described, 120–34, 125*f*
  insecure anxious attachment and, 124–25
  internalized aggression in, 126–27
  shame in, 132
  therapeutic goal of, 134–35

Walker-Andres, A. S., 13–14
Wampold, B. E., 259
Wass, S. V., 235
Watt, D. F., 97
Weber, A. M., 241
Weinberg, I., 120, 121, 138, 148–49, 151, 156–57, 173, 245

Weise, K. L., 131
Welch, M. G., 6
well-being
  "a background state of," 29
  child. *see* child well-being
  emotional, 12
Welling, H., 151
"well-kept secrets of the right hemisphere," 111
"we-mode"
  of cognition, 270
Weston, D. R., 106
Whitehead, C. C., 158
wholeness
  psychotherapy as growth of, 222
Williamson, P. A., 127
Winnicott, D. W., 9, 60, 73, 83, 135–36, 218, 249–50
witnessing
  "embodied," 47
Wolberg, L. R., 101–3
Wolf, E. S., 129–30
Wolitzky, D. L., 135
Woll, B., 182
word(s)
  attachment. *see* attachment words
  as "a weapon," 121

Yamada, H., 203

Zeigler-Hill, V., 122
Zeki, S., 214–15
Zhang, Y., 282–26, 284*f*, 285*f*, 288
Zhao, N., 316–17, 317*f*
Zoom
  face-to-face communication vs., 314–23
  limitations of, 321–25
"Zoom fatigue," 322–23

About the Author

Over the last three decades **Allan Schore's** interdisciplinary studies have been directed towards integrating psychological and biological models of emotional and social development across the human lifespan. His work in regulation theory on the development, psychopathogenesis, and treatment of the right brain subjective self focuses on implicit emotional regulation and unconscious right-brain-to-right-brain communication in both the psychotherapy relationship first described by Sigmund Freud, and the attachment relationship, first elaborated by John Bowlby. Overviewing and evaluating the body of his work on the interpersonal neurobiology of attachment, his son (and Schore's dear friend) Sir Richard Bowlby has asserted: "All human achievement is built on the shoulders of giants, and just as John Bowlby and Allan Schore have stood on 'giant's shoulders,' so future generations of scientists will in turn be standing on their shoulders. In his books he has integrated a vast array of scientific advances and organized it in an overarching way that deserves the deepest acknowledgment and gratitude."